Dental Materials

**Clinical Applications for
Dental Assistants and
Dental Hygienists**

Dental Materials

Clinical Applications for Dental Assistants and Dental Hygienists

CAROL DIXON HATRICK, CDA, RDA, RDH, MS
Lead Instructor, First Year Dental Hygiene
Santa Rosa Junior College
Santa Rosa, California

W. STEPHAN EAKLE, DDS
Professor and Chair, Division of Preclinical General Dentistry
Department of Preventive and Restorative Dental Sciences
School of Dentistry
University of California, San Francisco
San Francisco, California

WILLIAM F. BIRD, DDS, MPH, DR PH
Vice Chair Department of Preventive and Restorative Dental Sciences
Associate Dean, Clinical Administration
University of California, San Francisco
School of Dentistry
San Francisco, California

With 360 illustrations, 10 Color Plates

SAUNDERS
An Imprint of Elsevier
Philadelphia   London   New York   St. Louis   Sydney   Toronto

SAUNDERS
An Imprint of Elsevier Science

11830 Westline Industrial Drive
St. Louis, Missouri 63146

Dental Materials: Clinical Applications for Dental Assistants and Dental Hygienists   ISBN 0-7216-8583-8

NOTICE

Dentistry is an ever-changing field. Standard safety precautions must be followed, but as new research and clinical experience broaden our knowledge, changes in treatment and drug therapy may become necessary or appropriate. Readers are advised to check the most current product information provided by the manufacturer of each drug to be administered to verify the recommended dose, the method and duration of administration, and contraindications. It is the responsibility of the licensed health care provider, relying on experience and knowledge of the patient, to determine dosages and the best treatment for each individual patient. Neither the publisher nor the editor assumes any liability for any injury and/or damage to persons or property arising from this publication.

Library of Congress Cataloging-in-Publication Data

Hatrick, Carol Dixon
   Dental materials : clinical applications for dental assistants and dental hygienists /
Carol Dixon Hatrick, W. Stephan Eakle, William F. Bird.
     p. ; cm.
   Includes bibliographical references and index.
   ISBN 0-7216-8583-8
    1. Dental materials. 2. Dental materials—Examinations, questions, etc. I. Eakle, W. Stephen,
II. Bird, William F. III. Title.
   [DNLM: 1. Dental Materials. 2. Dental Materials—Examination Questions. WU 190
B618d 2003]
   RK652.5 .B58 2003
   617.6'95—dc21   2002075764

Acquisitions Editor: Shirley Kuhn
Developmental Editor: Helaine Tobin
Publishing Services Manager: Pat Joiner
Project Manager: Maureen Niebruegge
Designer: Mark Oberkrom
Cover Art: WT Design

GW/QWF
Printed in United States of America

Last digit is the print number: 9 8 7 6 5 4 3 2 1

REVIEWERS

Joseph Elmer Baughman, DDS
Oral Pathology Certification
Lanier Technical Institute
Oakwood, Georgia

Karen Castleberry, CDA, RDA, BS
Chattanooga State Technical Community College
Chattanooga, Tennessee

Susan J. Cochran, CDA, RDH, BS, MS
Florence Darlington Technical College
Florence, South Carolina

Alison Collins, CDA, MS
Northwestern Michigan College
Traverse City, Michigan

Cynthia S. Cronick, CDA, AAS, BS
Southeast Community College
Lincoln, Nebraska

Candida J. Ditzler, CDA, RDA
Coordinator of Dental Assisting Program
Cape May County Technical School
Cape May Court House, New Jersey

Manville G. Duncanson, Jr., DDS, PhD, FADM, FACD
Professor Emeritus of Dental Materials
Department of Dental Materials
University of Oklahoma College of Dentistry
Oklahoma City, Oklahoma

Carol Anne Giaquinto, CDA, RDH, MEd
Program Coordinator, Dental Assisting
Springfield Technical Community College
Springfield, Massachusetts

Terry Sigal Greene, RDH, BSeD, MEd
Northampton Community College
Bethlehem, Pennsylvania

Paulette Susan Kehm-Yelton, CDA, MPA
East Tennessee State University
Elizabethton, Tennessee

Stella Lovato, CDA, MS, MA
San Antonio College/ACCD
San Antonio, Texas

Elizabeth A. McClure, RDH, MEd
Raymond Walters College
University of Cincinnati
Cincinnati, Ohio

Thomas F. McDaniel, DMD, FAGD
Floyd College
Rome, Georgia

Diana L. Olsen, CDA, CDPMA, RDH, MS
University of Maine at Augusta
Bangor, Maine

Vickie Parrish Overman, RDH, MEd
Clinical Associate Professor
University of North Carolina at Chapel Hill
School of Dentistry
Chapel Hill, North Carolina

M. Elaine Parker, RDH, MS, PhD
Associate Professor and Graduate Program Director
University of Maryland
Department of Dental Hygiene
Baltimore, Maryland

Cynthia Rietkerk, CDA, RDA, AS
Chaffey College
Rancho Cucamonga, California

Debbie Robinson, CDA, MS
Co-Author Modern Dental Assisting/Essentials of
   Dental Assisting
Hillsborough, North Carolina

Juanita Robinson, CDA, EFDA, LDH, MSEd
Program Director of Dental Education
Indiana University Northwest
Gary, Indiana

Naomi L. Smith, CDA, MEd
Western Piedmont Community College
Morganton, North Carolina

PREFACE

Life-Long Learning

The subject of dental materials is rapidly changing as researchers and manufacturers develop new materials and improve those currently in use. Consequently, dental hygienists and dental assistants are challenged to keep up with the new materials, their physical properties, and their handling characteristics. As important members of the dental team, they must be adept at placing or assisting in the placement of dental materials, and they play a valuable role in the maintenance of dental materials once they are placed in the mouth. Dental hygienists and dental assistants also are instrumental in educating patients in the home maintenance of restorations and prostheses. As allied oral health providers, dental hygienists and dental assistants play major roles in preventive education and therapy in most practices. In order to stay current, they must be life-long learners who know how to use available resources to update their knowledge. *Dental Materials: Clinical Applications for Dental Assistants and Dental Hygienists* will provide the foundation for that life-long learning for the new student and will serve as an important update on new materials or improvements in materials for the practicing assistant or hygienist.

Goals

The goal of *Dental Materials: Clinical Applications for Dental Assistants and Dental Hygienists* is to provide students with:
- The principles of dental materials so they can understand the rationale for their use
- The opportunity to apply their knowledge through clinical and laboratory procedures
- The opportunity to test their knowledge and prepare for board examinations
- The resources they will need in order to obtain updates on dental materials and contact dental manufacturers
- Contact information for dental agencies so they have access to the wealth of information available regarding career opportunities, testing boards, personal safety and ergonomics, dental organizations, and a multitude of other dental topics.

Features

Chapters have the following components:
- **Chapter outline** of the subject matter
- **Learning and performance objectives** to guide students in learning
- **Key terms** listed and defined in the order of their presentation in the chapters and highlighted in the chapters in bold print.

- **Basic principles and applications, physical properties, and handling characteristics** of the dental materialspresented in each chapter
- **Helpful clinical tips or precautions** regarding the use of the materials, highlighted in boxes set apart from the main text for emphasis.
- **Illustrated clinical and laboratory procedures** presented in step-by-step instructions so that students can practice common applications of the materials. Icons placed at the top of the procedure sheets guide the clinician as to precautions for patients or clinicians and alert the clinician when procedures may not be allowed by all state dental boards.
- **Review questions** to enable students to test their comprehension of the subject matter and prepare for examinations; answers are provided at the end of the text.
- **Case-based discussion topics** that encourage students to relate what they have learned to the actual application in the dental office. Instructors may want to use them as topics for group discussions.
- **Reference lists** at the end of each chapter to help students find additional information about the principles and properties of the dental materials discussed.
- A **resource appendix** at the end of the text to guide students in their efforts for life-long learning. In addition to information on how to contact dental organizations and manufacturers, a section is devoted to the use of the Internet to access information. Most international, national, state and local dental organizations maintain websites with valuable information concerning the organization, continuing education and patient education materials as well. For those students who want to delve deeper into a subject, information is provided for conducting a MEDLINE literature search. Most manufacturers have their own web sites, and many of these have continuing education materials in addition to information about their materials. By using these resources the students will enrich their educational experiences.
- **Competency evaluations** for each procedure in an appendix at the end of the text to allow students to gauge their own level of learning; these can also be evaluated by an instructor for valuable feedback.

Explanation of Icons

Easily recognizable icons appear at the top of each procedure sheet to give you important information at a glance. The icons represent cautions on patient and clinician safety and alert you to functions that may or may not be allowed by your state dental board. The icons alert the clinician to the following:

 Icon for patient safety: It is recommended that the patient wear safety glasses for this procedure

 Icon for operator safety: The clinician must wear personal protective equipment such as mask, safety glasses, and gloves when performing this procedure.

 Icon for hazard sign: This procedure may present a hazardous working environment to the clinician if appropriate safety protocol is not followed.

 Icon for legal functions: This procedure may or may not be allowable for allied oral health professionals in your state. Please check your state dental practice act *before* performing this procedure.

A Note to Educators

Dental Materials: Clinical Applications for Dental Assistants and Dental Hygienists is written to be easily comprehended by students with varying amounts of science in their educational backgrounds. Learning and performance **objectives** draw the students' attention to the important concepts and features of the materials. **Key terms** are not only listed but also defined at the start of each chapter. Helpful **clinical tips** are used throughout the chapters to call attention to clinical points the student may not have been exposed to, and **cautions** are noted where appropriate for both patient and clinician safety.. The text is generously illustrated to help with comprehension of clinical and laboratory **procedures**, especially for our visual learners. The procedures help the students to see how the materials are actually used, and by applying their newly gained knowledge they reinforce learning. **Competencies** are included for each procedure in an appendix at the back of the book so that students can evaluate their own efforts and also receive feedback from their instructors. **Review questions** help reinforce what the students have learned and help prepare them for boards. **Case-based discussion topics** can be used for group discussions and bring the flavor of real-life dentistry to the application of dental materials. The **resource appendix** makes use of the Internet and creates a very dynamic learning opportunity. It can be used to give assignments for students to retrieve information for patient education regarding the use of fluorides, sealants, and a variety of other materials, and to view on-line continuing education materials offered by dental organizations and manufacturers. Once the students gain some experience searching these sites, they likely will continue to do so when they are in practice.

Your Comments, Please

The authors would appreciate suggestions or comments regarding this text, because it is written with your needs in mind. We hope instructors and students will enjoy this textbook and gain as much from it as we have intended.

ACKNOWLEDGEMENTS

The authors would like to thank the many people whose contributions were instrumental in the completion of this text.

We wish to thank the staff at W.B. Saunders, especially Shirley Kuhn, Senior Acquisition Editor, and Helaine Tobin, Senior Developmental Editor, for their excellent assistance, guidance, prodding, nagging and, above all, patience during the development of this text.

We want to acknowledge our reviewers who took the time to carefully evaluate our work and provide us with constructive criticism and helpful suggestions.

We are deeply indebted to our many colleagues and to dental materials manufacturers who generously provided their expertise, support and clinical illustrations to enhance the quality of this text and make it "user friendly."

We would like to give special thanks to our photographer, Dr. Mark Dellinges, for his technical assistance and talent in transforming our thoughts into pictures and for providing numerous photographs from his collection.

We would especially like to thank our significant others, Doni Bird, Sheila Eakle and Michael Steinert, and our families and friends for their ongoing patience when we sequestered ourselves away from human kind for seemingly endless hours and for their understanding on the many occasions when we needed their encouragement to forge ahead with our best efforts to complete this text for our students.

CONTENTS

LIST OF PROCEDURES

Dental Materials

Clinical Applications for Dental Assistants and Dental Hygienists

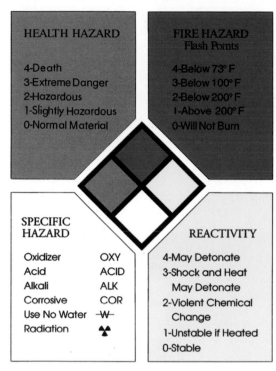

Color Plate 1

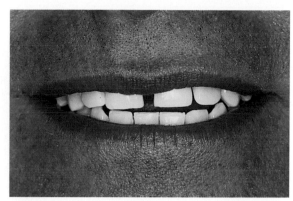

A

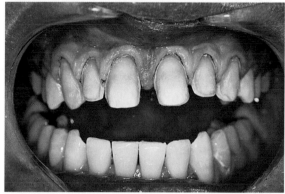

B

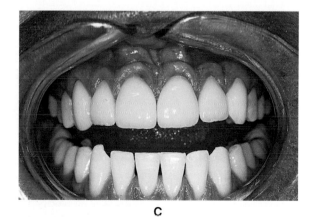

C

Color Plate 2

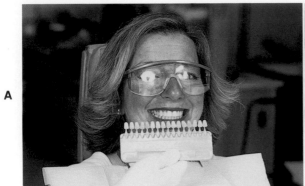

A

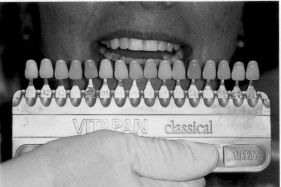

B

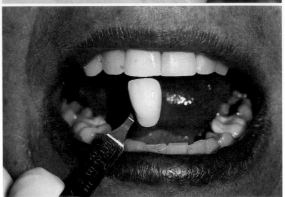

C

Color Plate 3

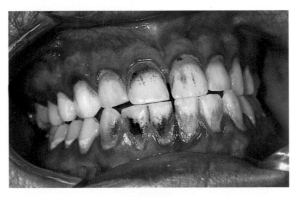

Color Plate 4

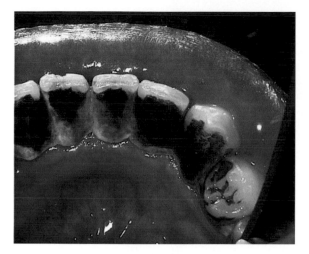

Color Plate 5

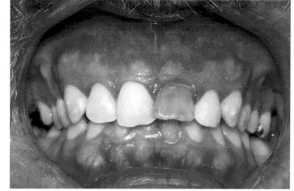

Color Plate 6

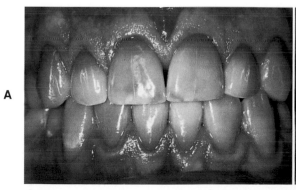

A

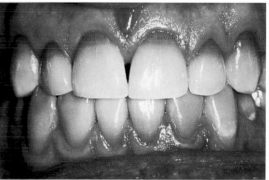

B

Color Plate 7

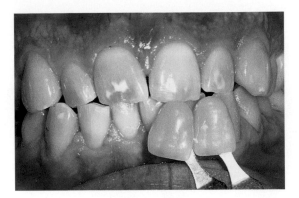

Color Plate 8

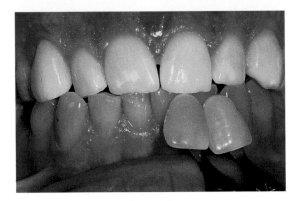

Color Plate 9

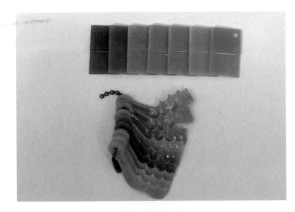

Color Plate 10

INTRODUCTION TO DENTAL MATERIALS

OBJECTIVES

On completion of this chapter the student will be able to:

1. Explain the importance of the study of dental materials for the allied oral health practitioner.
2. Explain why it is necessary that the allied oral health practitioner have an understanding of dental materials for the delivery of dental care.
3. Review the historical development of dental materials.
4. List the agencies responsible for setting standards and specifications of dental materials.
5. List the requirements necessary for a product to qualify for the ADA Seal of Acceptance.

The study of dental materials is a science dealing with the development, properties, manipulation, care, evolution, and evaluation of materials used in the treatment and prevention of dental diseases. Specifically, it includes principles of engineering, chemistry, physics, and biology. Through the understanding of how these basic principles affect the choice, manipulation, patient education, and care of all materials used to assist in rendering dental services, the dental assistant, dental hygienist, and dentist can help ensure the ultimate success of a patient's dental work.

Role of the Allied Oral Health Practitioner and Dental Maretials

Since 1970 efforts have been made to utilize allied oral health practitioners (also referred to in the text as dental auxiliaries) in the performance of intraoral tasks to efficiently deliver health care and enhance the productivity of the dentist. Until 1970 only the dental hygienist was allowed to perform intraoral functions in all states. Although laws vary from state to state, virtually every state has modified, updated, and made changes to its state restrictions to allow for the performance of intraoral procedures by all allied oral health practitioners. Currently several states allow for the placement and care of restorative and other therapeutic agents in the patient's mouth. The dental assistant is most directly responsible for the delivery of dental materials within specific guidelines outlined by the dental manufacturer. The dental hygienist's responsibilities more frequently include the care of the restorative material once it has been placed and the application of some therapeutic and preventive agents. All allied oral health practitioners must have a complete understanding of the potential hazards in the manipulation and disposal of materials and be trained to handle them safely. Background knowledge in the basic principles of dental materials is also essential to the appreciation of the selection of a particular restoration or treatment procedure for individual patient application. It also becomes, in many circumstances, the auxiliary's role to advise the patient why the dentist has recommended a particular restorative or therapeutic material or the choices the patient may have for a particular circumstance.

All of this may seem an overwhelming task given the ever-growing variety of materials available, recommendations for their use or disuse, and rapidly developing techniques in manipulation, placement, and care. Professional journals, dental materials manufacturers and manufacturer's representatives, Internet links, and other resources can provide valuable information. The knowledgeable allied oral health practitioner reviews products used and recommended by the practitioner's office to provide a reliable resource for the patient and the dentist.

Historical Development of Dental Materials

The concept of using materials for restoration, replacement, or beautification to change the appearance or function of the natural dentition predates the Christian era by several generations. Just as today, the diet of our distant ancestors was a chief contributor to dental disease. Although rarely afflicted with dental caries, due to a lack of refined sugars, excessive wear from a diet containing sand, dirt, and grit from grain ground on rough stones produced occlusal surfaces of teeth often worn to the pulp with resultant abscess formation. Examination of mummies has shown loss of teeth because of abscess and periodontal disease from as early as 2500 BCE. Much is found in the literature about treatment options, including remedies of potions and prayer, but no evidence of restorative dentistry exists until around 600 to 300 BCE. The Etruscans, who occupied a nation in the area of present-day Tuscany, created bridges of gold rings and natural teeth. By the Christian Era the Romans had become skilled at restoring teeth with gold shells, fixed bridges, and partial and full dentures, although through the Middle Ages and into the mid-1800s most dental treatment consisted of extraction and artificial replacements.

Casts constructed of plaster from wax impressions were developed in Prussia in the middle of the eighteenth century. Hippopotamus ivory bases with human and animal teeth replacements were popular. However, because it was so difficult to carve ivory, retention of dentures was accomplished by joining the maxillary and mandibular dentures with springs forcing the two parts against the arches. Pierre Fuchard, considered the "father of modern dentistry," devotes a portion of his 1728 book *The Surgeon-Dentist* to this technique. George Washington had several sets of such dentures, losing one tooth after another until at the time of his inauguration in 1790 he had only one tooth left (Figure 1-1). In France in the late 1700s, work was done to improve denture teeth by firing them from porcelain. In 1788 King Louis XVI bestowed on a Parisian dentist an inventor's patent for porcelain teeth. For denture bases the Goodyear brothers gained a patent for rubber called Vulcanite in 1844, and this remained the primary denture base material until World War II (Figure 1-2).

Silver paste is first mentioned by the Chinese in 659 AD; more than 1000 years later, in 1800, it was produced in France from "shavings from silver cut from coins mixed with enough mercury to form a sloppy paste" (Ring, 1993). Health problems arising from the high mercury content of this early amalgam prompted the American Society of Dental Surgeons in 1846 to pass a resolution not to use amalgam under any circumstances. The disagreement over the

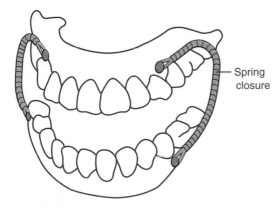

FIGURE 1-1 ■ A denture with spring closure, much like those worn by George Washington.

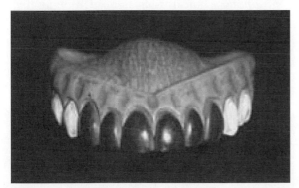

FIGURE 1-2 ■ A denture carved of wood with black and white overlays of materials covering the facial surfaces of teeth. This denture was hand-carved in Japan in the middle 1800s. Notice the detailed carving of the palatal tissues.

(Courtesy Dr. Mark Dillinges)

value and safety of amalgam came to be called the "Amalgam War," and it did not end until 1895 when G.V. Black developed an acceptable amalgam formula.

Gold remained popular for the restoration and decoration of teeth and gained in popularity in 1855 when cohesive gold foil, which could be condensed directly into the cavity preparation, was introduced. At the same time dental cements were introduced. Patterned after a technique for cementing tiles to floors, the first mixtures of cements using zinc oxide with a weak phosphoric acid were developed. In 1907 Dr. William Taggart demonstrated a casting method to produce gold inlays. In 1932 synthetic resins were introduced; these resins soon replaced rubber as the denture base of choice. At this time synthetic resins also became a popular tooth-colored alternative, and, together with the introduction of the acid-etch technique in 1955, they have evolved into one of the most popular of the restorative materials, composite resins.

Preventive dentistry had an early beginning as well, with the first mention of fluoride introduced in 1874 and dispensed in England at this time for the prevention of caries. In 1901 Dr. Frederick McKay is credited with noting dental fluorosis in Colorado Springs, and McKay and G.V. Black determined that drinking water was the factor. These caries-free but mottled teeth prompted McKay to suggest changes in the water supply leading to the first community water fluoridation program in 1945.

Whether through the desire for a natural look or more ornamentation, history shows that the appearance of the teeth was important to our early ancestors. King Solomon is said to have complimented Sheba on her teeth: "Thy teeth are like a flock of sheep that are even shorn, which come up from the washing" (Wynbrandt, 1998). Empress Josephine used a handkerchief to conceal her bad teeth, turning the hankie into a fashion accessory. In 1295 Marco Polo wrote of the people of southern China covering their teeth with thin plates of gold. This use of gold may have suggested the socioeconomic status of the individual, as well as serving a protective purpose. In the mid-1800s, California railroad king Charles Crocker had a gold crown imbedded with diamonds forming the cusps placed on one of his molars.

The history of dental materials and techniques in the restoration, replacement, and beautification of our teeth is full of ingenuity. Even early man knew the importance of maintaining these important structures and more often than not suffered the pain associated with their neglect.

Agencies Responsible for Standards

Most of the triumphs and atrocities of dentistry were discovered by trial and error, mainly at the expense of the patient. It is only in recent times that the study of dental materials includes standards set forth to evaluate a material or technique before it is tried in the patient's mouth. In 1839 the first such attempt was made when the American Society of Dental Surgeons was formed to fight against the use of amalgam.

AMERICAN DENTAL ASSOCIATION

Dentistry continued to try to elevate and regulate the practice of the profession with the establishment of the American Dental Association (ADA) in 1859. In 1866 an ADA committee prepared a statement on a toothpaste claiming that "it cut teeth like so much acid" (Wynbrandt, 1998). By 1930 the ADA had established guidelines for testing of products and awarded the first ADA Seal of Acceptance in 1931 (Figure 1-3). Today members of the ADA's Council on Scientific Affairs and ADA staff scientists review dental drugs, materials, instruments, and equipment for safety and effectiveness before awarding the ADA Seal of Acceptance. Although a strictly voluntary program, today more than 1300 dental products carry the ADA

Seal of Acceptance. Approximately 45% of these products are sold to consumers; most common among these are toothpastes and toothbrushes. The consumer and dentist alike recognize this important symbol of a dental product's safety and effectiveness. The ADA outlines a broad spectrum of requirements that must be met to qualify for the ADA Seal of Acceptance. A list of products qualifying for the ADA Seal of Acceptance is available online at www.ada.org.

The ADA Council on Scientific Affairs also assumes the responsibility of formulating standards and specifications for mechanical, physical, and chemical properties of dental materials to ensure their quality.

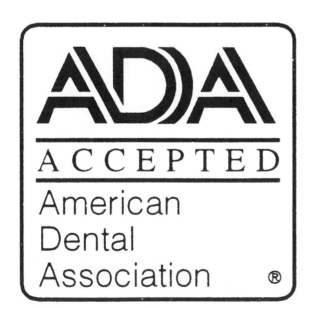

FIGURE 1–3 ■ The ADA Seal of Acceptance.

QUALIFYING FOR THE ADA SEAL OF ACCEPTANCE

Not every dental product qualifies for the ADA Seal of Acceptance. The process typically requires at least 3 months for completion. The ADA Seal of Acceptance is usually awarded for a period of 5 years, at which time it is reevaluated. Products are also reevaluated any time the composition of a previously Accepted product is changed.

Certain requirements must be met. A manufacturer who applies for the ADA Seal of Acceptance must do the following:

- Supply objective data from clinical or laboratory studies that support the product's safety, effectiveness, and promotional claims
- Conduct clinical trials as needed in strict compliance with ADA guidelines and procedures
- Provide evidence that manufacturing and laboratory facilities are properly supervised and adequate to ensure purity and uniformity of the product and that the product is manufactured in compliance with the Good Manufacturing Practice Code
- Submit all advertising, promotional, and patient education materials for review and approval by the ADA and comply with the ADA's Advertising and Exhibiting Standards
- Submit patient information, ingredients lists, and other pertinent product information for review and approval

FOOD AND DRUG ADMINISTRATION

The Food and Drug Administration (FDA) is one of the oldest consumer protection agencies and is charged with protecting the public by ensuring that products meet certain standards of safety and efficacy. The original Food and Drug Act of 1906 did not include provisions to ensure medical and dental device safety or claims. In 1976 the Medical Device Amendment was signed to give the FDA regulatory authority over medical and dental devices, which are now classified and regulated according to their degree of risk to the public. Dental materials, considered devices by the FDA, as well as over-the-counter products sold to the public, are subject to control and regulation by the FDA Center for Devices and Radiological Health.

INTERNATIONAL AGENCIES

Internationally two agencies, the International Dental Federation and the International Standards Organization (ISO), represent the standards used to develop specifications and testing in other countries.

SUMMARY

The dental materials used today are much better than those used in the past, but they are still far from being ideal. Materials continue to be developed and techniques in their manipulation improved. The ADA and FDA are committed to continue to evaluate, test, monitor, assess risks, and review claims and labels of all materials used in dentistry. Current research is concentrating in the areas of composites, adhesives, and ceramics with an emphasis on bringing technology to the dental office and therefore making dental appointments shorter and more comfortable for the patient. The allied oral health practitioner will continue to play an important role in the successful delivery, manipulation, and maintenance of these and other materials as we look forward to the future.

CASE-BASED DISCUSSION TOPICS

◉ Compile a list of 5 to 10 dental products displaying the ADA Seal of Acceptance found in your local drugstore or supermarket. *How is the seal displayed on these items? Ask family and friends if the ADA Seal of Acceptance is important in their selection of a dental product. How does a product carrying the ADA Seal of Acceptance affect your recommendation of that product?*

◉ Research a dental product using the Internet or by contacting a manufacturer's representative. *What information is available? What type of research has been done? How is the product marketed? What assistance is available to the consumer or dental office?*

REFERENCES

American Dental Association: *Dentist's desk reference: materials, instruments and equipment,* ed 2, Chicago, 1983, American Dental Association.
American Dental Association: *Clinical products in dentistry, a desktop reference,* Chicago, 1993, American Dental Association.
Ring ME: *Dentistry: an illustrated history,* New York, 1993, Harry N Abrams.
Wynbrandt J: *The excruciating history of dentistry,* New York, 1998, St Martin's Press.
ADA Online: A list of products qualifying for the ADA Seal of Acceptance. Available at www.ada.org.

2 ORAL ENVIRONMENT AND PATIENT CONSIDERATIONS

OBJECTIVES

On completion of this chapter the student will be able to:

1. List the qualities of the oral environment that make it challenging for long-term clinical performance of dental materials.
2. Describe the long-term clinical requirements of therapeutic and restorative materials.
3. List the three types of biting forces and the tooth structures most ideally suited to them.
4. Define *stress, strain,* and *ultimate strength* and compare the ultimate strength of restorative materials during each type of stress to tooth structures.
5. Describe the effects of moisture and acidity on dental materials.
6. Describe the clinical significance of galvanism and how it can be prevented.
7. Define *thermal conductivity* and *thermal expansion and contraction* and compare the values of thermal expansion and conductivity of restorative materials with those of tooth structures.
8. Describe the process used to achieve mechanical, chemical, and bonding retention.
9. Describe the factors that determine successful adhesion, including wettability, viscosity, film thickness, and surface characteristics.
10. Describe microleakage and how the results of this process can lead to recurrent decay and postoperative sensitivity.
11. Define *biocompatibility* and discuss why requirements for biocompatibility may fluctuate.
12. List the three visible light wavelengths that are sensed when recognizing color.
13. Describe tooth color in terms of hue, value, and chroma.
14. Discuss the importance of detection of restorations and methods for detection.

KEY TERMS ▰▰▰▰▰▰▰▰▰▰▰▰

Therapeutic agents—Items used to treat disease.

Restorative agents—Items used to reconstruct tooth structure.

Compressive force—Pressure applied to compress/condense.

Tensile force—Pressure applied in opposite directions to stretch an object.

Shearing force—Pressure applied when two surfaces slide against each other or in a twisting or rotating motion.

Stress—Pressure or tension exerted on a material object.

Strain—Distortion or deformation occurring when an object cannot resists a stress.

Flexural stress—Bending stress, a combination of tension and compression.

Fatigue failure—Repeated stresses resulting in fractures.

Solubility—Susceptibility to being dissolved.

Water sorption—The ability to absorb moisture.

Corrosion—To wear away, especially by a chemical reaction.

Tarnish—Discoloration caused by oxidation of a metal surface.

Galvanism—An electric current transmitted between two dissimilar metals.

Dimensional change—Expansion and contraction of matter when heated.

Coefficient of thermal expansion—Measurement of expansion and contraction.

Percolation—Space between restoration and tooth caused by continual shrinkage and expansion of restoration.

Thermal conductivity—The rate at which heat flows through a material.

Insulators—Matter that prevents the passage of electricity, heat, or sound through an object.

Exothermic reaction—The reaction of certain components when they are mixed, resulting in the production of heat.

Retention—The ability of a material to maintain its position without displacement under stress.

Adhesion—Ability to stick tightly to another surface.

Bonding—Ability to hold together.

Wetting—The degree to which a liquid adhesive is able to spread over the surface of a tooth and restorative material.

Viscosity—The ability of a liquid material to flow.

Film thickness—The minimum thickness obtainable by a layer of material.

Surface energy—The attraction of atoms to a surface.

Interface—The space between the walls of the preparation and the restoration.

Microleakage—The seepage of harmful materials.

Biocompatible—Materials that do not impede or adversely affect living tissue.

Hue—The dominant color of the wavelength detected.

Chroma—The intensity or strength of the color.

Value—How light or dark a color is.

Transparent—An object that one can see through.

Opaque—An object that completely absorbs light.

Translucency—The balance of transparency and opaqueness in an object.

Vitality—Lifelike appearance.

In the selection, manipulation, and handling of dental materials it is important that the student have an appreciation for the complexity and challenges of the oral environment. The materials placed and used within the oral cavity must be biocompatible, durable, nonreactive in acid or alkaline conditions, compatible with other materials, and esthetically acceptable. All of these factors must be considered within a unique environment. The oral environment produces many limitations: limitations in what can and cannot be used safely, limitations in the type and long-term clinical needs of the treatment, and limitations in the conditions of the oral cavity. These limitations may vary somewhat from patient to patient or in specific circumstances.

The materials must be compatible in an environment of moisture and differing stresses, temperatures, and acid levels. The degree of compatibility may depend on how and how long the materials are expected to be used. Therapeutic agents are generally used for short periods of time whereas restorative agents are expected to remain in contact with tissues for indefinite periods of time. Consider the following cases. If a therapeutic agent is being used to treat a specific condition, such as a denture sore, it would need to be biocompatible with the tissues but would not require an extreme amount of longevity. If the material were being placed as a permanent restoration, such as a gold crown, biocompatibility and longevity would be of great concern.

Patient concerns, questions, and demands must also play a part in the decision process. The patient should be brought into the decision process very early. Tooth-colored materials are frequently requested by the patient, but they may present limitations in their use under certain circumstances. The patient needs to be educated in the limitations of his or her particular situation and the appropriate restorative choices. The allied oral health care practitioner is frequently involved in this education.

Force and Stress

Materials must withstand varying degrees of force through the muscular action of pushing or pulling an object during mastication and for some patients from bruxism or clenching as well. Normal biting force varies among individuals and from one area of the mouth to another. Biting force is largely a mea-

surement of the strength of the muscles of mastication during the normal chewing of foods. When clenching or grinding, this force is increased because of the lack of food cushion and the resultant direct contact of tooth surfaces. Normal masticatory forces on the occlusal surface of molar teeth average 90 to 200 pounds and can increase to as much as 28,000 pounds per square inch on a cusp tip. Masticatory forces decrease in incisor areas and can increase during bruxism or clenching. A study of the anatomy of teeth reveals that each tooth is more ideally suited for specific types of force. The three basic types of force are as follows (Figure 2-1):

Compressive force. Posterior teeth are ideally suited for this type of force. The large occlusal surface and multirooted base will resist a crushing force.

Tensile force. When biting forces are used to stretch a material, the tooth is exerting tensile force.

Shearing force. An incisor used for cutting is an example of shearing force.

When a force is exerted on a tooth, the tooth or material creates resistance to counteract the force. The internal force, which resists the applied force, is called **stress.** If the stress within the object cannot resist the force, distortion or deformation occurs and the object has undergone **strain.** Stress is the amount of force exerted from within an object, and strain is the amount of change that the force has produced. The normal process of chewing rarely involves only one type of stress; these combinations of stresses form complex-stress combinations. Dental bridges are subject to **flexural stress** when compressive forces placed on the occlusal surface of the bridge bend the bridge downward and tensile forces on the tissue side of the bridge stretch upward in response.

Materials may be suited to one type of stress but fail during another. If the force is exerted over a large area, the tooth structures can more adequately

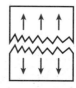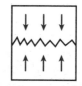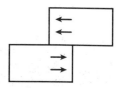

FIGURE 2-1 ■ Types of stress and strain. Tensile stress pulls and stretches a material. Comprehensive stress pushes it together. Shear stress tries to slice it apart.

(From Bird D, Robinson D: *Torres and Ehrlich modern dental assisting,* ed 6, Philadelphia, 1999, WB Saunders, p 370.)

handle the stress. When the force is exerted over a small area, the increase in pressure may result in fracture. Consider a woman wearing flat shoes or spike heels. The weight supported by both is the same, so there is no difference in force. However, because the area of shoe contacting the ground is very different, the pressure on the ground is drastically different. This is the reason that teeth may fracture when biting into small, hard objects, such as a piece of nutshell or a cherry pit.

Values of compressive, tensile, and shearing forces are expressed in Table 2-1. Compare tooth structures, the type of force most predominantly associated with that structure, and the different restorative materials to understand why a material may be better suited in a specific area or situation. For example, amalgam and composite resins more closely replicate enamel in compressive strength, whereas porcelain falls short. Porcelain is more likely to fracture under compressive stresses.

During mastication, stresses occur repetitively over time. Failures rarely occur in a single-force application; they occur when stress is frequently repeated. These repeated stresses may produce microscopic flaws that grow over time, resulting in fracture known as **fatigue failure.** A metal wire bent repeatedly will eventually break; this is an example of fatigue failure. Restorative materials are subject to repeated fatigue testing for all forces. Conditions of the oral cavity such as humidity and temperature and pH fluctuations may also increase fatigue failure.

Moisture and Acid Levels

The oral cavity is continually in contact with moisture. This moisture can vary from acid to alkaline depending on foods, beverages, medications, and the amount of acid-producing bacteria present (plaque). Normal resting pH of saliva ranges from 6.2 to 7.0 (neutral), but it can fluctuate higher or lower by several points during the course of a day. Many materials that would be compatible in a neutral environment will not be compatible in an acidic one. Most materials are adversely affected by moisture, either during placement or over time. The breakdown of most restorative materials is directly related to the effects of moisture, acid, and stress. Materials intended for long-term retention in the mouth must not deteriorate rapidly.

Desirable materials should have low **solubility.** Gold and porcelain are retained in the oral environment for many years because of their insoluble nature. Materials frequently used as tooth-colored restorations are more soluble. They tend to "wash out" or change in mass rather rapidly, requiring their replacement (Figure 2-2). Some materials also have the undesirable characteristic of **water sorption,** which may result in staining or a slight enlargement of the material. The staining of resins and acrylics from repeated exposure to coffee, tea, and other dyed beverages is due to water sorption. Dentures placed in a glass of water will take up the liquid and become slightly larger. Some acrylics will absorb both odors and tastes from foods. Although restorations are not large enough to perceptibly take up the odor or taste of a fluid, the larger surface area of a denture or an orthodontic retainer can absorb enough to take on the odor or taste of foods and fluids. Directions on routine home care can help alleviate this problem.

Metals suffer the effects of moisture and acidity, with the exception of noble metals such as gold. The deterioration of the metal to a chemical attack (acid)

TABLE 2-1

Ultimate Compressive and Tensile Strengths of Tooth and Restorative Structures

Structure	Ultimate Compressive Strength (lbs/in^2)	Ultimate Tensile Strength (lbs/in^2)
Enamel	56,000	1500
Dentin	43,000	4500
Amalgam	45,000-64,000	7000-9000
Porcelain	21,000	5400
Composite resins	30,000-60,000	6000-9000
Acrylic	11,000	8000

or an electrochemical reaction with other metals caused by the moisture and acid present in the oral environment is called **corrosion.** Metals such as steel cannot be used in the oral cavity without first coating them with a barrier to corrosive components; this barrier gives steel its stainless quality. Dental amalgams are particularly susceptible to corrosion. Surface **tarnish** can accelerate in crevices between tooth and restoration and on rough surfaces. Polishing of amalgams to produce a smooth surface has been recommended to help delay this process. In newer high-copper amalgams, this may not be as critical to their longevity.

Galvanism

An environment containing moisture, acidity, and dissimilar metals makes the generation of electric current possible. The salts of the saliva facilitate the movement of electric current from one type of metal to another. The phenomenon of electric current being transmitted between two dissimilar metals is called **galvanism.** The current may result in stimulation to the pulp, called *galvanic shock.* The classic example of a metal fork touching a metal restoration will be familiar to anyone with metal restorations and unfamiliar to those who have no metal in their mouth. Some patients may even feel galvanic shock or report a metal taste when instruments are used against the surface of a restoration. When it becomes necessary to place differing types of metal restorations such as a gold crown in contact with an

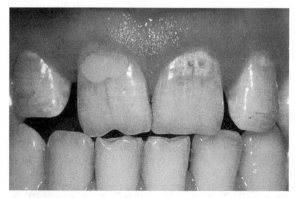

FIGURE 2-2 ■ "Washed out" composite restorations on teeth 8 and 9 are stained as a result of solubility of this restorative material.

amalgam restoration, insulation of the restorations can help lessen the stimulation. In time the galvanic stimulation will decrease as oxides form on the surface of the metal, acting as an insulator against the galvanic current.

Temperature

The ingestion of foods and beverages and smoking may alter the temperature of the oral environment. With few exceptions, all forms of matter expand when they are heated and contract when cooled, resulting in **dimensional change.** Acceptable materials used as restorations and replacement of tooth structure should have characteristics of expansion and contraction similar enough to tooth structures to maintain them within the preparation. Excessive expansion may result in fracture of cusps, and excessive contraction may result in leakage of fluids and bacteria into the open gaps, resulting in sensitivity. Expansion and contraction are measured using the **coefficient of thermal expansion** (CTE), the measurement of change in volume or length in relationship to change in temperature. Materials such as composites and amalgam have rates of expansion and contraction that differ enough from tooth structures that the marginal integrity of the restoration may be compromised. The repeated shrinkage and expansion of the restoration during ingestion of cold and hot fluids and foods produces the opening and closing of a gap between the restoration and the tooth surface; this is called **percolation.** Percolation allows the ingress of bacteria and oral fluids and may lead to recurrent caries, staining, and pulpal irritation.

Thermal conductivity is the rate at which heat flows through a material. Metals are excellent thermal conductors. Gold is one of the best thermal conductors, whereas nonmetals such as ceramics, resins, cements, enamel, and dentin are poor conductors. Poor conductors can be used as **insulators;** dentin is a natural insulator. When metal restorations conduct temperature changes from the foods and beverages taken into the oral cavity, the stimulation may be felt by the pulp of the tooth, causing sensitivity. A piece of ice placed on an amalgam restoration may conduct stimulation to the pulp in as little as 2 to 3 seconds. When metal restorations are placed close to the pulp of the tooth, an insulating cement or material is often placed between the tooth structure and the restoration to delay and absorb the transfer of temperature. Metals placed against tissue such as partial denture framework and some orthodontic appliances can have the same effect.

Table 2-2 gives values of thermal expansion and thermal conductivity. Compare values with tooth structures to determine the potential marginal leakage through percolation or the need for insulation. When there is a large difference between the CTE and the restorative material, as for amalgam and tooth structure, the percolation will be greater. Although composite has a larger CTE than tooth structure, bonding it to the tooth structure helps prevent percolation. Amalgam and gold have much higher values of thermal conductivity than dentin and enamel; hot coffee may transmit heat readily through these metals, resulting in pulpal stimulation. The use of insulating materials such as an insulating base is recommended when these materials are placed near the pulp.

In addition to temperature considerations for materials already present in the mouth, it is important to consider the temperature of materials as they are placed into the mouth. The reaction of the components of some materials when they are mixed results in the production of heat. This **exothermic reaction** must be minimized by proper mixing to prevent excess heat from coming in contact with susceptible tooth surface.

Retention

An important factor in the selection of a material is how it will be retained within or on the tooth. **Retention** may be secured through mechanical or chemical **adhesion** or **bonding** mechanisms between materials. Mechanical retention involves the use of undercuts or other projections into which the material is locked in place. The undercuts used in a typical amalgam preparation are an illustration of mechanical retention (Figure 2-3). Notice that the opening is smaller than the internal floor of the preparation. Once the material is hardened in place, it is retained through this design. When a significant amount of tooth structure has been removed, undercuts can no longer be successfully used. At this time the clinician may wish to place a restoration over the remaining tooth structure (a crown) and hold it in place with a chemical adhesive. Adhesives used in dentistry are commonly called *dental cements*. Dental cement retains the restoration by chemically and mechanically connecting the two surfaces.

TABLE 2-2
Thermal Properties of Tooth and Restorative Structures

Structure	Coefficient of Thermal Expansion ($\times 10^{-6}$/°C)	Thermal Conductivity (k [mcal cm]/cm² sec °C)
Enamel	11	2.0
Dentin	8	1.30
Amalgam	20-28	54
Gold	15	350
Porcelain	15	2.5
Composite resin	26-40	2.6

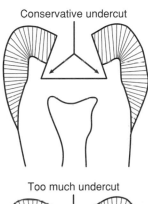

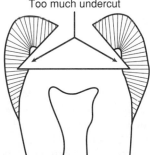

FIGURE 2-3 ■ The retentive undercuts of a conservative preparation and an excessively undercut preparation that compromised the remaining tooth structure.

Bonding is a term also commonly used when describing the retention of materials. Bonding of materials occurs when the tooth surface is prepared with an acid etch technique to create microscopic pores in enamel and dentin. A fluid bonding material is then allowed to flow into these pores and mechanically lock into the tooth structure. Restorative materials are then placed that adhere chemically to the bonding material. This technique in producing retention has several advantages. It requires less removal of tooth structure, because no undercuts are necessary; it produces a stronger retentive force between tooth and restoration; and it can seal the margin of the restoration to prevent the seepage of bacteria and fluids through percolation.

Most of today's restorative materials use a combination of mechanical and chemical or bonding adhesion for optimum retention. Retention by mechanical undercuts alone will not adequately seal the margins of the restoration and will frequently place tooth structure in jeopardy of fracture when undercuts leave vulnerable areas of tooth structure unsupported. Adhesion and bonding require the intimate contact of surfaces to produce the best bond strength. The strength of the bond is measured by applying shear and tensile stresses.

Several factors affect the bond strength or the success of a material as an adhesive. These include wetting; viscosity; film thickness; and the surface characteristics of the tooth, the restoration, and the adhesive.

Wetting is the degree to which the liquid adhesive is able to spread over the surface of the tooth and restorative material. The Teflon surface of cooking equipment has poor wetting; that is, liquids bead up on the surface rather than spreading out. The better the adhesive is able to spread on the surface of the tooth and restoration, the more retentive it is. This ability may be hindered or enhanced by the material's **viscosity,** the ability of a liquid material to flow. Materials with high viscosity are thicker and do not flow well and therefore may not be effective in wetting an area. Viscosity also can affect the film thickness of the adhesive. **Film thickness** is particularly important to dental cements. When cementing a crown, if the film thickness of the cement is too great, it may keep the crown from seating completely. A thin film of cement is desirable to allow the cement to completely wet the surfaces and for excess material to flow from under the crown when it is seated under pressure during cementation.

Surface characteristics are the final factors that affect the adhesive retention of a material. They include the cleanliness of a surface, moisture contamination, surface texture, and surface energy of the restoration and tooth. As mentioned, adhesion is dependent on intimate contact of surfaces. Even slight contamination can prevent contact. Debris from the tooth preparation, microorganisms in plaque, and products of saliva are often impossible to completely eliminate.

Surface irregularities may prevent complete wetting of the surfaces. Microscopic surface irregularities trap air as the adhesive flows over them, resulting in an incomplete wetting of the surface. The **surface energy** of the surfaces involved determines the attraction of the atoms to them. When liquids bead up on a surface, the surface has low surface energy, such as on wax or many plastics. Liquids generally wet or spread over materials with high surface energy better; metals, ceramics, and enamel have high surface energies.

Many situations present conditions that are not favorable for retention of materials. The dentist is responsible for the mechanical design of the preparation but is not solely responsible for other factors. In many states, allied oral health care practitioners routinely place therapeutic and restorative materials. In addition, the dental assistant plays an essential role in delivering materials and controlling the conditions of the oral environment during their delivery. An understanding of the factors that influence retention is essential to achieving a successful restoration.

Microleakage

The need for replacement of restorative materials can be significantly influenced by microleakage. The space between the walls of the preparation and the restoration is called the **interface.** If this interface is not sealed, fluids and microorganisms can penetrate between tooth structure and restorative material. This seepage of harmful materials is called **microleakage** and is frequently responsible for recurrent decay, marginal staining, and postoperative sensitivity. It is easy to understand why the seepage of bacteria and other fluids between preparation and restoration sets up an environment for recurrent

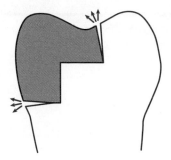

FIGURE 2-4 ■ Microleakage allows the seepage of fluids and microorganisms into the restoration/tooth structure interface.

decay and staining. Postoperative sensitivity maybe due to microleakage as well (Figure 2-4). The tubules, which make up the hard tooth structure, are filled with fluids under pressure from the pulp. When the enamel of the tooth is removed, fluids can flow out of the much larger dentinal tubules and outside chemicals can flow in. Both the movement of fluids out of the tubules and the movement of chemicals into the tubules, as well as air trapped in the tubules, can cause postoperative sensitivity. Procedures for ensuring the proper seal of the dentinal tubules are described in Chapter 5.

Biocompatibility

Materials must be **biocompatible;** that is, they must not impede or adversely affect living tissue. However, all materials contain potentially irritating ingredients. A material may be acceptable for use or fabrication on hard tissues (tooth structure) but may not be acceptable for use on soft tissues. Some materials may be therapeutic in small quantities or if in contact with tissues for short periods of time, but may be irritating or toxic with longer or larger doses. Topical fluoride is of great benefit when used according to the manufacturer's directions, but it can be irritating to soft tissues and can even excessively etch enamel if used improperly. The limitations and precautions for the use of each material are outlined in later chapters.

Adverse responses may be due to the material itself or due to the breakdown of its components in the oral environment. Frequently materials are used in combination to produce the restoration, such as a porcelain-fused-to-metal crown cemented with glass ionomer cement. The use of multiple materials makes adverse responses more difficult to evaluate. It is now reported that significant percentages of people have skin allergies or hypersensitivity to some metals, particularly nickel and acrylics, and should avoid these materials. A complete health history and questioning of the patient can help identify such individuals. In general, materials intended for permanent replacement of tooth structures should exhibit no adverse biologic responses.

Esthetics

Materials used in dentistry must be esthetically acceptable. Esthetic dentistry is a growing priority, and esthetics may be of great concern to the patient. The human eye senses light through the cone cells in the retina in three different ranges of wavelength: red, green, and blue. Having three types of color-sensing cells does not limit the human eye to three colors. The stimulation of two or more types of cone cells, the amount of light they detect, and the interpretation of that light by the brain determine the overall response to a particular color. Mixtures of red, green, and blue light allow one to see any color. A color television mixes these primary colors of light to produce full-color pictures.

Three components describe the resultant color: hue, chroma, and value. **Hue** is the dominant color of the wavelength detected. Tooth colors are predominantly seen in the yellow and brown range. The **chroma** refers to the intensity or strength of the color; teeth are rather pale in color. **Value** describes how light or dark the color is; teeth have value ranges in the light scale.

The color of teeth is also determined by the way they reflect light. If light passes directly through an object it is **transparent;** if light is completely absorbed by the object it is **opaque.** Usually both of these processes occur in varying degrees, reflecting light and giving the tooth **translucency.** This lifelike quality is called **vitality.**

Individuals see these many colors, components, and reflections of color somewhat differently and in different situations. It is important that we have a standardized measure of color such as a shade guide to provide an objective measure. It is also important that we produce an environment that reduces the

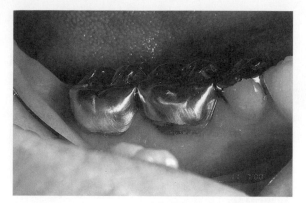

FIGURE 2-5 ■ The scratched surface of these gold crowns may be due to inappropriate use of polishing agents.

possibility of extraneous color reflection, producing an inaccurate color. A detailed discussion of shade selection is presented in Chapter 6.

Detection of Restorative Materials

It is important that oral health care professionals are able to identify restorative materials within the oral environment to treat them appropriately. Heavy pressure during scaling, the use of sonic and ultrasonic scaling or air polishing, and inappropriate use of polishing agents may gouge or scratch the surface of a restoration (Figure 2-5). The placement of therapeutic agents such as fluoride may erode the surface of the restoration.

Identification of restorative materials—although often obvious, such as with amalgam materials—may be difficult when identifying tooth-colored materials. In addition, restorations may be composed of different materials, such as a porcelain inlay cemented with resin-based cement. Tooth-colored restorative materials may be identified by appearance, location, tactile sensitivity, and radiography. The appearance of a well-matched tooth-colored restoration may be difficult to distinguish from natural tooth structures. Adequate illumination, liberal use of air, and even magnification may be needed to identify these restorations. The location of margins, especially those placed subgingivally, makes visual inspection of many materials impossible.

Tactile evaluation of the tooth surface may be the most reliable means of clinical assessment. The surface of some composite and glass ionomer restorations may have a rougher surface than enamel. Tracing the enamel surface onto the restoration with the sharp tip of an explorer is the best way to distinguish this difference. Once the presence of a restoration is identified, the entire cavosurface margin may be evaluated. Sealants have a smooth, glassy surface covering the anatomic pits and fissures of the tooth surfaces.

Radiographs are a valuable tool for detection of restorations and the assessment of restorative components. Composites may be radiopaque or radiolucent; glass ionomers are radiopaque, as are many resin-based cements and porcelain (Figures 2-6 and 2-7).

For most difficult to detect restorations, it is necessary to use a combination of methods to determine the presence and type of material before clinical procedures are performed.

SUMMARY

The oral environment presents unique obstacles to the success of dental materials used as restorative and therapeutic agents. An understanding of the limiting factors in this environment and an appreciation for how these limitations affect the selection of materials is essential to the study of dental materials. Materials used must be biocompatible, exhibit long-term clinical durability, and be esthetically acceptable. No one material is superior in all of these areas. The allied oral health care practitioner must have an understanding of the limitations and the criteria for selection of therapeutic and restorative materials. With this knowledge, the practitioner can inform the patient about the materials used in the patient's mouth, as well as select and properly manipulate materials to ensure their ultimate success.

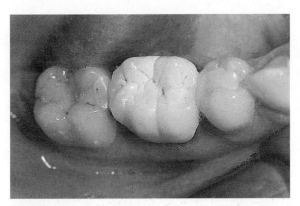

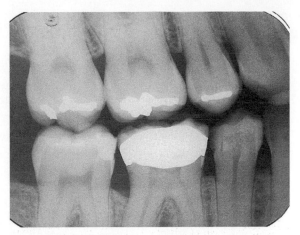

FIGURE 2-6 ■ Tooth-colored restorative materials may be difficult to detect: number 29 distal occlusal (DO) composite, number 30 porcelain fused to metal crown, number 31 mesial occlusal (MO) composite restoration.

FIGURE 2-7 ■ Radiograph of the restorations in Figure 2-6. Note the radiopacity and radiolucency of the restorative materials.

CHAPTER REVIEW

Select the one correct response for each of the following multiple-choice questions:

1. **Materials that require long-term clinical biocompatibility include**
   a. Therapeutic agents
   b. Restorative agents

2. **Which of the following restorative materials is most likely to fracture under compressive stress?**
   a. Amalgam
   b. Composite resin
   c. Porcelain

3. **Which of the following restorative materials is the least soluble?**
   a. Amalgam
   b. Composite resin
   c. Porcelain

4. **Corrosion is of greatest concern for which of the following restorative materials?**
   a. Gold
   b. Composite resin
   c. Amalgam

5. **Restorative materials with values of thermal conductivity similar to enamel include**
   a. Gold
   b. Composite resin
   c. Amalgam

6. **An example of galvanism is**
   a. Amalgam contacting gold
   b. Amalgam contacting composite
   c. Amalgam contacting porcelain

7. **Microleakage may be responsible for**
   a. Recurrent decay   c. Postoperative sensitivity
   b. Marginal staining   d. All of the above

8. **An excessive film thickness may cause**
   a. An increase in retention
   b. A decrease in marginal leakage
   c. Improper seating of the restoration

9. **Materials used for the restoration of enamel need high**
   a. Opacity
   b. Chroma
   c. Vitality

10. **Conditions necessary to adequately identify tooth-colored restorations include all of the following EXCEPT:**
    a. Natural lighting   c. Magnification
    b. A sharp explorer   d. Dry field

CASE-BASED DISCUSSION TOPICS

◉ A 45-year-old businessman comes to your dental office with the chief complaint of having to wear a maxillary removable partial denture. He wishes to have this removable prosthesis replaced with a fixed bridge. Examination reveals that the partial denture replaces teeth numbers 6 through 11. *Discuss the stresses that would be placed on this bridge and the indications and contraindications for a bridge replacing this many teeth and replacing teeth in this location.*

◉ A 25-year-old schoolteacher comes to your office with the chief complaint of losing a distal-incisal class IV composite from tooth number 9. She explains that this restoration has been in place for only a few days. *Discuss the factors that might affect the bond strength of this restoration and what you can do to help prevent this from happening again.*

◉ Stand looking into a mirror or position yourself to examine someone else's mouth. Check how tooth surfaces contact on the posterior, middle, and anterior teeth when in normal occlusion, biting edge-to-edge on anterior teeth, and moving the jaw laterally and front to back. *Which forces are being exerted by these teeth and when?*

◉ Stand looking into a mirror or position yourself to examine someone else's mouth. Check for metal and resin restorations. Place a piece of ice on the enamel of a tooth, on the metal, and on the resin restoration. *How long does it take to feel sensation to the pulp for each? What is this property called?*

◉ Stand looking into a mirror or position yourself to examine someone else's mouth. Look at the gingival, middle, and incisal/occlusal third of the anterior and posterior teeth. *How does the color of the area change? Is there a change in translucency or opacity? Place something bright red close to the teeth. Then direct the dental lamp or other bright light onto the teeth. How do these factors affect the color?*

REFERENCES

Anusavice KJ: *Phillips' science of dental materials,* ed 10, Philadelphia, 1996, WB Saunders.

Bird D, Robinson D: *Torres and Ehrlich modern dental assisting,* ed 6, Philadelphia, 1999, WB Saunders.

Craig RG: *Restorative dental materials,* ed 10, St Louis, 1997, Mosby.

Ferracane JL: *Materials in dentistry,* Philadelphia, 1995, Lippincott.

Gladwin M, Bagby M: *Clinical aspects of dental materials,* Philadelphia, 1999, Lippincott.

Introduction to biomaterials properties. Biomaterials properties table listing. Available at www.lib.umich.edu/dentlib/Dental_tables/toc.html.

3 PHYSICAL PROPERTIES OF DENTAL MATERIALS

CHAPTER OUTLINE

Physical Structure
Solids
Liquids

Application

Composition

Reaction

Manipulation

Summary

Chapter Review

Case-Based Discussion Topics

References

OBJECTIVES

On completion of this chapter the student will be able to:

1. List the three forms of matter and give a defining characteristic of each.
2. Define *density* and explain the relationship of density, volume, and crystalline structure.
3. Define *hardness* and describe how it contributes to abrasion resistance.
4. Define *elasticity* and give an example of when elasticity is desirable in dental procedures.
5. Relate stiffness and proportional limit and how these properties apply to restorative dental materials.
6. Define *ductility* and *malleability* and how these characteristics contribute to the edge strength of a gold crown.
7. Differentiate between toughness and resilience.
8. Define *brittleness* and how this property applies to restorative dental materials.
9. Define *viscosity* and *thixotropic materials* and give the clinical significance of each.
10. Differentiate among therapeutic, preventive, and restorative materials.
11. List the component classifications that may make up a dental material.
12. Describe the reaction stages a material undergoes to acquire its final state.
13. Describe the variables in the manipulation of a material.

KEY TERMS

Density—Measure of weight of a material as compared with its volume.
Hardness—The resistance of a solid to penetration.
Ultimate strength—The maximum amount of stress a material can withstand without breaking.
Elasticity—The ability to stretch and not break.
Stiffness—The resistance to deformation of a material.
Proportional limit—The greatest stress a structure can withstand without permanent deformation.
Resilience—The resistance of a material to permanent deformation.

Toughness—The ability of a material to resist fracture.

Ductility—The amount of dimensional change a material can withstand without breaking.

Malleability—The ability for a material to be compressed without breaking.

Edge strength—The combination of ductility and malleability gives metal the ability to resist fracture or abrasion even at fine margins.

Viscosity—The ability of a liquid material to flow.

Thixotropic materials—Liquids that flow more easily under mechanical forces (e.g., fluoride gel).

Direct restorative materials—Materials that can be applied directly in the mouth, such as amalgams.

Indirect restorative materials—Materials that must be fabricated outside of the mouth, such as porcelain.

Mixing time—The amount of time the auxiliary has to bring the components.

Working time—The time permitted to manipulate the material in the mouth.

Initial set time—The time that begins when the material can no longer be manipulated in the mouth.

Final set time—The time when the material has reached its ultimate state.

Chemical-set materials—Materials that set through a timed chemical reaction with the combination of a catalyst and base.

Light-activated materials—Materials that require a blue light source to initiate a reaction.

Dual-set materials—Materials that begin with the initiation of a blue light source and continue with a chemical-set reaction.

Shelf life—The deterioration and change in quality of a material over time.

To predict how a material will react under oral conditions, it is necessary to have an understanding of its physical properties. Chapter 2 discusses how the oral environment can affect and challenge the properties of dental materials. This chapter discusses how those properties are achieved, how they influence the clinician's choice of a material, and how and when properties can be manipulated.

To begin a discussion of the physical properties of dental materials, it is necessary to categorize materials by classification. Their physical structure, application, manipulation, composition, and reaction can classify materials.

Physical Structure

The physical structure of a material may take on three basic forms: solid, liquid, or gas. Solids have both shape and volume; liquids have volume but no shape; and gases have neither definite shape nor volume. Most materials are mixtures of more than one state of matter. For example, plaster is a mixture of both a solid and liquid, and fluoride foams are a mixture of a liquid and gas (air). This chapter explores the general characteristics common to each form of matter.

SOLIDS

Primary bonds hold solids together, giving them strength and stability. The most stable have a regular crystalline structure with molecules in a regularly spaced pattern. If these molecules are arranged in a random form with no regular pattern, the solid is less stable and is termed *amorphous*. Solids are described by their density, hardness, elasticity, stiffness, ductility, malleability, and brittleness.

Density is a measure of the compactness of matter, or how much mass is squeezed into a given space. The denser a material is, the less air or spacing there is between atoms. If you take a marshmallow and flatten it, the volume of the marshmallow is decreased and the density increased. The close spacing of the crystalline structure gives the greatest density. Enamel is the densest of the tooth structures, and gold is a dense restorative material.

Hardness is used to define a material's resistance to wear and abrasion. The hardness of a material is used to determine the ability of an abrasive to scratch or resist scratching the substrate to which it is applied. Enamel and porcelain are two of the hardest materials and are more resistant to being scratched than are cementum on the root or composite resins or gold crowns.

When a solid is subjected to an external force, it undergoes change in size and shape. Chapter 2 discusses the effects of compressive, shearing, and tensile forces on oral structures and restorative materials. The maximum amount of stress a material can withstand without breaking is known as the **ultimate strength.** A material does not necessarily have to break when subjected to an external compressive, shearing, or tensile force; it may deform. If this deformation is not permanent and the material recovers from the force completely, it has good **elasticity.** A rubber band is an example of a material with elasticity. Not all materials return to their original shape when the deforming force is removed. Materials that do not return to their original shape have exceeded their elastic limit. Rubber can be deformed quite a bit before undergoing permanent deformation. The elasticity of a material is important for impression materials, which must be stretched over tooth or bony undercuts without permanent deformation. It is important for orthodontics because wires and springs are deformed and the force they generate in returning to their original shape moves teeth.

The **stiffness** of a material is its resistance to deformation and is measured by Young's elastic modulus. Stiffer materials have a higher modulus; for example, enamel has a high modulus. Restorative materials should have a modulus that is compatible with tooth structure. Although it is usually not desirable for dental restorations to bend or compress when a force is applied, this is a desirable characteristic for impression materials and orthodontic wire. When enough force is applied to a structure it may not be able to recover from this force, and the structure may become permanently deformed. This material has reached its limit of elasticity, or **proportional limit.** Below the proportional limit no permanent deformation occurs, and the structure returns to its original shape. **Resilience** is the resistance of a material to permanently deform. Impression materials and orthodontic wire must be resilient to be successful. **Toughness** is the ability of a material to resist fracture; restorative materials must exhibit toughness.

The orthodontic wire being pulled or stretched under tension is a measure of its **ductility.** Materials with poor ductility are classified as *brittle.* These materials are much weaker when subjected to tensile forces than when subjected to compressive forces. Porcelain is brittle and cannot undergo much tensile stress without fracture; its ultimate strength is approximately equal to its elastic limit.

Gold is highly ductile and **malleable,** easily compressed and formed into a thin sheet. The combination of malleability and ductility gives a metal the ability to resist fracture or abrasion even at fine margins, giving the metal **edge strength.** These characteristics allow for the superior edge strength of gold crowns. In most cases metals tend to be ductile and malleable whereas ceramics are brittle.

LIQUIDS

Unlike the molecules of a solid, molecules in a liquid state are not confined to patterns; they can flow. The study of this flow is the science of rheology. Fluid flow can be steady or unsteady. The movement of a liquid will depend on the characteristics of the liquid and the surface on which it is placed. Chapter 2 defines these characteristics and their relationship in the discussion of bonding.

The **viscosity** of a liquid is its resistance to flow. Values of viscosity depend on the nature of the fluid—thin fluids have low viscosity whereas thicker fluids have high viscosity. Usually the viscosity of liquids decreases as the temperature increases. **Thixotropic materials** are liquids that flow more easily under mechanical forces. Fluoride gels are often advertised as thixotropic. This gives the operator control of the gel while in the delivery tray so that it does not drip out when being inserted into the mouth. Once the material is in the mouth, the patient is instructed to chew on the tray, decreasing the material's viscosity and allowing it to flow into pits and fissures and interproximally to improve penetration into all surfaces.

Application

Materials are classified by their application, how they will be used and fabricated. They may be preventive, therapeutic, or restorative. Preventive materials are directed toward preventing the occurrence of oral diseases and promoting oral health. Fluorides and pit and fissure sealants are preventive materials. Therapeutic materials are used in the treatment of disease and include materials such as medicated bases or topical treatments for periodontal disease. Restorative materials make up the largest classification. This classification applies to any filling, inlay, crown, bridge, implant, partial denture, or complete denture that restores or replaces lost tooth structure, teeth, or oral tissue. These restorations may be further classified as **direct restorative materials** or **indirect restorative materials.** Some materials may be fabricated directly in the mouth, such as amalgams and composites. Other materials, because of convenience or toxic or other physically harmful characteristics, must be fabricated indirectly outside the mouth and then placed into the oral environment. For example, porcelain must be fired to temperatures of over 1000° F, making it necessary to be fabricated indirectly.

Composition

Components and the reaction of those components may classify materials. Most materials combine two components at chairside to form the resulting material. These initial two components may begin as water and powder, liquid and powder, paste and liquid, paste and paste, or paste and initiator (blue light). Dental plaster begins with water and powder components; composite restorations may use a paste and blue light as an initiator. Many components are classified as catalyst and base; the catalyst is responsible for the speed with which the reaction occurs and is often the liquid component. Components may be measured and dispensed as catalyst and base or prepackaged in predosed amounts. The standardization of measurements in predosed packages eliminates the errors produced in measuring.

Reaction

When components are mixed together, a reaction occurs. That reaction may be physical, such as the evaporation or cooling of liquid, or it may be chemical, creating new primary bonds. Most reactions of the two components result in a solid structure. This process goes through stages before the material reaches its ultimate state: the manipulation stage and the reaction stage. Both stages are defined in units of time. The manipulation stage includes the mixing time and working time; the reaction stage includes the initial set and final set times. **Mixing time** is the amount of time the auxiliary has to bring the components together into a homogeneous mix. Mixing times must be strictly adhered to in order to allow the clinician the full **working time.** The working time is the time permitted to manipulate the material in the mouth. The **initial set time** begins when the material no longer can be manipulated in the mouth, and the **final set time** is when the material has reached its ultimate state. The mixing and working time often offer some control variables. Mixing slowly and cooling the components may increase the working time; the addition of more catalyst may decrease the working time. The control of these variables is important for some situations. When working with pediatric patients, or patients who have limited opening, decreasing the working time would be desirable. When working with a large amount of restorative material, an increase in the working time may be required so that the material can be manipulated for a longer amount of time.

The amount of working time may also be controlled by how the reaction stage is initiated. **Chemical-set materials** are those that set through the timed chemical reaction of the catalyst and base. Once the two components come in contact with each other, the chemical reaction begins and continues through the reaction stage. **Light-activated materials** use a blue light source to initiate the reaction stage. Both components are present in the material but do not react until the material comes in contact with the blue light source, thus giving the clinician unlimited working time. **Dual-set materials** begin with the initiation of the blue light source and then continue with a chemical-set reaction; this also gives the clinician much more control of the working time.

The setting times, initial and final, are also important to the auxiliary. Through the end of the initial set the material must not be disturbed. Moisture and pressure controls are frequently important during initial set. Moisture contamination, from saliva and blood, during initial setting time may have an adverse effect on many dental materials, causing them to fail. Continued firm pressure from biting force, or by holding the material firmly in the mouth, is essential for materials needing intimate contact with the tooth, such as dental cements. The final set of the material may occur while the patient is still in the office or several hours later. Many amalgam restorations reach their final set 6 to 8 hours after placement. Appropriate patient postoperative instructions on when and what to eat or to place pressure on the restoration are essential to avoid fracture of these materials. The accompanying box gives manipulation instructions for a dental cement indicated in units of time.

Manipulation

The manipulation of the material's components is an important consideration for the dental auxiliary. It is through this manipulation that the final characteristics of the material are achieved. Some materials offer some variation in their manipulation; others are highly technique-sensitive, and even the slightest variation will have a detrimental affect on the final product. Variables in the manipulation of the material begin with the ratios of the components. The manufacturer, using the weight or volume of the components, recommends specific ratios. Many materials are produced as separate components that must be measured and dispensed according to the manufacturer's recommendations. Manufacturers

also produce materials in predosed units, eliminating the need to measure and dispense the components and thus standardizing the ratios. Changing the ratios of the materials by adding more catalyst may result in a faster reaction; increasing the amount of water or liquid component may also result in a less dense, weaker material. These ratio changes are variables that permit the clinician to alter manipulation and reaction times for some materials but are contraindicated with other materials because of adverse effects. Manufacturers give direction as to when and how much variation in ratio the material can withstand without adverse results.

External variables such as the temperature of the material and the room temperature and humidity can also play an important part in the manipulation of materials. In general, high temperatures and humidity will accelerate the reaction of the material, and low temperatures and humidity will retard the reaction.

How the materials are mixed—quickly or slowly, on a paper pad or a glass slab, or by hand mixing or using automix dispensers—will affect the final material and its consistency (Figure 3-1). Materials mixed slowly on glass will usually result in a slower reaction; automix materials will give a more consistent result, because the materials are mixed by equipment in a standardized manner, eliminating the variables of human error.

The **shelf life** of a material refers to the deterioration and change in quality of the material over

---

MANIPULATION OF A DENTAL CEMENT FOR CEMENTATION OF A CROWN EXPRESSED IN UNITS OF TIME

- *Liquid/powder ratio:* 2 scoops of powder to 4 drops of liquid.
- *Mixing time:* Mix all of the powder aggressively into the liquid, about 30 seconds.
- *Working time:* Spread the cement over all of the internal surfaces of the crown; working time is 2.5 minutes.
- *Initial setting time:* Wait 2 minutes after placement, then remove the excess cement with an appropriate instrument. Knotted floss can be used in the interproximal areas.
- *Final setting time:* Oral set time is approximately 6 minutes.

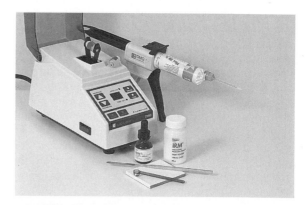

FIGURE 3-1 ■ Hand-mixed materials include a powder and a liquid mixed together on a mixing slab; equipment used in mixing materials includes the dental amalgamator. Automix dispensers will mix materials as they are expressed out of the gun-type applicator.

time. Attention to the date of expiration is important for consistency in the optimum characteristics of the product. Conditions of storage such as temperature and humidity, as well as type of storage container, may directly affect the material's shelf life. Some materials require refrigeration to prolong their useful life; some must be protected from direct light and may be packaged in light-blocking containers. Always refer to manufacturers' directions to determine conditions of storage and expiration.

SUMMARY

The physical structure of a material helps define the characteristics expected from that material. The success of dental materials is directly related to the choices the auxiliary makes in selecting and manipulating the components while keeping in mind those variables that cannot be altered. Controlling variables of manipulation and reaction stages has become increasingly important with more sophisticated materials and challenging clinical situations. Hand mixing of materials allows for some control of manipulation and reaction stages. However, inconsistencies in mixing and time demands have become problematic in many clinical situations. Manufacturers produce materials in a variety of forms to address these concerns. Predosed materials are manufactured to standardize the amount of catalyst and base included in the mix, thus preventing inconsistencies in resultant physical properties. Automix materials standardize the amount of catalyst and base and produce a consistent homogeneous mix. It is important to refer to the manufacturer's directions for instruction in the storage, proportioning, mixing, and variables that may be changed to produce the best final results.

CHAPTER REVIEW

Select the one correct response for each of the following multiple-choice questions:

1. **A defining characteristic of a solid is that it has**
   a. Shape and volume
   b. Shape only
   c. Neither shape nor volume
   d. Volume but no shape

2. **The most stable primary bonds**
   a. Have random form
   b. Have regular crystalline structures
   c. Are amorphous
   d. Have mixed physical structure

3. **When the weight of a material increases in relationship to its volume, it is described as**
   a. Elastic
   b. Resilient
   c. Dense
   d. Hard

4. **Hardness determines the material's ability to**
   a. Deform an object
   b. Break an object
   c. Be easily compressed
   d. Resist wear

5. **When deformation is not permanent and a material recovers, it has good**
   a. Toughness
   b. Elasticity
   c. Malleability
   d. Ductility

6. **If a material becomes permanently deformed, it has exceeded its**
   a. Ultimate strength
   b. Stiffness
   c. Proportional limit
   d. Toughness

7. **Thixotropic materials are those that**
   a. Have poor viscosity
   b. Flow under mechanical forces
   c. Flow at higher temperatures
   d. Flow at lower temperatures

8. **Indirect restorative materials would include all of the following EXCEPT:**
   a. Porcelain crowns
   b. Amalgam restorations
   c. Gold crowns
   d. Porcelain veneers

9. **Mixing time is the length of time from**
   a. The beginning of mixing to the end of setting time
   b. The beginning of mixing to the initial set time
   c. The beginning of mixing to the beginning of working time
   d. The beginning of mixing to the end of working time

10. **A material mixed slowly on a cooled glass surface will**
    a. Have a shorter working and setting time
    b. Have a longer setting and working time
    c. Have a shorter working and longer setting time
    d. Have a longer working and shorter setting time

CASE-BASED DISCUSSION TOPICS

◉ Mary Smith has come to your office for a crown preparation on tooth number 18. The dentist has recommended a porcelain-fused-to-metal crown for this area. The tooth is prepared with tapered, feather-edge margins, and a final impression is taken. *How would the stiffness of the impression material affect the accuracy of the final impression? If Mary grinds or clenches her teeth, how will this affect the new restoration and restorations on the opposing teeth? Why is gold's edge strength an important characteristic for this preparation?*

◉ Bill Miller is scheduled for an orthodontic appointment; he has been in full orthodontic treatment for several months, resulting in the alignment of most of his teeth. *Give two important properties of the orthodontic wire used in this movement. How do these properties contribute to this movement?*

◉ You have been asked to prepare cement for a final cementation appointment. *What control variables would be desirable if this was a multiunit bridge? How might these variables be manipulated?*

◉ While attending your state dental convention, you find a great deal on dental plaster. To take advantage of this offer you must buy five 25-pound containers. When the plaster is delivered to the office, you find that there is not enough space to store the material, so it is decided to store it in the dentist's garage. The material in the first container used has normal setting reactions. However, material in containers opened later is inconsistent in its working and setting time. *What may account for these inconsistencies?*

REFERENCES

Anusavice KJ: *Phillips' science of dental materials,* ed 10, Philadelphia, 1996, WB Saunders.
Craig RG: *Restorative dental materials,* ed 10, St Louis, 1997, Mosby.
Darby ML: *Comprehensive review of dental hygiene,* ed 4, St Louis, 1998, Mosby.
Ferracane JL: *Materials in dentistry,* Philadelphia, 1995, Lippincott.
Introduction to biomaterials properties. Biomaterials properties table listing. Available at www.lib.umich.edu/dentlib/Dental_tables/toc.html.

4 GENERAL HANDLING AND SAFETY

OBJECTIVES

On completion of this chapter the student will be able to:

1. Identify five job-related health and safety hazards for employees in dental offices, and explain the methods of prevention of each one.
2. Explain the components of the Occupational Safety and Health Administration Hazard Communication Standard.
3. Describe the ways that chemicals can enter the body.
4. Describe the employee and employer responsibility for safety training.
5. Describe the basic infection control methods for the handling of dental materials in the treatment area.

KEY TERMS

Particulate matter—Extremely small particles (e.g., dust from dental plaster or stone).

Personal protective equipment (PPE)—Gloves, masks, gowns, eyewear, and other protective equipment for the employee.

Hazardous chemical—Chemical that can cause burns to the skin, is poisonous, or can cause fire.

Toxicity—The strength of a product or of a chemical that can cause poisonous substances to spread throughout the body.

Flash point—The lowest temperature at which the vapor of a volatile substance will ignite with a flash. A low flash point means that a substance can catch fire easily.

Ignitable—A material or chemical that can erupt into fire easily.

Corrosive—Usually an acid or strong base that can cause damage to skin, clothing, metals, and equipment.

Reactive—The reaction of opposing chemical substances, thus creating a different end product.

Material Safety Data Sheet (MSDS)—Printed product reports from the manufacturer containing important information about the chemicals, hazards, handling, clean-up, and special PPE related to a product.

Bio-aerosol—A cloudlike mist containing droplets, tooth dust, materials dust, and bacteria of a particle size less than 5 microns in diameter.

The dental office uses a wide variety of materials that contain chemicals used for patient treatment and laboratory procedures. All chemicals are capable of causing harmful effects if they are absorbed into the human body in large enough amounts. The dental assistant and dental hygienist must understand the safe use, cleanup, and disposal methods for all of the materials used in the dental office. This chapter also discusses compliance with governmental regulations and explains health and safety procedures.

Materials Hazards in the Dental Environment

EXPOSURE TO PARTICULATE MATTER

During the manipulation of many dental materials, **particulate matter** can be generated. Items such as gypsum products, alginate, microblasting materials, and pumice may generate dust during handling. Gypsum models, processed acrylic, porcelain, and various restorative materials may generate dust during the grinding and polishing processes. It is important for each person handling and manipulating these materials to have and use the proper **personal protective equipment (PPE)** such as dust or surgical masks, eyewear, gowns, and (when appropriate) hair covering or tieback.

> **MATERIALS HAZARDS IN THE DENTAL OFFICE**
>
> - Exposure to particulate matter
> - Exposure to mercury
> - Exposure to toxic effects of chemicals
> - Exposure to airborne contaminants
> - Exposure to biologic contaminants

EXPOSURE TO BIOLOGIC CONTAMINANTS

Dental personnel are exposed to a variety of microorganisms via exposure to blood, body fluids, or oral and respiratory secretions. These microorganisms may include hepatitis B virus (HBV), hepatitis C virus (HCV), human immunodeficiency virus (HIV), and other viruses and bacteria. Dental personnel can be protected from the occupational transmission of infectious diseases through strict adherence to the requirements of the Occupational Safety and Health Administration (OSHA) Bloodborne Pathogen Standard and to the infection control guidelines issued by the Centers for Disease Control and Prevention (CDC). The dental assistant/hygienist must be familiar with these guidelines. In addition, some states have regulations specific to infection control for dentistry. Dental personnel must consider the possibility of any container or piece of equip-

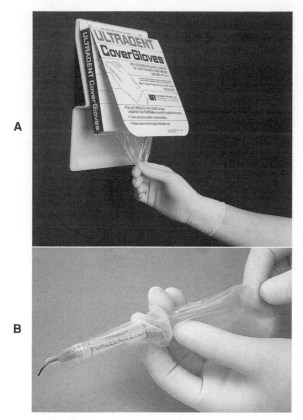

A

B

FIGURE 4-1 ■ A, Overgloves for use to prevent cross-contamination when handling multiple-use dental material containers and dispensers. **B,** Syringe is barrier protected with a disposable plastic cover.
(Courtesy of Ultradent Products Inc., South Jordan, UT.)

ment or dental material becoming contaminated during handling. Thus it is important to use proper barrier protection such as overgloves or plastic covers when handling the bottles, cans, or tubes that contain many of the dental materials in a modern dental practice (Figure 4-1).

Chemical Safety in the Dental Office

HAZARDOUS CHEMICALS

A **hazardous chemical** is defined as any chemical that has been shown to cause either a physical or health hazard. It can be any substance that can catch fire, can react or explode when mixed with other

> **HOW CHEMICALS ENTER THE BODY**
> 1. Inhalation
> 2. Absorption through the skin
> 3. Ingestion (eating or drinking)
> 4. Invasion directly through a break in the skin

substances, or is corrosive or toxic. It is the chemical manufacturers' responsibility to assess the hazards of their products and pass this information on to consumers. Many dental materials contain more than one chemical.

SKIN

The skin is an effective barrier for many chemicals; however, some chemicals are absorbed through the skin. Generally the skin must be in direct contact with the chemical for this to happen. Absorption also may occur directly through breaks in the skin such as cuts, open sores, or inflamed hands. After repeated contact with some chemicals, a skin disease called *dermatitis* may occur. Other chemicals, such as acids, can cause skin burns and are extremely harmful to the eyes.

INHALATION

Inhalation of the gases, vapors, or dusts of materials is a common route of chemical exposure to dental personnel. Some chemicals can cause damage directly to the lungs. Other chemicals may not affect the lungs, but are absorbed by the lungs and sent via the bloodstream to other organs such as the brain, liver, or kidneys where they may cause damage.

INGESTION

Ingestion (swallowing) is another way that chemicals can enter the body. Eating in an area where chemicals are used or eating with hands that are contaminated with chemicals is a common way of ingesting harmful chemicals. In the dental laboratory, many procedures are done that produce contaminants such as metal grindings and gypsum products. It is important to wash your hands thoroughly after contact with any chemical. In many cases the use of special protective gloves is indicated, and they must be removed and the hands washed before handling food.

Acute and Chronic Chemical Toxicity

The **toxicity** of a chemical, and thus its harmfulness, depends directly on the dose, length, and frequency of the exposure.

ACUTE CHEMICAL TOXICITY

Acute chemical toxicity results from high levels of exposure over a short period of time. This is frequently caused by a chemical spill in which the exposure is sudden and often involves a large amount of the chemical. The effects of this type of toxicity are felt right away. The symptoms of acute overexposure to chemicals include dizziness, fainting (syncope), headache, nausea, and vomiting.

CHRONIC CHEMICAL TOXICITY

Chronic chemical toxicity results from repeated exposures, generally to lower doses, over a much longer time period. The time period can be months or even years. The effects of chronic toxicity can include cancer, neurologic deficits, or infertility.

For example, a single exposure to a high concentration of benzene may cause dizziness, headache, and unconsciousness; a long-term, daily exposure to low levels of benzene may eventually cause leukemia. Another example is that some of the metals used in partial denture frameworks contained beryllium. When grinding these frameworks for adjustment, inhaling of the dust must be avoided because it is a toxic hazard that can lead to lung disease. A proper mask or respirator must be worn.

Personal Chemical Protection

HAND PROTECTION

The latex gloves worn during patient care do *not* provide adequate protection when handling chemicals. When exposed to chemical disinfectants, the latex in the gloves degrades and can actually pull contaminants and chemicals through the glove like a wick and onto the hands. Chemical-resistant gloves

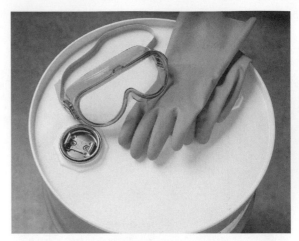

FIGURE 4-2 ■ Chemical-resistant polyvinyl chloride (PVC) goggles are soft and lightweight for comfortable fit and seal. Nitrile gloves are chemical-resistant for handling acids and hazardous chemicals.
(Courtesy of Lab Safety Supply Inc., Janesville, WI.)

such as nitrile gloves are recommended for wear when handling chemicals.

EYE PROTECTION

Serious damage to the eyes, including blindness, can result from chemical accidents. It is necessary to protect the eyes from fumes and splashes while pouring chemicals such as alcohol or methyl methacrylate monomer or other solvents. The acids used for bonding procedures can be splashed into the eyes during rinsing from the etched teeth. Safety eyewear should always be used, such as goggles with soft vinyl flanges at the top and bottom that fit the face snugly (Figure 4-2).

PROTECTIVE CLOTHING

The type of chemical being used should guide the selection of protective wear. A rubber or neoprene apron should be worn when mixing or pouring chemicals that are caustic and can stain or would saturate and penetrate regular fabric.

INHALATION PROTECTION

Masks worn during patient care may or may not provide adequate protection when working with

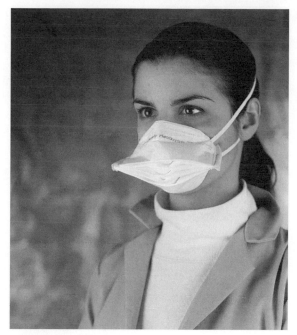

FIGURE 4-3 ■ Disposable N-95 respirator with tapered angle to fit facial contours around nose and chin. Protects against dusts and chemical mists.

(Courtesy of Lab Safety Supply Inc., Janesville, WI.)

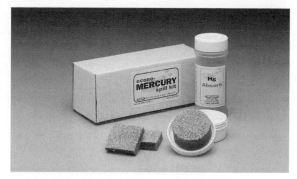

FIGURE 4-4 ■ Mercury spill kit. Note compact size for convenient storage.

(Courtesy of Lab Safety Supply Inc., Janesville, WI.)

chemicals, depending on their quality. The facemask should be fluid repelling and provide respiratory protection. If the job requires pouring or mixing chemicals frequently, sensitive or allergic individuals might need a National Institute of Occupational Safety and Health (NIOSH)–approved mist respirator facemask (Figure 4-3).

Control of Chemical Spills

MERCURY SPILL

Mercury spill kits should be available in all dental offices that use amalgam for restorations. Exposure to even small amounts of mercury is very hazardous to workers' health. Mercury can be absorbed through the skin or by the inhalation of mercury vapors.

The spill kit for small amounts of mercury should contain mercury absorbing powder, mercury sponges, and a disposal bag. A mask and utility-type gloves should be worn whenever cleaning a mercury spill (Figure 4-4).

PRECAUTIONS WHEN WORKING WITH MERCURY

- Work in a well-ventilated space.
- Avoid direct skin contact with mercury.
- Avoid inhaling mercury vapor.
- Store mercury in unbreakable, tightly sealed containers away from heat.
- When preparing amalgam for restorations, use preloaded capsules. (This avoids exposure while measuring mercury.)
- When mixing amalgam, always close the cover before starting the amalgamator.
- Reassemble amalgam capsules immediately after dispensing the amalgam mass. (The used amalgam capsule is highly contaminated with mercury and is a significant source of mercury vapor if left open.)
- Leftover scrap amalgam (i.e., unused amalgam) is stored under water in a tightly closed container.
- Scrap amalgam (amalgam that has been retrieved from dental unit traps) is disinfected in a solution of bleach and water. Then it is placed in the container with other scrap alloy.
- Clean spills, using appropriate procedures and equipment; do NOT use a household vacuum cleaner OR the HVE. (Dangerous fumes from the mercury can be released into the air.)
- Place contaminated disposable materials in polyethylene bags and seal and dispose of them according to state and local regulations.

FLAMMABLE LIQUIDS

Many of the solvents used with dental materials have a very low **flash point** and can easily ignite when used near open flame such as from a Bunsen burner or an alcohol torch. Use extreme caution when using flammable products (e.g., the liquid monomer for acrylic or acetone). The Material Safety Data Sheet (MSDS) for each product will describe the flammability of that product. See how to read the MSDS later in this chapter.

ACIDS

Acids such as phosphoric, hydrofluoric, and hydrochloric acid are used during manipulation of various dental materials. Splashing any of these acids on the skin, eyes, or clothing can cause severe burns or damage. Flushing with water immediately is essential to prevent severe injury.

> **CAUTION**
> - *Skin: Immediately rinse with copious amounts of water. Seek medical attention if a burn or wound has occurred.*
> - *Eyes: Immediately use the nearest eyewash station and flush the eyes with water for at least 5 minutes. Seek medical attention immediately.*

EYEWASH

OSHA regulations require an eyewash unit to be installed in every place of employment where chemicals are used. A wide variety of styles are available. The standard eyewash unit attaches directly to existing faucets for emergencies, yet still allows normal faucet use. When turned on, the eyewash unit will irrigate the eyes with a soft, wide flow of water necessary to bathe away contaminants without causing additional damage. As an employee, you must be trained in the proper use of the eyewash station. A nearby posting of the directions for the proper use of the particular type of eyewash unit is recommended (Figure 4-5).

VENTILATION

Good ventilation is a necessity when dealing with any type of chemical. Dental offices should be equipped with special exhaust systems in the laboratory and

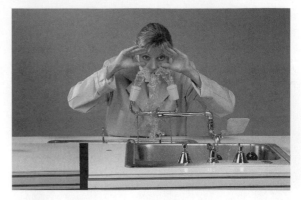

FIGURE 4-5 ■ Countertop eye and eye/face wash station. (Courtesy of Lab Safety Supply Inc., Janesville, WI.)

radiographic areas for fumes and dust. For example, vapors from chemicals used in radiographic processing can cause contact dermatitis and irritation of eyes, nose, throat, and respiratory tract. Other laboratory areas may have fine dust particles from grinding or chemical vapors such as from acrylic monomer or pickling acid (used for removing oxides from cast metals).

General Precautions for Storing Chemicals

All dental materials contain chemical components, and some are more hazardous than others. The careful use and storage of dental materials is important to ensure that these products retain their therapeutic activity and identity. Changes in chemical composition of materials can occur for many reasons. When changes take place, the product may no longer retain its effectiveness. A basic "safe" policy for the storage of dental medications and chemicals is to keep them in a dry, cool, dark place where they are not exposed to direct sunlight.

Disposal of Chemicals

EMPTY CONTAINERS

Even empty containers can be hazardous because they often hold residues that can burn or explode. Never fill an empty container with another substance because a dangerous chemical reaction could occur.

> ### TIPS TO AID IN THE SAFE USE AND EFFECTIVENESS OF DENTAL MATERIALS
>
> 1. **Follow instructions.** The manufacturer has determined the best methods of protective packaging and storage. Therefore manufacturer's instructions for storage, manipulation, and protection should be followed.
> 2. **Light, heat, and air.** Exposures to light, heat, and air are the prime factors in the deterioration of many bonding solutions. Changes in color, viscosity, or curing time are the most common signs of deterioration.
> 3. **Expiration date.** The substance's expiration date should always be noted. To maintain the proper chemical reactions, materials should be replaced when the expiration date is reached. Also, new supplies should always be stocked behind the current inventory so that the oldest product is used first.

Follow the label and the MSDS on how to dispose of empty containers. (Material Safety Data Sheets are discussed later in this chapter.)

HAZARDOUS WASTE DISPOSAL

A waste is considered hazardous if it has certain properties or chemicals that could pose dangers to human health and the environment after it is discarded. Generally waste is classified as hazardous if it has any of the following characteristics:

1. **Ignitable:** The substance is flammable or combustible.
2. **Corrosive:** The substance is either highly acidic or basic with a pH less than 2.0 or greater than 12.5. (Water has a pH of 7.0, which is neutral.)
3. **Reactive:** The substance is chemically unstable or explosive, reacts violently with water, or is capable of giving off toxic fumes when mixed with water.
4. **Toxic:** The substance contains amounts of arsenic, barium, chromium, mercury, lead, silver, or certain pesticides. (NOTE: Dental amalgam, asbestos, and lead foil from laboratory procedures are examples of hazardous waste and are regulated by individual states.)
5. **Listed by the Environmental Protection Administration (EPA):** Several hundred chemicals are listed by the EPA as being hazardous chemicals.

> ### GUIDELINES FOR MINIMIZING EXPOSURE TO CHEMICAL HAZARDS IN THE DENTAL OFFICE
>
> * Keep a minimum of hazardous chemicals in the office.
> * Read the labels and use only as directed.
> * Store according to the manufacturer's directions.
> * Keep containers tightly covered.
> * Avoid mixing chemicals unless consequences are known.
> * Wear appropriate PPE when handling hazardous substances.
> * Wash hands immediately after removing gloves.
> * Avoid skin contact with chemicals; immediately wash skin that has come in contact with chemicals.
> * Maintain good ventilation.
> * Do not eat, drink, smoke, apply lip balm, or insert contact lenses in areas where chemicals are used.
> * Keep vaporizing chemicals away from open flames and heat sources.
> * Always have an operational fire extinguisher handy.
> * Know and use proper cleanup procedures.
> * Keep neutralizing agents available for strong acid and alkaline solutions.
> * Dispose of all hazardous chemicals according to MSDS instructions.

Regulations for hazardous waste disposal vary among states, and there can be heavy fines for those individuals who knowingly violate regulations. More important than the legal penalties are the environmental damage and pollution of surface and ground water that can result from improper handling and disposal of hazardous wastes.

Occupational Safety and Health Administration Hazard Communication Standard

OSHA issued the Hazard Communication Standard because employees have both the right and the need to know the *identity and the hazards* of chemicals that they use in the workplace. The Hazard

Communication Standard, also known as the Employee Right To Know Law, requires employers to implement a hazard communication program.

HAZARD COMMUNICATION PROGRAM

A chemical hazard communication program has five parts: the written program, the chemical inventory, the Material Safety Data Sheets, labeling of containers, and employee training.

Written Program The written program must identify the employees by name who are exposed to hazardous chemicals. It must describe how chemicals are handled in the workplace, including a description of all safety measures and how to respond to chemical emergencies such as spills or exposures.

Chemical Inventory The chemical inventory is a comprehensive list of every product used in the office that contains chemicals, including amalgam, bonding agents, disinfectants, and impression materials. Each time a new product containing a hazardous chemical is added to the office, it must be added to the chemical list, and the MSDS for that product is placed in the MSDS file.

The office will frequently appoint a staff member to be the hazard program coordinator. This person will be responsible for maintaining the chemical inventory and updating the MSDS file.

Material Safety Data Sheets Material Safety Data Sheets contain health and safety information about each chemical in the office. MSDSs provide comprehensive technical information and are a resource for employees/providers working with chemicals. They describe the physical and chemical properties of a chemical, health hazards, routes of exposure, precautions for safe handling and use, emergency and first aid procedures, and spill-control measures (Figure 4-6).

MSDSs must be provided by the manufacturer of products that contain hazardous chemicals, and there must be an MSDS for every chemical used in the office. MSDSs are often enclosed in the box with the product. The MSDSs should be organized in binders so that the employees/providers have ready access to them and can easily locate a particular MSDS (Table 4-1).

Labeling of Chemical Containers Containers must be labeled to indicate what chemicals they contain and any hazards that may be present (Figure 4-7).

TABLE 4-1
Explanation of the Material Safety Data Sheet*

SECTION I	Product information	Identifies the name of the material, manufacturer, date MSDS was prepared, and person or agency to call in case of an emergency.
SECTION II	Hazardous ingredient	Identifies the hazardous ingredient. Product identity must match the label. It must also include the permissible exposure limit (PEL) and short-term exposure limit (STEL) in the air.
SECTION III	Physical hazard data	Identifies how the material will look or smell and some of its physical characteristics.
SECTION IV	Fire and explosion data	Indicates the ignition or flash point and tells how to put out any fire containing that material or any explosion or reactivity hazard.
SECTION V	Health hazard information	Indicates symptoms of overexposure, health effects, emergency procedures, cancer-causing agents, etc.
SECTION VI	Reactivity data	Describes the stability of the product.
SECTION VII	Spill or leak procedures	Describes disposal of product and how to deal with a spill or leak.
SECTION VIII	Special protection information	Identifies control measures, such as ventilation, gloves, respirator, etc., when handling the product.
SECTION IX	Special precautions	Cautions of special handling or storage precautions to be taken with the material and any protective measures.

Sample of OSHA Form 20 for MSDS.

IDENTITY/ PRODUCT NAME: ABC LIQUID

SECTION I

MANUFACTURER'S NAME: ABC Manufacturing Company

ADDRESS: 8800-B Oakdale Office Park, Chicago, IL 60666

EMERGENCY TELEPHONE NUMBER: 1-800-224-5681

TELEPHONE NUMBER FOR INFORMATION: 1-800-341-9000   Date prepared: 1/25/19XX

SECTION II - HAZARDOUS INGREDIENTS/IDENTITY INFORMATION

HAZARDOUS COMPONENTS:	OSHA PEL	OTHER LIMITS
Eugenol	–	–
Acetic acid	10 ppm	

SECTION III - PHYSICAL/CHEMICAL CHARACTERISTICS

BOILING POINT: 491°F/255°C   SPECIFIC GRAVITY: Above 1.0

VAPOR PRESSURE: 0.1Hg@20°C   MELTING POINT: -9°C

VAPOR DENSITY: N.E.   EVAPORATION RATE: N.E.

SOLUBILITY IN WATER: Slightly soluble

APPEARANCE AND ODOR: Colorless or pale yellow liquid. Odor is oil of cloves.

SECTION IV - FIRE AND EXPLOSION HAZARD DATA

FLASH POINT (Method Used): Approx 250°F Closed cup

FLAMMABILITY (Explosive Limits): N.E.   LEL: N.E.   UEL: N.E.

EXTINGUISHING MEDIA: Carbon dioxide, dry chemical, or foam-type extinguishers.

SPECIAL FIRE FIGHTING PROCEDURES: Fire fighters should wear full protective clothing, including self-contained breathing apparatus. Cool containers exposed to flame with water.

UNUSUAL FIRE AND EXPLOSION HAZARDS: None

SECTION V - REACTIVITY DATA

STABILITY: Unstable _____   Stable __X__

CONDITIONS TO AVOID: Excessive heat, strong oxidizing agents.

INCOMPATIBILITY (Materials to Avoid): Ferric chloride, potassium permanganate.

HAZARDOUS DECOMPOSITION OR BYPRODUCTS: Forms carbon monoxide and/or carbon dioxide upon burning.

HAZARDOUS POLYMERIZATION: May Occur _____   Will Not Occur __X__

CONDITIONS TO AVOID: None

FIGURE 4-6 ■ Simulated Material Safety Data Sheet.
(From Bird D, Robinson D: *Torres and Ehrlich modern dental assisting,* ed 6, Philadelphia, 2002 (Revised), WB Saunders.)

SECTION VI - HEALTH HAZARD DATA

ROUTES OF ENTRY: **Inhalation?** Yes   **Skin?** Yes   **Ingestion?** Possible

HEALTH HAZARDS (Acute and Chronic): Liquid irritating to skin and eyes. Repeated contact may cause allergic dermatitis. Repeated daily oral dosing of large amount to rats caused liver damage. The effects in humans are unknown. Excessive exposure may result in similar effects.

CARCINOGENICITY: **OSHA REGULATED:** No

SIGNS AND SYMPTOMS OF EXPOSURE: Redness or irritation of eyes or skin.

MEDICAL CONDITIONS GENERALLY AGGRAVATED BY EXPOSURE: Known sensitization to eugenol.
Open sores or wounds of the skin.

EMERGENCY AND FIRST AID PROCEDURES:

EYE CONTACT: Rinse with plenty of water for at least 15 minutes and seek medical attention.

SKIN CONTACT: Wash with soap and water.

INHALATION: Remove person to fresh air. Seek medical attention if irritation persists.

INGESTION: Seek medical advice.

SECTION VII - PRECAUTIONS FOR SAFE HANDLING AND USE

STEPS TO BE TAKEN IN CASE MATERIAL IS RELEASED OR SPILLED: Soak material up by using sand or vermiculite, then scoop up material and place in a closed metal waste container.

WASTE DISPOSAL METHOD: Dispose of in accordance with all federal, state, and local regulations.

PRECAUTIONS TO BE TAKEN IN HANDLING AND STORING: Store in tight full containers, well sealed, protected from light. Keep away from foodstuffs and beverages. Do not expose to temperatures above 35°C.

OTHER PRECAUTIONS: Eugenol darkens and thickens upon exposure to air. Observe normal warehousing and handling precautions.

SECTION VIII - CONTROL MEASURES

RESPIRATORY PROTECTION (specify type): As with all materials, avoid casual breathing of vapors. No special respiratory protection required for the intended use of this product.

VENTILATION: Local Exhaust ___X___   Special _____

PROTECTIVE GLOVES: Clinical Worker Gloves (Rubber)

EYE PROTECTION: Chemical Worker Goggles

OTHER PROTECTING CLOTHING OR EQUIPMENT: None

WORK/HYGIENIC PRACTICES: Observe normal care when working with chemicals.

FIGURE 4-6 ■ *Continued.*

All chemicals in the dental office must be labeled. In many cases the manufacturer's label is suitable. However, when the chemical is transferred to a different container, the new container must also be labeled. For example, when a concentrated chemical such as acrylic monomer is transferred to a small bottle for use in the treatment area or laboratory, it must be labeled. There is no official labeling system that must be used, and there are a variety of styles on the market. Even a photocopy of the label from the

OUTLINE FOR A HAZARD COMMUNICATION TRAINING PROGRAM

1. Requirements of the Hazard Communication Standard
2. Written communication plan for the office (location, use, etc.)
3. Understand the hazards of the chemicals
4. Be able to interpret warning labels and MSDS
5. Know how to obtain more information
6. Measures to protect themselves and others:
   * Office safety procedures
   * Available PPE
   * Instructions for reporting accidents and emergencies
   * Information about first aid
7. Methods and observations to detect the presence or release of a hazardous chemical
8. Question-and-answer opportunity
9. On completion, ask employees to sign a training record that will remain in their personnel file

original container affixed to the new container is acceptable. The most important things are that the labeling system is easy to use and that employees are properly trained to understand and read the labels.

National Fire Protection Association Labels The National Fire Protection Association (NFPA) has a labeling system that is frequently used to label containers of hazardous chemicals. This system consists of a blue, red, yellow, and white diamond filled with numerical ratings from 0 to 4. The categories are identified as follows: health (blue); flammability (red); reactivity (yellow); and special hazard symbols, such as "OXY" for oxidizers (white) (Figure 4-8; see also Color Plate 1 at the front of the book.).

Exemptions to Labeling Requirements Certain chemicals are exempted from the Hazard Communication Standard. These products include

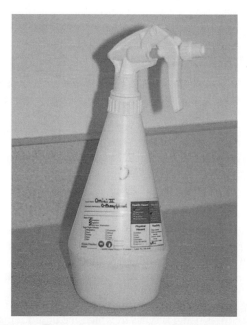

FIGURE 4-7 ■ Secondary chemical container labeling.
(From Bird D, Robinson D: *Torres and Ehrlich modern dental assisting,* ed 6, Philadelphia, 2002 (Revised), WB Saunders.)

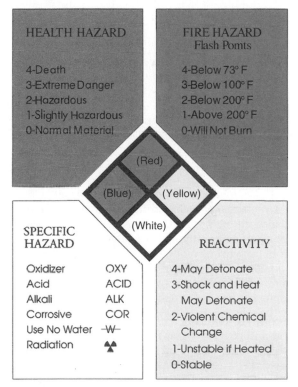

FIGURE 4-8 ■ NFPA hazard labeling system. See also Color Plate 1 at the front of the book.
(Copyright © 1990, National Fire Protection Association, Quincy, Mass., 02269. From Bird D, Robinson D: *Torres and Ehrlich modern dental assisting,* ed 6, Philadelphia, 2002 (Revised), WB Saunders.)

NECESSARY PARTS OF A HAZARD COMMUNICATION PROGRAM

- Written hazard communication program
- Inventory of hazardous chemicals
- MSDS for all chemicals
- Labeling
- Employee training
- Record keeping

GUIDELINES FOR CHEMICAL LABELING

The label must contain the following information:
- Identity of the hazardous chemical(s)
- Name and address of the manufacturer or responsible party
- Appropriate warnings

RESPONSIBILITIES OF THE HAZARD PROGRAM COORDINATOR

- Read and understand the Hazard Communication Standard
- Implement the written hazard communication program
- Compile a list (chemical inventory) of products in the office that contain hazardous chemicals
- Obtain MSDSs
- Update the MSDS file as new products are added to office inventory
- Inform other employees of the location of the MSDS file
- Label appropriate containers
- Provide training to other employees

The chemical training program for employees must include the following:
- The use of hazardous chemicals
- All safety practices, including all warnings
- Required personal protective devices
- Safe handling and disposal methods

Bio-aerosols in the Dental Setting

A **bio-aerosol** (*bio* = living and *aerosol* = mist) is a cloudlike mist containing microbes such as bacteria, viruses, molds, fungi, and yeast. Airborne microorganisms can be found in any building. Air-conditioning systems, humidifiers, carpets, wall coverings, and plants can easily become microbial breeding grounds.

DENTAL BIO-AEROSOLS

In addition to the usual sources of airborne microorganisms, bio-aerosols in the dental office are even more complex. This is because the aerosols created during many dental procedures contain oral fluids, blood, dental materials, powder, latex particles, and dust from metal composites and hygiene procedures. (Figure 4-9). The bio-aerosols created by the dental handpiece and air abrasion procedures alone can contain particles of human teeth, oral fluids, bacteria and viruses, old restorations, lubricating oil, and abrasive powder. The use of certain air-water powder slurry products during hygiene procedures has also been implicated in the creation of bio-aerosols. Aerosols can also be generated in the laboratory during grinding and polishing procedures.

Chemical contamination of the air can result from procedures using acrylics in which the liquid remains uncovered. When the amount of bio-aerosol in the environment exceeds the capacity of the air-filtering

tobacco and tobacco products, wood and wood products, food, drugs, cosmetics, and alcoholic beverages sold and packaged for consumer use. Drugs dispensed by a pharmacy to a health care provider for direct administration to a patient are also exempt from the labeling requirement. In addition, over-the-counter drugs and drugs intended for personal consumption by employees while in the workplace (e.g., aspirin or first aid supplies) are exempt.

Employee Training Employee training is essential for a successful hazard communication program. Staff training is required (1) when a new employee is hired, (2) when a new chemical product is added to the office, and (3) once a year for all continuing employees. Records of each training session must be kept on file and retained for at least 5 years. Although the dentist is responsible for providing the training, the hazard program coordinator is responsible for routinely following these safety precautions.

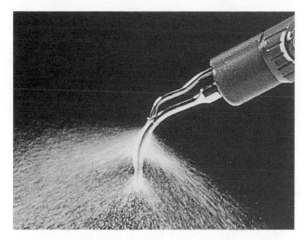

FIGURE 4-9 ■ Aerosol and droplets generated from dental equipment and procedures.

(Photo is © Hu-Friedy Mfg. Co., Inc., and is used with permission.)

system, allergens, toxins, irritants, and infectious agents will continue to build up. Employees can suffer from allergic responses, infectious diseases, and respiratory problems as a result of prolonged exposure to bio-aerosols and chemical irritants.

MANAGEMENT OF BIO-AEROSOLS

The effects of bio-aerosols in dental offices can be minimized by the following procedures:
- Frequently cleaning the air-filtration system
- Using proper oral and laboratory evacuation techniques during bio-aerosol–producing procedures
- Wearing the appropriate PPE
- Keeping all containers of chemicals tightly covered

Patient Safety

It is extremely important for the provider to consider the safety of the patient while care is given and the various materials and chemicals are used. The first consideration should be given to protection of the patient's eyes. It is recommended that protective eyewear be supplied to the patient if he or she does not wear glasses. The same type of general eyewear as used by the practitioner will do. Eyewear should be washed and disinfected between patients. Although some patients prefer dark glasses to shield their eyes from the dental unit light, most providers prefer clear

---

MANAGEMENT OF AEROSOLS IN THE DENTAL OFFICE

- Use high-volume suction during all procedures that produce aerosol
- Use rubber dams (minimizes exposure to oral fluids)
- Pour chemicals rather than spraying
- Clean air and vacuum filters frequently
- Use lids on ultrasonic cleaners and other chemical containers
- Minimize the use of latex products
- Use powder-free gloves
- Use a vacuum dust collection system during dust-producing laboratory procedures
- Wear appropriate PPE

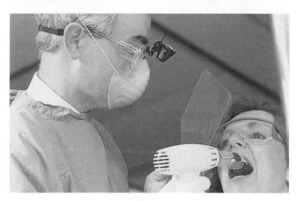

FIGURE 4-10 ■ Patient and clinician wearing protective eyewear and use of the protective curing light shield.

lenses so that they can observe the patient's eyes and facial expressions during treatment as a clue to the patient's level of comfort (Figure 4-10).

Another vital safety consideration is the patient's airway. The use of high-velocity evacuation (HVE) and rubber dam whenever possible is excellent practice. During rinsing of chemicals such as acid for etching, the patient can experience an unpleasant, bitter taste and may experience a gagging reaction. The patient should be warned of this taste, and the rinse should be controlled to minimize the discomfort.

Patients are more aware of the various chemicals and filling materials that are being used in dental practice than ever before. It behooves the allied oral health practitioner to be as familiar as possible with the hazards and reactions that can occur with these materials and chemicals. The MSDS can be the best source of this information, as well as the directions for use supplied with the product by the manufacturer.

SUMMARY

The management of a safe environment in the dental office is the responsibility of the employer and all who work there. The safe use of any chemical or material is the responsibility of the user at the time. The safety of the patient is the responsibility of the solo provider or the provider team. Familiarity with each material or chemical used by the dental team is a must. This text provides general and technical information, but the specific hazards are best determined by referring to the manufacturer's instructions and the MSDS.

CHAPTER REVIEW

Select the one correct response for each of the following multiple-choice questions:

1. **When working with dental materials, the most common work-related health and safety hazards are**
   a. Exposure to mercury, exposure to particulate matter, exposure to perfume, exposure to airborne contaminants
   b. Exposure to particulate matter, exposure to biologic contaminants, exposure to noise, exposure to perfume, exposure to airborne contaminants
   c. Exposure to particulate matter, exposure to biologic contaminants, exposure to perfume, exposure to airborne contaminants
   d. Exposure to mercury, exposure to particulate matter, exposure to biologic contaminants, exposure to perfume, exposure to toxic effects of chemicals

2. **The proper PPE to be worn during the handling of dental materials that can generate particulate matter are**
   a. Safety glasses, surgical or special dust mask, heavy-duty utility gloves, overgloves
   b. Lab coat or clinic gown, surgical or special dust mask, heavy-duty utility gloves, vinyl examination gloves
   c. Safety glasses, lab coat or clinic gown, surgical or special dust mask, heavy-duty utility gloves
   d. Safety glasses, lab coat or clinic gown, surgical or special dust mask

3. **During the use of acrylic monomer in the lab, the hazards are**
   a. Skin contact, inhalation of vapors, fire
   b. Inhalation of vapors, particulate matter inhalation, fire
   c. Skin contact, particulate matter inhalation, fire
   d. Skin contact, inhalation of vapors, particulate matter inhalation

4. **The ways in which chemicals can enter the body are**
   a. Inhaling, through cuts in the skin, through touching the result of a reaction product
   b. Swallowing, inhaling, through touching the result of a reaction product
   c. Swallowing, inhaling, through cuts in the skin
   d. Swallowing, through cuts in the skin, through touching the result of a reaction product

5. **When storing leftover amalgam scrap,**
   a. It should be stored in the x-ray fixer solution
   b. It is to be kept in a dry container

   c. It is to be kept under water in a tightly closed container
   d. It can be collected in the trap of the HVE and recovered later because this is a
      wet environment and vented

6. Eyewash stations are
   a. Never to be tested because they create a mess
   b. Best used at the end of the day for tired eyes
   c. Required to have a posted set of instructions
   d. Best used in an emergency if the employee has had training in their use

7. What are the best ways to minimize exposure to chemical hazards in the dental office?
   a. Read the label, place in a secondary container to keep the original fresher
   b. Place in a secondary container to keep the original fresher, keep a log of all chemicals ever purchased
   c. Read the label, store according to the manufacturer's directions
   d. Place in a secondary container to keep the original fresher, store according to the manufacturer's directions

CASE-BASED DISCUSSION TOPICS

◉ Discuss the various items in an MSDS. Take out an MSDS for a sealant kit and identify all of the precautions needed in handling the various components. *What if it is light-cured versus chemical-cured?*

◉ Regarding secondary labeling: *Discuss the requirements and exceptions to the use of secondary labels.*

◉ Discuss some of the aerosols and bio-aerosols in the dental office. *Give examples of procedures that are most likely to generate these areosols, and describe how they can be eliminated or reduced. (Hint! Don't forget about disinfecting and sterilizing procedures, as well as the treatment done on patients.)*

◉ Patient safety: *Discuss the various procedures that must be in place to ensure patient safety.*

◉ Cross-contamination: *Describe the procedures used to control cross-contamination of the various materials used at chairside. Be specific for each. For example, what can you do to prevent cross-contamination of the composite dispensing device?*

REFERENCES

American Dental Association regulatory compliance manual, Chicago, 1990, American Dental Association.

Bird D, Robinson D: *Torres and Ehrlich modern dental assisting,* ed 6, Philadelphia, 2002 (Revised), WB Saunders.

MacDonald G: Chemical hazards: regulations, identification and resources, *Journal of the California Dental Association* 17:12, 1989.

Miller C, Palenik C: *Infection control and management of hazardous materials for the dental team,* St Louis, 1994, Mosby.

Mount G, Hume W: *Preservation and restoration of tooth structure,* Appendix 1, St Louis, 1998, Mosby.

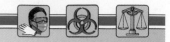

PROCEDURE 4-1

MSDS Labeling Exercise

Using the information found on the MSDS for acrylic monomer, create a label for a secondary container that is being filled from the manufacturer's original bulk container.

EQUIPMENT/SUPPLIES

- MSDS for product to labeled
- Ballpoint pen
- National Fire Protection Association chemical label

PROCEDURE STEPS

1 Write the manufacturer's name and address on the label. (This information is found in the product information section of the MSDS.)

2 Write the name of the chemical(s) on the label. (This information is found in the product information section of the MSDS.)

3 Write the appropriate health hazard code in the blue triangle. (This information is found in the health hazard data section of the MSDS.)

4 Write the appropriate flammability and explosion code in the red triangle. (This information is found in the fire and explosion section of the MSDS.)

5 Write the appropriate reactivity code in the yellow triangle. (This information is found in the reactivity data section of the MSDS.)

6 Write the appropriate specific hazard warning in the white triangle. (This information is found in the precautions for safe handling and use section of the MSDS.)

7 Affix the National Fire Protection Association chemical label (see Figure 4-8).

5 PRINCIPLES OF BONDING

CHAPTER OUTLINE

OBJECTIVES

On completion of this chapter the student will be able to:

1. Discuss the effects of acid etching on enamel and dentin.
2. Describe the basic steps of bonding.
3. Describe the agents used for bonding.
4. Discuss the factors that interfere with good bonding.
5. Define the correct terms used to describe the various bonding procedures.
6. Describe the amalgam bonding technique.
7. Describe the bonding of orthodontic brackets.
8. Describe the bonding of endodontic posts.
9. Explain the differences in bonding to enamel, dentin, metal, and porcelain.
10. List the factors that contribute to tooth sensitivity after bonding.

KEY TERMS

Bond or **bonding**—To connect or fasten; to bind (*Webster's New World Dictionary*). Basically, there are two ways that items are joined together at the surface: by mechanical adhesion (physical interlocking) and by chemical adhesion.

Adhesion—The act of sticking two things together. In dentistry it is frequently used to describe the bonding or cementation process. Chemical adhesion occurs when atoms or molecules of dissimilar substances bond together. *Adhesion* differs from *cohesion*, in which attraction among atoms and molecules of like (similar) materials holds them together.

Etching or **conditioning**—Terms used interchangeably to describe the process of preparing the surface of a tooth or restoration for bonding. The most common etching material (etchant) is phosphoric acid.

Cure or **polymerization**—A reaction that links low molecular weight resin molecules (monomers) together into high molecular weight chains (polymers) that harden or set. The reaction can be initiated by strictly a chemical reaction (self-cure), by light in the blue wave spectrum (light-cure), by a combination of the two (dual-cure), or by heat.

Wetting—Ability of a liquid to wet or intimately contact a solid surface. Water beading on a waxed car is an example of poor wetting.

Wet dentin bonding—Bonding to dentin that is kept moist after acid etching to facilitate penetration of bonding resins into etched dentin.

Bonding agent—A low-viscosity resin that penetrates porosities and irregularities in the surface of the tooth or restoration created by acid etching for the purpose of facilitating bonding.

Smear layer—A tenacious layer of debris on the dentin surface resulting from cutting the tooth during cavity preparation. It is composed of fine particles of cut tooth structure, bacteria, and salivary components.

Hybrid layer—A resin/dentin layer formed by the intermixing of the dentin bonding resin with collagen fibrils exposed by acid etching. It serves as an excellent resin-rich layer onto which the restorative material, such as composite resin, can be bonded.

Microleakage—Leakage of fluid and bacteria that occurs at the interface of the tooth and the restoration margins and is caused by microscopic gaps.

Percolation—Movement of fluid in the microscopic gap of the restoration margin as a result of differences in the expansion and contraction rates of the tooth and the restoration with temperature changes.

Hydrodynamic theory of tooth sensitivity—Pain caused by movement of pulpal fluid in open (unsealed) dentinal tubules. Actions that cause a change in the pressure on the fluid within the dentinal tubules stimulate nerve fibers in the processes of odontoblasts in the pulp to send out a pain response.

Contamination—Contact with a substance that changes the chemical or mechanical properties (e.g., contamination of the etched surface of the tooth with saliva before bonding).

The modern dental practice uses bonding for a wide variety of dental procedures. The dental assistant and dental hygienist must be familiar with the terms and processes used in bonding of the various restorative and preventive materials to be knowledgeable, effective members of the dental team. The dental assistant will be involved in helping the dentist perform bonding procedures many times each day, and the dental hygienist may place sealants and perform prophylaxis procedures that might affect bonded restorations. Therefore it is important that the allied oral health practitioner understand the properties and handling characteristics of the bonding materials and the processes involved in their use.

Basic Principles of Bonding

In dentistry the term **bond,** or **bonding,** is used to describe the process of attaching restorative materials, such as a bonded amalgam or a bonded composite resin, to the tooth by **adhesion**. When describing cosmetic restorations such as porcelain or composite veneers, patients often use the term *bonding;* for example, "The dentist is bonding my front teeth." Bonding also is the basis for several other dental procedures, such as the placement of resin-bonded bridges and orthodontic brackets and fixed retainers. It is also used to describe some of the materials used in the process of placing restorations. For example, the bonding resin is placed on the etched tooth surface before light-curing. Manufacturers often use the word "bond" in the trade names of their bonding resins, such as Prime & Bond NT (Dentsply/Caulk).

The basic principles in the bonding process involve preparing the surface of the tooth or the restoration (or both). Preparing the tooth surface usually involves removing plaque and debris, then **etching** or **conditioning** the enamel or dentin (or both) with an acid. The most commonly used acid is orthophosphoric acid in concentrations ranging from 10% to 40%. Acid removes mineral from the surface to create porosity. When a resin bonding agent is flowed over the surface, it penetrates into these microscopic pores. When it hardens (**cures** or **polymerizes**), it creates projections called *resin tags* that lock into the tooth, creating a mechanical bond called *micromechanical retention*. The resin bonding agent will then chemically bond to other resins placed over it, such as composite resin. The chemical bond, called a *primary bond*, is a true adhesion between atoms or molecules of the composite resin and the bonding resin. The chemical bond is stronger than a physical bond, called a *secondary bond*, which is a weak physical attraction between two surfaces such as the adhesion of paint to a metal surface. Roughening the metal surface by sandblasting increases the adhesion of the paint by mechanical retention, much like acid etching roughens the surface of the enamel. Acid etching also increases the ability of liquids to wet the surface of the tooth. **Wetting** increases the intimate contact of the bonding resin with the etched tooth structure, improving the penetration of resin to form tags and thereby improving the bond. Surfaces that are poorly wet will cause beading of the liquid, similar to water on a newly waxed car. The bead of water stands up on the surface of the car with a high angle of contact; on a nonwaxed car, the water easily spreads out and has a low angle of contact (Figure 5-1).

ENAMEL ETCHING

Dr. Michael Buonocore introduced etching of enamel into dentistry in the 1950s. Etching of enamel

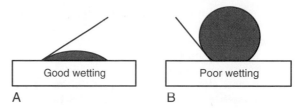

FIGURE 5-1 ■ Acid etching of enamel increases its ability to be wet by a resin bonding agent, resulting in a stronger bond. **A,** A low contact angle indicates good wetting as the liquid spreads over the surface. **B,** A high contact angle indicates poor wetting as the liquid beads on the surface like water on a waxed car.

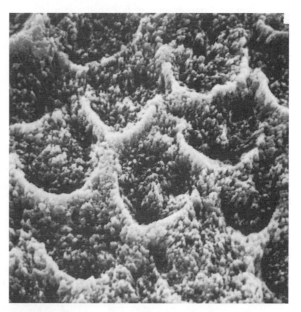

FIGURE 5-2 ■ An etched enamel surface as seen in this scanning electron micrograph has numerous peaks and valleys that provide retention and greatly increase the surface area for bonding.

(From Phillips RW, Moore BK. Synthetic resins. In *Elements of dental materials for dental hygienists and dental assistants,* Philadelphia, 1994, WB Saunders.)

removes a small portion of the surface, reduces enamel rods, and opens porosities among the rods (Figure 5-2). The enamel of permanent teeth is usually etched for 10 to 30 seconds. Although etching times as short as 10 seconds appear to give good clinical results in some teeth, some researchers suggest that 20 to 30 seconds is optimal. Some teeth may be more resistant to etching and may require up to 60 seconds of etching. The etched surface should have a frosty appearance when dried (see Figure 5-17 in Procedure 5-3). However, when a cavity preparation involves the etching of both enamel and dentin, and the preparation is left slightly moist for **wet dentin bonding,** it cannot be determined if the enamel has a frosty appearance or not. Primary teeth should be etched for longer periods of time (up to 60 seconds) because the enamel prism pattern is not as well structured, is considered amorphic (without a regular prism pattern), and is more resistant to deep resin tag formation. The acid etchant comes in a liquid or gel. Often coloring agents are added so the practitioner can see where the etchant is on the tooth. Liquid etchants are usually applied with a brush, small cotton pledget, or small sponge. Gels are usually applied by brush or dispensed from a syringe through a fine needle or brush tip. Recommended rinsing times for acid gels are from 10 to 30 seconds. Rinsing times under 5 seconds may not remove residual silica that is a component of most gels to make them thicker and prevent them from running onto tooth surfaces that should not be etched. Rinsing times for liquid etchants can be shorter, 5 to 10 seconds.

DENTIN ETCHING

The dentin structure has a higher water and organic content than enamel. It contains a collagen matrix woven throughout the mineral component (hydroxyapatite) and a system of dentinal tubules through which fluids from the pulp flow. Etching dentin removes some of the mineral from the surface and around the orifices of the dentinal tubules, exposing fibrils of the matrix (Figure 5-3). Because dentin is not as highly mineralized as enamel, it should be etched for shorter periods of time, typically for 10 seconds. Longer etching times on dentin will open the orifices of the dentinal tubules excessively and will remove more mineral from the dentin surface than is ideal. Overetching will expose too much col-

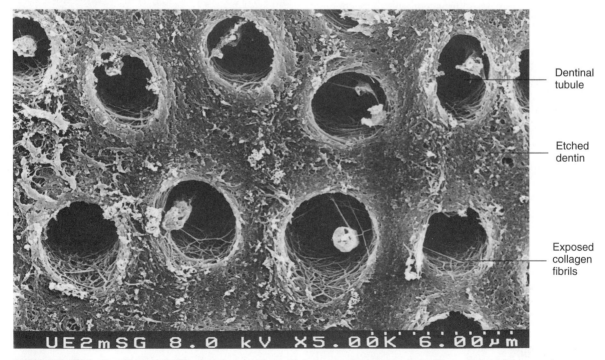

Dentinal tubule

Etched dentin

Exposed collagen fibrils

FIGURE 5-3 ■ Acid etching of the dentin removes some of the mineral exposing the collagen fibers of the matrix as seen in this scanning electron micrograph.

(Courtesy Dr. Jorge Peridigao, University of Minnesota School of Dentistry.)

lagen matrix, causing it to act as a thick barrier and making it more difficult to coat the dentin and seal the tubules with the resin bonding agents.

BONDING AGENTS

Bonding agents are low-viscosity resins dissolved in solvents that penetrate porosities in the tooth surfaces created by etching. The solvents are typically acetone or ethyl alcohol. Some water-based systems are also available. Bonding agents can be viewed as two components. The first is a resin primer that penetrates etched dentin and enamel and lays down a resin layer that subsequently bonds chemically with a resin adhesive that is applied over it. That is, the initial resin bonding material prepares (or primes) the tooth surface much like a primer is applied to wood before painting so the paint will adhere better. The second resin then chemically bonds to the primer. A primer is more important on dentin than enamel because it contains hydrophilic (water-loving) groups that penetrate wet, etched dentin. The resin adhesive bonds to the primer and contains hydrophobic (water-repelling) groups that will chemically bond to resin restorative materials such as composite resin. The variety of combinations of primers and adhesives can be confusing to the beginner until some experience is gained using the materials. In multiple-component systems, the primer and adhesive are bottled separately. Agents for bonding to enamel, dentin, and restorations have been rapidly changing. In response to practitioners' requests for simpler systems, some manufacturers have developed single-bottle systems that have incorporated both the primer and adhesive together.

Universal Bonding Agents   Many of the current generation of bonding agents are designated as universal bonding agents. This means that they are suitable for bonding on all enamel, dentin, and restoration surfaces. Many also have fluoride compounds in them that are claimed by manufacturers to be released over time to aid in the prevention of recurrent caries at the margins of restorations. However, the quantities of fluoride released are generally too small to have a therapeutic effect. Newer universal bonding resins may also have a small quantity of microscopic, inorganic filler particles added to increase the strength of the resin. These small filler particles are often composed of colloidal silica. The filler size is in a range of 0.8 to 0.0007 microns (μm). The extremely small filler sizes are sometimes referred to as *nano fillers*. To put the size of these nano fillers into perspective, the following comparisons are made: the diameter of a human hair is approximately 40 μm, a bacterium is about 2 μm, and a virus is about 0.1 μm.

Self-Etching Primers   Some two-component bonding agents have incorporated acidic groups in the primer that will etch enamel and dentin and allow penetration of the resin without the need for rinsing and drying. These are called *self-etching primers*. The acid component gradually shifts to neutral and is incorporated into the polymerized resin, as is the dissolved tooth mineral. A lightly filled light-curing adhesive resin is then placed over the primer. These self-etching primers have the advantage of eliminating the rinsing and drying steps that might introduce errors of overdrying or underdrying. Some self-etching primers do not etch uncut enamel and cannot be used in direct bonding to unprepared enamel such as for a direct composite veneer.

Modes of Cure   There are three modes of curing for the resin bonding agents. The first is a *self-cure* process in which a chemical reaction occurs when two resins, a base with chemical activators and a catalyst, are mixed together. The second is a *light-cure* process that uses a light in the blue wave range to activate a chemical (photoinitiator) that sets off the polymerization reaction or curing process. The third is a *dual-cure* process that uses a combination of self-cure and light-cure ingredients. Dual-cured resins can be activated by light or can cure chemically without the application of the curing light.

Bonding of Restoration   After the initial bonding resin is cured on the tooth, other adhesive bonding resins or cements can be used to attach restorations to the tooth by way of resin-to-resin chemical bonds. Restorations that are not made of resin such as metal or porcelain require treatment of their surfaces to allow them to bond to the resin on the tooth. Usually the metal or porcelain is roughened with a coarse diamond or sandblasted for mechanical retention of a resin that is coated on the surface. This resin will allow chemical bonding to the resin primer on the tooth. The resins then *chemically* bond to each other and *mechanically* bond to the tooth and the restoration.

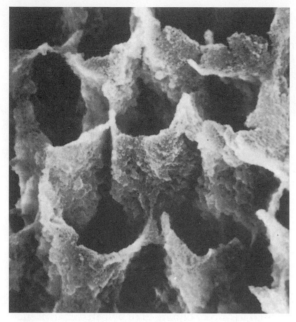

FIGURE 5-4 ■ A resin bonding agent placed on etched enamel penetrates the porous surface and forms resin extensions or tags that lock into the enamel and form a mechanical bond.

(From Phillips RW, Moore BK. Synthetic resins. In *Elements of dental materials for dental hygienists and dental assistants,* Philadelphia, 1994, WB Saunders.)

> ◤ **CAUTION**
> *A small portion of the population may have an allergic response to acrylate resins. Operator precautions are to be followed, because these resins may penetrate commonly used gloves.*

ENAMEL BONDING

Etching of enamel creates a high-energy, low-tension surface that makes the surface easier to wet. A high-energy surface attracts the atoms in the resin bonding agents to improve penetration into the porous etched enamel, resulting in resin tags that can be 10 to 50 μm long (Figure 5-4). The bond to enamel is very strong. However, contaminants on the surface, such as saliva or blood, can dramatically lower the strength of the bond to the enamel. If enamel becomes contaminated after etching, it must

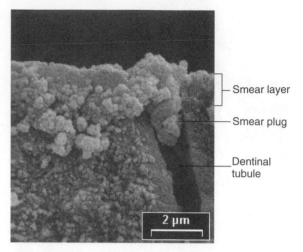

Smear layer
Smear plug
Dentinal tubule

2 μm

FIGURE 5-5 ■ Cutting of tooth structure with a rotary instrument forms a layer of cutting debris called the *smear layer,* as seen in this scanning electron micrograph. It is removed by acid etching so that it does not interfere with the formation of a bond.

(Courtesy Grayson Marshall, University of California School of Dentistry, San Francisco, Calif.)

be re-etched for 15 seconds before proceeding with the bonding process.

DENTIN BONDING

Formation and Removal of Smear Layer
Bonding to dentin is more complex than bonding to enamel. When the dentin is cut with the dental bur during tooth preparation, a **smear layer** is left on the surface of the dentin. This smear layer is composed of cut tooth debris created by the rotary cutting instruments and may also contain plaque, bacteria, pellicle, saliva, and even blood (Figure 5-5). It is best to isolate the tooth with a rubber dam to minimize sources of debris other than tooth debris. The smear layer adheres tenaciously to the dentin and occludes dentinal tubules and is not removed by vigorous rinsing. The smear layer interferes with the formation of a bond to dentin and should be removed so that the bonding resin can penetrate the open tubules and create a seal of the dentin for protection. A good dentinal seal helps eliminate bacterial leakage and postoperative sensitivity. Smear layer removal is achieved by etching with phosphoric acid for 10 seconds, followed by rinsing with water.

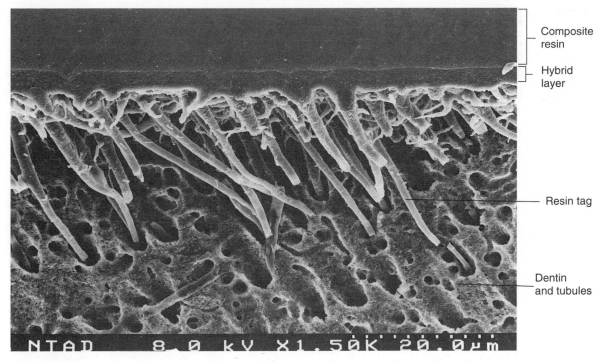

Composite
resin

Hybrid
layer

Resin tag

Dentin
and tubules

NTAD   8.0 kV X1.50K 20.0µm

FIGURE 5-6 ■ When a bonding resin is applied to etched dentin, it penetrates the exposed collagen matrix and dentinal tubules. An intermingling of resin with etched dentin forms a hybrid layer. This layer provides a resin-rich layer for bonding with other resins such as composite resin.
(Courtesy Dr. Jorge Peridigao, University of Minnesota School of Dentistry.)

Etching Dentin   Etching dentin with phosphoric acid dissolves hydroxyapatite mineral from the surface, creating a porous surface and exposing collagen fibrils that are part of the dentin matrix. When enamel and dentin are etched during the same acid application, it is commonly referred to as the "all etch technique." It is best to apply the acid to the enamel first for 10 seconds, then to the dentin for 10 seconds. Etching dentin for 20 seconds or more opens the tubules too wide and removes hydroxyapatite mineral to too great a depth. Overetched dentin can result in a weaker bond and posttreatment sensitivity. The acid is removed by rinsing for at least 10 seconds. The excess water is removed by gentle drying with air, but the dentin is left moist so that it glistens. It is critical at this stage not to overdry the dentin. The dentin surface must be moist to keep the collagen fibrils fluffed up. If the dentin is dried, the collagen fibrils collapse and totally occlude the tubules and block adequate penetration by the dentin bonding resins. A much weaker bond results because the dentin/resin interface will fracture more easily.

Formation of the Hybrid Layer   When dentin bonding resins are applied to moist dentin, the solvents in which the resins are dissolved allow the resins to penetrate through the water and around the fluffed-up collagen fibrils into the dentinal tubules and etched dentin surface. Drying with air is done at this stage to remove the volatile solvents from the resin and any remaining water. The layer that is formed by the dentin bonding resin and the collagen fibrils is called the **hybrid layer** (first described by Dr. Nakabyashi) because it is a combination (or hybrid) of dentin components and resin. The bond to the dentin and the restorative material is accomplished through the hybrid layer (Figure 5-6).

MICROLEAKAGE

When restorations are not completely sealed at their margins (junction of the restoration with the tooth surface), they can leak. Leakage is usually at the microscopic level (called **microleakage**) and permits fluids, bacteria, and debris to enter the cavity preparation. (Figure 5-7). Microleakage can contribute to decay under the restoration and sensitivity of the tooth. *Contaminants* are substances that interfere with the enamel or dentin bonding, such as saliva, blood, smear layer, or oils from the dental handpiece or from prophy pastes. Contaminants can contribute to microleakage when they are not properly removed before and during the bonding process. Microleakage can have other causes, such as shrinkage of composite resins when they cure (see Chapter 6), or restorations placed without bonding, such as conventional amalgam restorations (see Chapter 8). When restorative materials expand and contract with temperature variations (the change in volume of the restoration is called the coefficient of thermal expansion) at a different rate than the tooth structure, **percolation** can occur, in which fluids percolate or flow in and out of the gap at the interface of the restoration and the tooth. Cold foods or beverages such as ice cream will cause contraction of the restoration and widening of the gap, and hot foods or beverages will cause expansion of the restoration and reduction of the gap.

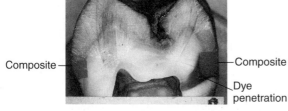

Composite — Composite

Dye penetration

FIGURE 5-7 ■ Seen is a longitudinal section through a molar that has cervical restorations on the right- and left-hand sides. When a good bond is not formed between the tooth and the restorative material, fluids and bacteria can seep between them, a process called *microleakage*. The tooth was soaked in a dark dye to show areas of microleakage. The restoration on the right shows leakage, as indicated by dye penetration; the one on the left does not.

(Courtesy Larry Watanabe, University of California School of Dentistry, San Francisco, Calif.)

FACTORS THAT PREVENT GOOD BONDING

- A surface that is overly wet does not allow good penetration of the bonding agent into the etched enamel and dentin.
- An overly dry dentin surface causes the collagen fibrils to collapse and cover the dentin surface so that the resin primer cannot penetrate to reach the etched dentin and the tubules.
- Blood or saliva on the etched enamel or dentin will interfere with the ability of the bonding agent to penetrate the surface.
- Failure to saturate dentin with bonding agent will result in voids and an incompletely sealed dentin. This can result in reduced bond strength and sensitivity because tubules are open.
- Failure to adequately cure the bonding resin will cause the resin to separate from the enamel or dentin.
- Moisture from the air/water lines can wet the enamel and dentin at the wrong step in the bonding process and result in a loss of a proper bond and seal.
- Oil lubricants expelled from the handpiece onto the tooth during preparation will prevent the resin primer from adhering to the etched enamel and dentin.
- Recently applied bleaching or topical fluoride agents can affect the enamel so that it is more difficult to etch or to bond to. Studies have shown that the bond to recently bleached enamel is not as strong. Fluoride makes the surface of the enamel more resistant to being etched by acid.
- Eugenol in cements for provisional restorations will interfere with the set of resin bonding agents and composite resins.
- Ferric sulfate–containing astringents (Astringedent or Viscostat) used to control gingival bleeding will interfere with the set of the bonding agents.
- Antimicrobial agents applied to disinfect the dentin might contaminate the surface and interfere with the resin primer

Clinical Applications of Bonding

PORCELAIN BONDING AND REPAIR

Porcelain restorations are retained much better if they are bonded to the tooth than if they are merely cemented. Bonding also helps minimize microleakage that can contribute to sensitivity or recurrent caries. Occasionally, porcelain restorations will chip and need repair instead of replacement. Techniques have been developed to permit repair of the porcelain in the mouth.

Clinical Technique   The process of bonding composite to porcelain is similar to bonding to enamel or dentin. The difference is in the etchant used and the surface preparation before the application of the bonding resin. Some operators prefer to roughen the surface of the porcelain with a diamond bur or by sandblasting before applying the acid. To bond to porcelain, the acid most commonly used is hydrofluoric acid in a syringe designed for intraoral or extraoral use. After the surface of the porcelain is etched, a solution of silane is placed for 30 seconds and then dried to evaporate the solvent. Silanes are coupling agents that react with the porcelain and leave a coating of vinyl that will bond to the resin in the bonding agent. Next, the resin bonding agent is placed and light-cured, and the final composite restorative material is placed and finished (see Chapter 6).

> ▶ **CAUTION**
> *Hydrofluoric acid is a highly caustic solution. Take precautions to properly isolate the area to be bonded. Protect the tissues and restorations adjacent to the area being etched. Hydrofluoric acid can etch porcelain, composite, and glass ionomer restorations, as well as tooth structure and can burn soft tissues.*

METAL BONDING

Metal bonding is used to create better retention of the metal to the tooth during the cementation (luting) of a restoration, such as a crown. (See Chapter 8 for a description of metals and Chapter 6 for porcelain-bonded-to-metal restorations.) Metal bonding is also used for placement of a composite veneer over metal for cosmetic reasons or for covering metal exposed when porcelain fractures from a porcelain-bonded-to-metal crown.

Laboratory and Clinical Techniques   To bond to the metal of a crown or resin-bonded (Maryland) bridge, the metal surface is roughened by sandblasting or with a coarse diamond to create micromechanical retention. The surface of the metal could also be treated by electrochemical etching in the laboratory or by depositing a thin layer of tin by an electroplater. The latter two methods are often used for metal preparation before cementation of a resin-bonded bridge. Noble metals such as gold particularly need to be tin-plated for an effective bond to the resin. Once the metal surface is prepared, it is cleaned and dried before it is coated with the bonding resin for cementation. These cements are usually self-cured or dual-cured (see Chapter 10). For repair of a porcelain-bonded-to-metal crown or bridge with fractured porcelain and exposed metal (see Figure 6-13 in Chapter 6 for an example), the porcelain and metal are prepared as previously described. Next, a one-step bonding resin is applied, thinned with air, and light-cured for 20 seconds. Then an opaque masking resin is applied to the metal to keep it from showing through and causing a gray appearance of the overlying composite. It is light-cured for 20 seconds. Finally, a composite resin that matches the color of the porcelain is selected, applied, light-cured, finished, and polished.

AMALGAM BONDING

Conventional amalgam restorations leak at the interface between the tooth and the amalgam. Freshly placed amalgams leak more than older amalgams. As amalgam ages, it begins to corrode and form corrosion products along the interface between the tooth and the amalgam (see Chapter 8). The corrosion products help reduce microleakage. Microleakage may contribute to tooth sensitivity and to recurrent caries. Many clinicians prefer to bond their amalgam restorations to increase the seal between the amalgam and the tooth structure and to reduce the potential for microleakage. Bonding of amalgams has been shown in laboratory studies to aid in the fracture resistance of the remaining tooth structure and to help retain the restoration.

Clinical Technique   After cavity preparation, isolation of the tooth is confirmed. If walls of the tooth are missing, a metal matrix band may be needed. If so, the inner metal surface of the band that will contact the amalgam should be coated with a thin layer of wax by rubbing it with a piece of baseplate wax, inlay wax, or crayon. This prevents amalgam from being bonded to the band by the bonding agent and causing a chunk of amalgam to be pulled away from the restoration when the band is removed. After the waxed band is placed on the tooth, the enamel and dentin are etched by 35% phosphoric acid—enamel for 20 seconds and dentin for 10 seconds. The acid removes the smear layer and prepares the surfaces for bonding. The acid is rinsed off, and the tooth is lightly dried to leave a slightly moist and glistening surface. Next, a dentin-enamel primer is applied, dried, and light-cured. Then, a self-cured or dual-cured bonding resin is applied in a thin coat to the entire cavity preparation. Immediately, freshly mixed amalgam is condensed into the preparation while the resin is still wet. The amalgam is bonded to the resin by physically mixing with the wet resin. When the resin cures it locks the amalgam in place. Although bonded amalgams help strengthen the tooth to a degree, they are not substitutes for stronger materials such as crowns or onlays when the remaining tooth structure is severely weakened.

ORTHODONTIC BRACKET BONDING

Orthodontic brackets have replaced bands for many uses, especially in the anterior part of the mouth. Because brackets cannot be used with conventional cements, they must be bonded to the enamel using adhesive materials. Bonding of orthodontic brackets is done with either metal brackets, which have a retentive mesh (see Figure 5-19 in Procedure 5-3) or series of knobs to lock in the resin adhesive, or ceramic brackets, which have a preetched bonding surface. The adhesive bonding resins are either self-cured or light-cured. Because the metal or ceramic material will not allow light to reach and cure the resin cement under the bracket directly, the light is cast from mesial, distal, and lingual, as well as facial, directions to cure the resin by light that has passed through the enamel.

Clinical Technique   Some clinicians use an indirect method of application of brackets. With the indirect method, brackets are aligned on the diagnostic cast in the same position as they will be placed on the teeth and held with sticky wax. Then a matrix, often constructed from impression putty, is formed over the brackets and the teeth on the cast. The brackets are picked up in the matrix and at the time of bonding are oriented in the same manner on the teeth as they were previously on the cast. Direct bonding of orthodontic brackets is explained and illustrated in Procedure 5-3.

BONDING OF ENDODONTIC POSTS

A post is placed within the roots of endodontically treated teeth in order to retain dental materials used to build up the tooth when there is inadequate coronal tooth structure for restoration with a crown (core buildup). The posts are made of a variety of materials and can be categorized into two general types: metal and nonmetal. Metal posts are made of cast gold, stainless steel, titanium alloy, or pure titanium. Nonmetal posts are made of carbon- or glass-fiber–reinforced resin or zirconium-based ceramic. The posts are bonded to the root with dentin bonding agents and resin cements following the manufacturer's recommendations.

Clinical Technique   When it is determined that an endodontically treated tooth needs a post, the dentist prepares one or more roots with specially shaped drills that shape the root canal to the shape of the post. The prepared canal is etched with phosphoric acid (10% or 35% depending on the materials used) for 10 to 15 seconds. The acid is thoroughly rinsed off and excess water is removed with a paper point. The dentin is left slightly moist (glistening but without puddling). A dentin primer is placed in the canal and air-dried to drive off any remaining water and the volatile solvents in the primer. Next, self-curing composite resin cement is applied to both the canal and the post. The post is inserted into the prepared canal and held under hand pressure until the cement has cured. If the post is manufactured (preformed) rather than a cast metal dowel with a core already attached, the buildup of missing coronal tooth structure may be done using amalgam or one of the bonded core materials (see Chapter 6). The dentist will place the core buildup and prepare the tooth for a crown. Metal and ceramic posts may be sandblasted to enhance the bond of the cement to the roughened surface of the post. Fiber-reinforced resin posts chemically bond to the resin cement.

HYPERSENSITIVE TEETH

Some patients may experience transient tooth sensitivity after a bonded restoration is placed. This is

Resin cement remaining on the mixing pad cannot be reliably used as a guide for final set of the cement in the canal. Many of the resin cements will not set when they are in thin layers exposed to the oxygen in the air. The cement in the canal is not exposed to air and will set readily.

usually for only a short time, a few hours to a few days. The pain response comes from odontoblasts that lie in the pulp at its junction with the dentin. The odontoblasts have processes that extend about a third of the way up the dentinal tubules that also contain a column of pulpal fluid. These processes have pressure receptors that can only interpret in a painful response any change in pressure in this column of pulpal fluid. The primary reason for the sensitivity is unsealed dentinal tubules. Acid etching greatly opens the tubules. If they are not properly sealed during the dentin bonding process, a number of things can influence the pressure on the fluid in the tubules and elicit a pain response. This dentinal fluid movement caused by pressure changes is called the **hydrodynamic theory of tooth sensitivity** and was described by Brännstrom. The following conditions can contribute to this sensitivity:

1. The tooth has been overdried (desiccated) during the bonding process, trapping air in the dentinal tubules; when the patient bites down, the restoration compresses the dentin, putting pressure on the air in the tubules.
2. The dentin has been overetched and not adequately sealed with priming resin.
3. The composite resin restoration is cured in increments that are too large, causing contraction stress on the tooth cusps or causing the composite resin to leak as it pulls away from the walls of the cavity preparation (see Chapter 6). It is important that proper procedures be followed during the bonding process to ensure that the dentinal tubules are sealed and posttreatment sensitivity is avoided.

SUMMARY

Bonding has a wide variety of uses in the modern dental practice. Bonding resins permits restorative materials to stick to tooth structure by way of micromechanical retention or chemical bonds. Phosphoric acid etches enamel and dentin to create surface roughness and porosities into which the bonding resins can flow. The bonding resins micromechanically lock into the etched tooth surface and chemically bond to composite resins. Their setting reactions can be self-activated by mixing components together, light-activated by stimulating photoinitiators with high-intensity blue light, or dual-cured (a combination of the two processes). Nonresin materials such as metal restorations or posts, amalgam, or porcelain can also be bonded to the tooth by way of bonding resins, but their bond is micromechanical in nature. Obtaining a strong bond to dentin is more difficult than to enamel. Dentin has a greater organic component and has a positive flow of pulpal fluid through the dentinal tubules that complicates the ability to bond to it. "Wet" (moist) dentin bonding allows bonding resins dissolved in solvents to penetrate through the water and around fibrils of the collagen matrix exposed by etching to form a hybrid layer of resin and dentin. This resin-rich layer allows other resins to bond to it by chemical resin-to-resin bonding. Thus composite resins can be retained by bonding to the hybrid layer and to the enamel that has been primed with resin. Nonresin materials can be bonded to the hybrid layer and to resin-primed enamel by resin adhesives (cements). Tooth sensitivity following bonding procedures is often the result of an incomplete seal of the dentin, allowing pressure gradients to act on the column of fluid in the dentinal tubules and causing the odontoblastic processes in the dentinal tubules to react with a pain response (hydrodynamic theory). As with many aspects of dentistry, careful attention to the proper steps in the bonding technique can usually eliminate these sensitivity problems.

CHAPTER REVIEW

Select the one correct response for each of the following multiple-choice questions:

1. **The acid used most commonly for etching tooth structure for bonding procedures is**
   a. Phosphoric
   b. Hydrochloric
   c. Hydrofluoric
   d. Citric

2. **All of the following statements about bonding to enamel are true EXCEPT one. Which one is this EXCEPTION?**
   a. Achieved by chemical bonding
   b. Achieved by micromechanical retention
   c. Achieved by resin tags penetrating porosities in the enamel and by locking into surface roughness
   d. Stronger than bonding to dentin

3. **Bonding to dentin**
   a. Is best accomplished when the dentin is kept moist after etching
   b. Is stronger when the dentin is well dried after etching
   c. Is inhibited by formation of the hybrid layer
   d. Is best on dentin that has been etched with 35% phosphoric acid for 30 seconds

4. **All of the following statements about resin bonding agents are true EXCEPT one. Which one is this EXCEPTION?**
   a. They are dissolved in solvents that allow them to penetrate the water on the moist dentin.
   b. They seal the dentin by penetrating into etched dentin surfaces and tubules.
   c. They chemically bond to the dentin.
   d. They chemically bond to composite resins.

5. **Dentin sensitivity can be caused by**
   a. Pressure changes in the column of fluid within the dentinal tubules
   b. Stimulation of odontoblastic processes within the dentinal tubules
   c. Open (unsealed) dentinal tubules
   d. Overetching or overdrying the dentin
   e. All of the above

6. **The smear layer**
   a. Is a tenacious layer of cut tooth debris and contaminants from the saliva
   b. Is easily removed by rinsing with water
   c. Is necessary for good bonding
   d. Is left on the dentin when the bonding agent is applied

7. **All of the following statements about bonding to repair fractured porcelain on a crown are true EXCEPT one. Which one is this EXCEPTION?**
   a. The surface is cleaned and roughened.
   b. 10% phosphoric acid is used for etching it.
   c. Silane is applied after etching to enhance the bond of adhesive resins to the porcelain.
   d. Composite resin is usually used to restore the fractured portion.

8. Which one of the following does NOT interfere with the formation of a good bond?
   a. Saliva on the etched enamel or dentin
   b. Oil lubricant from the handpiece
   c. Moist dentin after rinsing etchant off and lightly drying
   d. Eugenol-containing temporary cements

9. Which one of the following is true regarding the bonding of amalgam to a cavity preparation?
   a. Only the enamel is acid-etched.
   b. Freshly mixed amalgam is condensed onto unset bonding resin.
   c. The bonding resin should be light-cured.
   d. Wax is rubbed on the inside of the matrix band to keep the band from being glued to the tooth by the bonding resin.

10. When bonding endodontic posts into root canals, the bonding agent should not be
    a. Self-curing
    b. Light-curing
    c. Dual-curing
    d. Applied in a thin layer

11. All of the following are correct steps for bonding orthodontic brackets EXCEPT one. Which one is this EXCEPTION?
    a. The tooth surface is cleaned with pumice.
    b. The enamel is etched with 35% phosphoric acid for approximately 30 seconds.
    c. The enamel is rinsed and left slightly moist.
    d. A resin adhesive is used to bond the bracket.

12. When bonding composite resin to metal that is exposed after the overlying porcelain has fractured, which one of the following is FALSE?
    a. Retention to the metal is enhanced by roughening the surface with a coarse diamond bur, by sandblasting, by electrochemically etching, or by tin-plating.
    b. Bonding agents are not needed because the composite resin sticks to the metal.
    c. An opaque resin is applied before the composite resin to mask the metal and prevents a gray color from showing through the slightly translucent composite resin.
    d. Light-curing materials can be used.

CASE-BASED DISCUSSION TOPICS

◉ A 24-year-old graduate student needs two occlusal sealants on his lower first molars and a composite resin restoration to repair toothbrush abrasion on the facial root surface of his maxillary left canine. *Discuss the similarities and differences in bonding to enamel for the sealants and to dentin for the composite resin.*

◉ A 50-year-old female attorney is in need of a porcelain onlay on her mandibular left first premolar. *Discuss the differences in the mechanisms and the procedural steps that are used to adhere the bonding agent to the tooth as opposed to adhering the bonding agent to the porcelain onlay.*

◉ A 42-year-old male factory worker comes to the dental office with a chief complaint of tooth sensitivity after the recent placement of a class II posterior composite resin restoration on the lower right second molar. He complains that the tooth hurts when he bites on it and when cold drinks or cold air hit the tooth. *Discuss the likely causes for the sensitivity and the measures that can be taken to prevent postoperative tooth sensitivity after bonding procedures.*

◉ A 65-year-old retired schoolteacher needs the restoration of both mandibular first molars that have root caries on the facial root surfaces. The caries extends slightly beneath the crest of the gingiva, which is inflamed and bleeds easily. The patient wants tooth-colored restorations. She has an allergy to latex, so you will not be using a rubber dam. *Discuss the requirements for ensuring a good bond.*

◉ A 35-year-old female stockbroker comes to the dental office with a chief complaint of having chipped the mesial corner off her right maxillary central incisor porcelain-fused-to-metal crown by accidentally biting on a fork. Examination reveals a 2 mm by 1 mm loss of porcelain without the exposure of underlying metal. *Discuss the materials and procedures in their proper sequence of use to repair the crown in the office.*

REFERENCES

Albers HF: Resin bonding. In *Tooth-colored restoratives,* ed 8, Santa Rosa, CA, 1996, Alto Books.

Craig RG, Powers JM, Wataha JC: Direct esthetic restorative materials. In *Dental materials: properties and manipulation,* ed 7, Philadelphia, 2000, Mosby.

Eakle WS, Staninec M, Lacy AM: Effect of bonded amalgam on the fracture resistance of teeth, *J Prosthet Dent* 68:257, 1992.

Gladwin MA, Bagby MD: Adhesive materials. In *Clinical aspects of dental materials,* Philadelphia, 2000, Lippincott Williams & Wilkins.

Nakabayashi N, Nakajima K, Masuhara E: The promotion of adhesion by resin infiltration of monomers into tooth structure, *J Biomed Mat Res* 16:265, 1982.

Phillips RW, Moore BK: Adhesion and elasticity. In *Elements of dental materials for dental hygienists and dental assistants,* Philadelphia, 1994, WB Saunders.

Retief DH: Effect of conditioning the enamel surface with phosphoric acid, *J Dent Res* 52(2):333, 1973.

Silverstone LM: The acid etch technique: in vitro studies with special reference to the enamel surface and the enamel-resin interface. In *Proceedings from the International Symposium on Acid Etch Technique,* St Paul, MN, 1975, North Central Publishing Co.

Staninec M, Holt M: Bonding of amalgam to tooth structure: tensile adhesion and microleakage tests, *J Prosthet Dent* 59:397, 1988.

PROCEDURE 5-1 (see p. 321 for competency sheet)

Enamel and Dentin Bonding

EQUIPMENT/SUPPLIES (Figure 5-8)

- Rubber dam setup or cotton rolls and bibulous pads
- Dappen dishes or wells for bonding agents
- Disposable brushes for applying bonding agents and acid (if not in a dispenser)
- Bonding agent, curing light
- Restorative material—composite or amalgam

PROCEDURE STEPS

1 Isolate the field.

NOTE: Rubber dam is preferred because it can provide the best isolation for the longest time. Cotton rolls and bibulous pads can also be used. Moisture interferes with the formation of a good bond.

2 Etch cavity preparation with acid 10 to 15 seconds for dentin and 20 to 30 seconds for enamel (Figure 5-9).

NOTE: Start applying the etchant to the enamel first, then to the dentin. Overetching dentin will open the tubules too much and remove too much mineral (hydroxyapatite) from the dentin surface.

3 Rinse with water for at least 10 seconds.

4 Blot or gently air-dry enamel and dentin for 2 seconds.

NOTE: Do not overdry the dentin, because the collagen matrix will collapse and prevent adequate penetration of the bonding agent into the tubules and etched dentin. Dentin should be glistening (moist) with no puddles. If only enamel is etched, it should be dried thoroughly and should appear frosty.

5 Saturate the etched surface with the resin bonding agent (Figure 5-10).

NOTE: Some bonding agents are one bottle/one step application and others are two bottles/two steps—each component applied separately. If the bonding agent contains acetone as its solvent, it is particularly volatile. Do not dispense it until you are ready to apply it to the etched tooth, or most of the solvent may have evaporated. Also, be sure to recap the bottle immediately to keep from changing the consistency of the bonding resin and its ability to penetrate moist etched dentin.

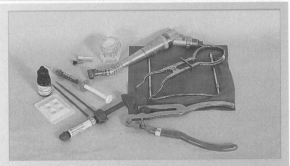

FIGURE 5-8

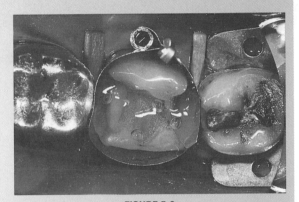

FIGURE 5-9
(Courtesy Dr. Alton Lacy, University of California School of Dentistry, San Francisco, Calif.)

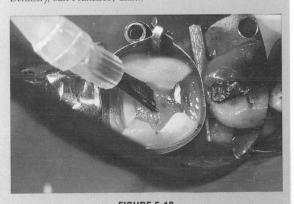

FIGURE 5-10
(Courtesy Dr. Alton Lacy, University of California School of Dentistry, San Francisco, Calif.)

Continued on following page

PROCEDURE 5-1 (Continued)

6 Apply a gentle air stream to thin the resin and to remove volatile solvents and water.

NOTE: The bonding resin is not as strong as the composite, so it should not be allowed to puddle in the preparation and cause weaknesses in the restoration. The solvent that the bonding resin was dissolved in must be removed by applying an air stream, otherwise the resin may not set completely. Likewise, air is used to evaporate any remaining water from the moist dentin.

7 Light-cure for 10 to 20 seconds. The cavity preparation is now ready for placement of a restoration.

NOTE: The tip of the light wand is usually held about 1 mm from the surface. The curing time may vary with newer, high-intensity curing lights. Follow manufacturers' recommendations. The enamel and dentin surfaces have been physically bonded with resin bonding agent and will bond to resin restorative materials such as composite placed on top of them by resin-to-resin chemical bonding.

PROCEDURE 5-2 (see p. 322 for competency sheet)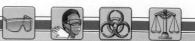

Surface Treatment for Bonding Porcelain Restorations or for Porcelain Repair

EQUIPMENT/SUPPLIES

- High- and low-speed handpieces with prophy attachment
- Dappen dish with flour of pumice and rubber prophy cup
- Isopropyl alcohol or acetone, hydrofluoric acid, silane, enamel, and dentin bonding agent
- 35% phosphoric acid, resin luting cement, curing light

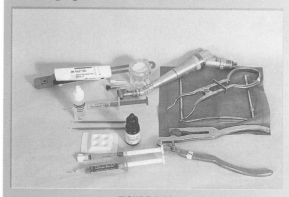

FIGURE 5-11

PROCEDURE STEPS

1 Isolate area to be bonded and clean tooth with wet flour of pumice. Try in porcelain restoration.

NOTE: Isolation is necessary to prevent moisture **contamination** of the surfaces during bonding. Pumice removes any plaque or pellicle that might interfere with etching and bonding.

2 Clean the internal surface of the porcelain with alcohol or acetone to remove salivary contaminants from the try in.

NOTE: For porcelain repair, roughen the surface with a coarse diamond or sandblasting to enhance the micromechanical retention.

3 Apply hydrofluoric acid to the cavity side of the porcelain for 1 minute to etch it.

4 Rinse with water for 10 seconds and dry with air (Figure 5-12).

5 Apply silane to etched porcelain for 30 seconds, and then dry with air to remove alcohol solvents.

NOTE: Silane allows bonding of resins to the treated porcelain surface.

Continued on following page

PROCEDURE 5-2 (Continued)

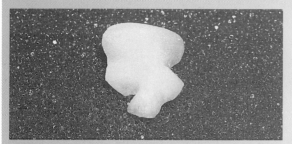

FIGURE 5-12
(Courtesy Dr. Alton Lacy, University of California School of Dentistry, San Francisco, Calif.)

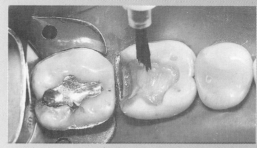

FIGURE 5-13
(Courtesy Dr. Alton Lacy, University of California School of Dentistry, San Francisco, Calif.)

6 Apply bonding agent to porcelain, but do not light-cure it.

NOTE: The thickness of the bonding resin will prevent proper seating of the restoration if cured at this stage. For porcelain repair, the bonding agent should be light-cured for 20 seconds.

7 *Steps 7 to 10 are the same as in Procedure 5-1 for enamel and dentin preparation for bonding.* Etch the tooth surfaces to be bonded with 35% phosphoric acid: 20 to 30 seconds for enamel and 10 seconds for dentin.

8 Rinse with water for 10 seconds.

NOTE: If surface is enamel only, dry thoroughly. If dentin is to be bonded, leave both enamel and dentin slightly moist.

9 Apply enamel-dentin bonding agent (Figure 5-13). Blow the bonding agent thin with air.

NOTE: Do not allow it to pool in the preparation or it will interfere with the seating of the restoration.

10 Light-cure for 20 seconds.

11 Apply resin cement to the restoration and seat it (Figure 5-14).

12 Remove gross excess cement, then light-cure for 3 seconds to cause the resin to partially set. Remove remaining excess resin (Figure 5-15).

13 Light-cure for 40 to 60 seconds or longer if needed for final set.

NOTE: Self-cured or dual-cured resins are used for cementation of inlays, onlays, or crowns, because the thickness of the restoration prevents adequate penetration of the light. With thin veneers, a light-cured resin can be

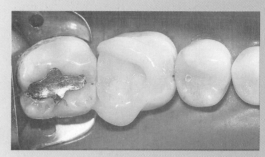

FIGURE 5-14
(Courtesy Dr. Alton Lacy, University of California School of Dentistry, San Francisco, Calif.)

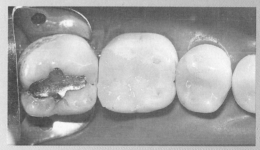

FIGURE 5-15
(Courtesy Dr. Alton Lacy, University of California School of Dentistry, San Francisco, Calif.)

used. For porcelain repair, apply composite resin and build up to full contour in increments. Light-cure each increment for 40 seconds. Newer curing lights with variable settings of light intensity might alter these recommended curing times. Check manufacturer's recommendations.

PROCEDURE 5-3 (see p. 323 for competency sheet)

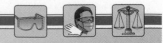

Bonding Orthodontic Brackets

EQUIPMENT/SUPPLIES (Figure 5-16)

- Basic setup
- Low-speed handpiece, prophy angle, rubber cup, and slurry of pumice
- Etchant (35% phosphoric acid), light-cured bonding resin
- Curing light, lip retractors
- High-volume evacuator (HVE) tip, cotton rolls
- Orthodontic brackets, bracket placement pliers, scaler

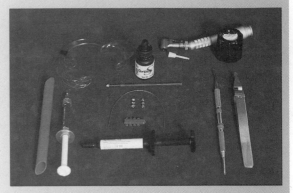

FIGURE 5-16

PROCEDURE STEPS

1 Inform the patient of the procedures to be done. Clean the facial surfaces of the teeth to be bonded with pumice slurry in a rubber cup.

NOTE: Pumice removes adherent plaque and organic pellicle that might interfere with proper etching and bonding.

2 Place lip retractors or cotton rolls to isolate the anterior teeth for bracket placement.

NOTE: Moisture from the lip mucosa will interfere with bonding.

3 Apply etching solution or gel for 30 seconds to that portion of the enamel that will receive the bracket.

4 Rinse the etchant off with water and thoroughly dry the enamel (Figure 5-17).

NOTE: Properly etched enamel should appear frosty or chalky white. Because no dentin is involved, the enamel is dried thoroughly.

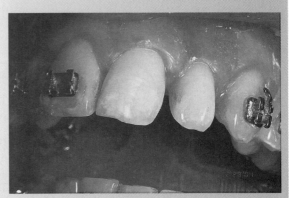

FIGURE 5-17

5 Apply a thin coating of liquid bonding resin to the etched enamel and light-cure for 20 seconds (Figure 5-18).

NOTE: This bonding resin acts to prepare or prime the enamel to allow the adhesion of the resin adhesive paste that holds the bracket in place. The bonding resin and the adhesive resin chemically bond to each other.

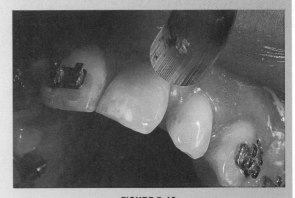

FIGURE 5-18

Continued on following page

PROCEDURE 5-3 (Continued)

6 Apply light-cured adhesive resin to the metal mesh on the back of the bracket (Figure 5-19), and place the bracket in the location prescribed by the dentist (or the dentist may place the bracket) using bracket-placement pliers. An orthodontic scaler can be used to adjust the position of the bracket and remove excess resin.

NOTE: The resin adhesive does not chemically bond to the bracket, but it will physically lock into the mesh on the back of the bracket. Some brackets are manufactured with the adhesive applied at the factory and covered with a plastic cover that is stripped away at the time of placement.

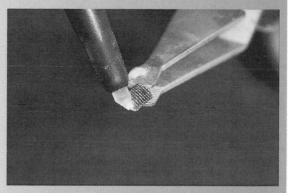

FIGURE 5-19

7 Light-cure the adhesive resin for 40 to 60 seconds.

NOTE: Although the metal of the bracket blocks the penetration of the light directly, the translucency of the enamel allows light to transmit through it to cure the resin underlying the bracket.

8 Repeat the procedure to complete the placement of all of the brackets (Figure 5-20).

NOTE: Typically, the six anterior teeth are all etched and primed at the same time. Brackets may be bonded individually or placed together and light-cured individually.

9 The arch wire and elastic or wire ligatures can be placed after all brackets are bonded.

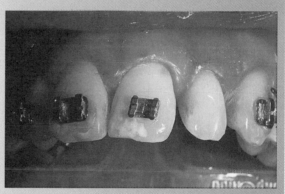

FIGURE 5-20

DIRECT AND INDIRECT ESTHETIC RESTORATIVE MATERIALS

OBJECTIVES

On completion of this chapter the student will be able to:

1. Describe the various types of composite resin restorative materials.
2. Discuss the uses, advantages, and disadvantages of each type of composite resin.
3. Compare and contrast the similarities and differences among chemical-cure, light-cure, and dual-cure composite resins.
4. Discuss the procedural differences between direct and indirect composite restorations.
5. Describe the composition of glass ionomer restoratives and their uses, advantages, and disadvantages.
6. Explain the effect of fluoride releasing, resin-modified glass ionomer restorations on prevention of recurrent caries.
7. List the components of compomers and their uses.
8. Describe how porcelain is bonded to metal.

9. Discuss the composition, uses, advantages, and disadvantages of an all-porcelain restorative material.
10. Describe steps to be taken to ensure proper conditions for shade taking.
11. Assist with placement of a composite resin restoration.

KEY TERMS

Direct-placement esthetic materials—Tooth-colored materials that can be placed directly into the cavity preparation without being constructed outside of the mouth first.

Composite resin—Tooth-colored material composed of an organic resin matrix and inorganic filler particles.

Organic resin (polymer) matrix—Thick liquids made up of two or more organic molecules that form a matrix around filler particles.

Inorganic filler particles—Fine particles of quartz, silica, or glass that give strength and wear resistance to the material.

Silane coupling agent—A chemical that helps bind the filler particles to the organic matrix.

Pigments—Coloring agents that give composites their color.

Self-cured composite—Composite that polymerizes by a chemical reaction when two resins are mixed together.

Light-cured composite—Composite that polymerizes when a chemical is activated by light in the blue wave range.

Dual-cured composite—Composite that contains components of light-cured and self-cured composites. When the two parts are mixed together, it polymerizes by a chemical reaction that can be accelerated by blue light activation.

Macrofilled composite—An early generation of composite that contained filler particles ranging from 10 to 100 μm.

Microfilled composite—Composite that contains very small filler particles averaging 0.04 μm in diameter.

Hybrid composite—Composite that contains both macrofill and microfill particles to obtain the strength of a macrofill and the polishability of a microfill.

Flowable composite—A light-cured, low-viscosity composite resin that contains fewer filler particles.

Packable composite—A light-cured, highly viscous, heavily filled composite resin for dentists who use a placement technique with composite that is similar to that of amalgam.

Glass ionomer—A self-cured, tooth-colored, fluoride-releasing restorative material that bonds to tooth structure without an additional bonding agent.

Hybrid (resin-modified) glass ionomer—A glass ionomer to which resin has been added to improve its physical properties.

Compomer—Composite resin that has polyacid, fluoride-releasing groups added.

Indirect-placement esthetic materials—Tooth-colored materials that are used to construct restorations outside of the mouth in the dental laboratory or at chairside on replicas of the prepared teeth. They are later cemented to the teeth.

Porcelain—A tooth-colored ceramic material composed of crystals of feldspar, alumina, and silica that are fused together at high temperatures to form a hard, uniform, glasslike material.

For the first half of the twentieth century amalgam and gold were the primary restorative materials for posterior teeth. Some anterior teeth also had metal in the form of gold margins of three-quarter crowns, class III gold foils, or class V inlays or amalgams that was visible when the patient smiled. In the latter half of the twentieth century a variety of direct-placement tooth-colored restorative materials were introduced. In the 1960s composite resins were introduced and have been continually improved on ever since by making them more durable and color stable. The use of porcelain has dramatically increased; currently porcelain is used in a variety of restorations made in the dental laboratory, such as crowns, inlays, onlays, and veneers. Other materials such as glass ionomer cements and compomers have also been developed, providing the dental team with a wide selection of esthetic materials for the restoration of damaged teeth and for cosmetic enhancement. Choosing the type of material depends, in part, on the extent of the damage to the tooth, the stresses that will be placed on the restoration, and the esthetic requirements of the patient. Because of the superior properties of the other esthetic materials, acrylic resin has been relegated primarily to use for denture bases and teeth (see Chapter 13) and for the fabrication of temporary or provisional restorations (see Chapter 14).

Now, with the ability to bond restorative materials to metal and tooth structure, advances in esthetic materials and techniques have improved the ability of the dental team to deliver the esthetic results that patients demand. The dental team must keep current with the rapid changes that occur with the materials and techniques. Good listening skills are needed to determine the types of esthetic services the patient is requesting so that the dental team and the patient are working in concert toward the same goal. Esthetic materials must be carefully selected so that their properties are compatible with the patient's oral condition and occlusion. Dental hygienists and dental assistants must understand the properties of these materials so that as important members of the dental team they can help the dentist to assess the performance of the restorations and alert the dentist when they perceive that a restoration may be failing. They need to be familiar with the physical properties of the materials so that they do not damage the restorations during routine oral hygiene, coronal polishing, and preventive procedures. Dental

assistants need to know the handling characteristics of the esthetic materials so that they can either assist the dentist in their placement or perform steps in their placement as permitted by state dental practice acts.

This chapter describes the physical properties, clinical applications, and shortcomings of directly placed and indirectly placed (constructed outside the mouth) esthetic materials. These materials include composite resins, glass ionomer cements, resin-modified glass ionomer cements, compomers, and porcelains. Guidelines for selection of the shade of these materials to obtain satisfactory cosmetic results also are discussed.

Direct-Placement Esthetic Restorative Materials

Direct-placement esthetic materials are those that can be placed directly into the cavity preparation or onto the tooth surface by the clinician without first being constructed outside of the mouth. Esthetic materials are those that are tooth colored. The direct-placement esthetic materials used most commonly are (1) composite resin, (2) glass ionomer cement, (3) resin-modified glass ionomer cement (also called hybrid ionomer), and (4) compomer. These are listed in their chronologic order of development.

COMPOSITE RESIN

A composite is a mixture of two or more materials with properties superior to any one component. **Composite resins** are tooth-colored materials that are used in both the anterior and posterior parts of the mouth. They are composed mainly of an **organic resin (polymer) matrix** and **inorganic filler particles** joined together by a **silane coupling agent** that sticks (adheres) the particles to the matrix. Also added are initiators and accelerators that cause the material to set and **pigments** that give color to the material and match tooth colors. Composite resins are commonly called *composites* and can also be referred to in the dental literature as *resin composites*.

COMPONENTS

Resin Matrix The most commonly used resin for the matrix of composites is bis-GMA, produced by reacting glycidyl methacrylate with bisphenol-A. Another resin that is used for the composite matrix is urethane dimethacrylate (UDMA). These resins are thick liquids made up of two or more organic molecules called *oligomers*. To reduce the viscosity and allow loading with filler particles, a low-molecular-weight monomer (molecules from which a resin or polymer is made) is added.

Filler Particles   Addition of filler particles makes the organic resin stronger and more wear resistant. Fillers are also added to control the handling characteristics of the composite resin and to reduce the shrinkage that occurs when the resin matrix polymerizes, or sets. The fillers used in composite resins are inorganic particles composed of a variety of materials including quartz, silica, and glasses composed of lithium, barium, strontium, or zinc. An important factor is the size of the filler particle and the ratio or weight of the filler to the matrix. As a general rule, the higher the filler content, the stronger the restoration and the more wear resistant it will be. There are differences in the filler size that affect the wear resistance and polishability (Figure 6-1). Wear of the composite is related to the filler particle size, the amount of filler in the resin, and the amount of resin between particles. Large filler particles tend to get pulled (called *plucking*) from the resin matrix at the surface when the restoration is under function or abraded by food and tooth brushing resulting in wear of the remaining resin matrix and leaving a rough surface. Smaller particles are not as easily plucked from the resin and therefore cause fewer voids that contribute to wear. Smaller particles can be packed closer together, thereby exposing less of the resin matrix to wear (Figures 6-2 and 6-3).

Coupling Agent   To provide a stronger bond between the organic fillers and the resin matrix, a coupling agent is used. This coupling agent is silane, which reacts with the surface of the inorganic filler and with the organic matrix to allow the two to adhere to each other. Good adhesion of the two is necessary to minimize loss of filler particles and to reduce wear.

Pigments   Inorganic pigments are added in varying amounts to develop a variety of colors that approximate the basic colors of teeth.

POLYMERIZATION

Polymerization is the chemical reaction that occurs when low-molecular-weight resin molecules called *monomers* join together to form long-chain, high-molecular-weight molecules called *polymers*. Chemicals that cause the polymerization reaction to begin are initiators and activators. *Activators* are organic molecules composed of tertiary amines.

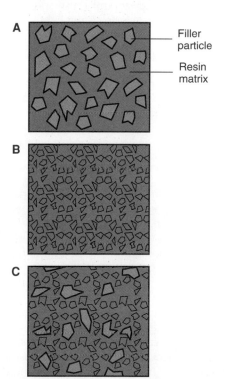

FIGURE 6-1 ■ Variety of filler sizes that are combined in the composite resins and contribute to their classification names. **A,** Macrofilled. **B,** Microfilled. **C,** Hybrid—a combination of the two.

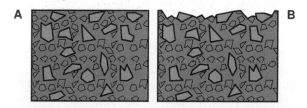

FIGURE 6-2 ■ Wear of composite surface. **A,** Smooth surface at the time of placement and surface polish. **B,** Rough surface caused by wear and loss of filler particles at the surface.

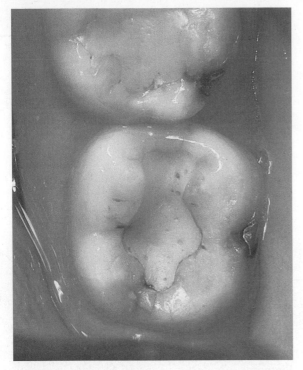

FIGURE 6-3 ■ Worn composite with staining at the margins indicative of microleakage. Opposing occlusion has worn the composite down, and numerous pits have developed as bits of the composite have fractured out.

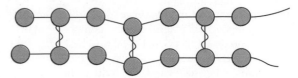

Diagramatical illustration
of cross linked polymer

FIGURE 6-4 ■ Cross-linking of adjacent polymer chains. Adjacent linear polymer chains are linked by covalently bonded atoms from short side chains.

The operator has a limited amount of time (working time) to place the restoration before it becomes too stiff to manipulate. Disposable mixing sticks are usually supplied with the material. Because the two pastes must be manually mixed, air can be incorporated into the material, causing voids or porosity in the restoration. Many clinicians prefer the light-cured composite resin because it requires no mixing, and the operator can control the working time by deciding when to apply the curing light.

CLINICAL TIP When dispensing the two pastes from jars the assistant must be careful not to use the same end of the stick in each jar because it will contaminate the materials and cause premature setting of a portion of the material still in the jar. For the same reason, when dispensing material from syringes it is important not to mix up the caps and put them on the wrong syringes.

Activators start a chemical reaction with the initiators to begin the process of linking monomers together one at a time (called *addition polymerization*) to form polymers. Polymer chains have small groups of atoms hanging off their sides. When side groups of adjacent polymers share electrons, they form covalent bonds that link (called *cross-linking*) the chains together (Figure 6-4). Cross-linking of polymers produces a much stronger, stiffer material than with single-chain polymers. (See Chapter 13 for a more detailed description of polymer formation and properties.)

Chemical Cure   Chemically cured composite resins, or **self-cured composite** resins, are two-paste systems supplied in jars or syringes. One paste, called the *base,* contains composite and benzoyl peroxide as an initiator. The other paste, called the *catalyst,* contains composite and a tertiary amine as an activator. Equal parts of these two pastes are mixed together, and the polymerization reaction begins.

Light Cure   **Light-cured composite** resins are the most common type of composite resin used in private practice. An intense visible light in the blue wave range activates these materials. Blue light with a wavelength between 400 and 500 nanometers (nm) activates a diketone that, in the presence of an organic amine, causes the resin to polymerize (cure or set). These components are both present in the composite and do not react until the light begins the reaction. If the composite resin is placed in too thick an increment, it may not cure all the way to the bottom. The depth of cure depends on the location and the color of the restoration. Interproximal areas may need additional time to cure completely because of the more difficult access of the area to the direct path of the light. Darker shades also have a longer curing time because the light is more readily absorbed by the dark color and does not transmit through the material as readily as through lighter-colored materials.

Dual Cure   Dual-cured composite resins are two-paste systems that contain the initiators and activators of both the light-activated and, to a smaller amount, the chemically activated materials. The advantage is that when the two pastes are mixed together and placed in the tooth, the curing light is used to initiate the setting reaction and the chemical setting reaction continues in areas not reached by the light to ensure a complete set (polymerization).

CLASSIFICATION OF COMPOSITES

Macrofilled Composites   The first generation of composite resins used relatively large particles as fillers, ranging in size from 10 to 100 microns (μm). These composites are called **macrofilled composites.** The large particles make these composites difficult to polish, and they become rough as filler particles are lost at the surface under function. They are generally stronger than composites with smaller particles. Because of their roughness, macrofilled composites are no longer widely used.

Microfilled Composites   Microfilled composites were developed to overcome the problems of the macrofills. As the name implies, microfilled composites have fillers that are much smaller than those in macrofilled composites. The filler particles average about 0.04 μm in diameter. Several small particles have a larger total surface area than one large particle of similar weight. It is difficult to load a large volume of microfillers in the resin matrix because of this large surface area. Therefore the volume of filler in microfilled composites is only 35% to 50% as opposed to 70% to 85% with many other composites. A lower filler volume results in a composite with poorer physical properties (i.e., weaker and less wear resistant). To help overcome these shortcomings, some manufacturers mix microfillers into a resin, polymerize (cure) it, and grind the hardened material into particles ranging from 10 to 20 μm. Then they use these particles (consisting of prepolymerized resin and microfillers) as the filler so that they can get more microfillers into the resin and improve its physical properties. Alternative methods to increase the numbers of microfillers that can be loaded into the resin include clumping the microfillers together by heating them or by condensing them into large clumps.

Small-Particle Composites   Small-particle composites have fillers 1 to 5 μm in size and are filled 80% to 85% by weight. Their physical properties lie between those of macrofills and microfills. They were produced for use as posterior composites but have been replaced by hybrid composites.

Hybrid Composites   Hybrid composites contain both macrofillers and microfillers in order to produce a strong composite that polishes well. Their filler content is 75% to 80% by weight. Microhybrid composites contain a mixture of small particles (0.5 to 3.0 μm) and microfine particles (0.04 μm). Microhybrids can contain a high filler content (70% by volume) because microfine particles fill in spaces between small particles. Hybrids are versatile because of their strength and polishability. They can be used in both the anterior and posterior parts of the mouth.

Flowable Composites   Flowable composites are low-viscosity, light-cured resins that may be lightly filled (about 40%) or more heavily filled (up to 70%). The particles generally average in size between 0.07 and 1.0 μm. These composites flow readily and can be delivered directly into cavity preparations by small needles from the syringes in which they are packaged. Because of their low viscosity, they adapt well to cavity walls and flow into microscopic irregularities created by diamonds and burs. They are well suited for use in conservative dentistry (i.e., preventive resin restorations), where they readily flow into the narrow preparations created with small burs and diamonds or air abrasion. Many dentists use them in place of conventional pit and fissure sealants, because their higher filler content makes them more wear resistant than most lightly filled sealants. They are useful as liners in large cavity preparations, because they adapt to the preparation better than more viscous materials such as hybrid and packable composites. Their low elastic modulus allows them to cushion stresses created by polymerization shrinkage or heavy occlusal loads when they are used as an intermediate layer under hybrid and packable composites. (The lower the elastic modulus, the more flexible the material; the higher the elastic modulus, the stiffer the material.) They are useful for restoration of class V noncarious lesions caused by toothbrush abrasion, acid erosion, or occlusal stresses, such as bruxing, that lead to flexing of the tooth (abfraction lesions). For toothbrush abrasion lesions, the patient should have the heavy toothbrushing habits corrected first. Otherwise, the flowable composites may wear too rapidly if the patient continues to brush too hard. The flowable composites shrink more when polymerized than the hybrid composites, wear more readily, and are weaker. However, they have many applications as liners, sealants, and restorative materials when they are not placed in areas under occlusal function or areas of high wear.

Pit and Fissure Sealants　Pit and fissure sealants are low-viscosity resins that vary in their filler content from no filler to more heavily filled resins that are essentially the same as flowable composites. They are used to prevent dental caries in pits and fissures of teeth (see Chapter 7). See Table 6-1 for classification of composites by four different criteria.

Packable Composites　Packable composites are highly viscous resins that contain a high volume of filler particles, which gives them a stiff consistency. They are used for restoration of posterior teeth in areas of high function, because they are stronger and more wear resistant than most hybrids that contain less filler. They are marketed as substitutes for amalgams, because they handle more like amalgam, due to their stiffness, than the hybrid composites. They are sometimes referred to as condensable composites, but they cannot truly be condensed (made more dense) but more correctly are packed into the cavity preparation. They shrink less when polymerized than less heavily filled composites, because there is less resin and more filler.

"Smart" Composites　The idea of restorative materials that would react to the oral environment to combat recurrent caries resulted in the introduction in 1998 of a "smart" composite resin. This composite releases fluoride, calcium, and hydroxyl ions when the acidity of the area around the restoration increases. If bacteria in plaque release acid as a by-product of their metabolism of sugars or cooked starches, the restoration is "smart" enough to release ions that will counteract the effects of the acid and remineralize the tooth. The effectiveness of this material has not yet been confirmed by clinical studies.

Core Buildup Composites　Core buildup composites are heavily filled composites used in badly broken-down teeth needing crowns. They replace missing tooth structure lost from dental caries or tooth frac-

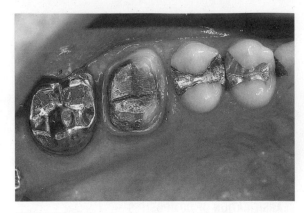

FIGURE 6-5 ■ Composite core material with color contrasting to the tooth structure for easy identification during crown preparation.
(Courtesy Dr. Dennis J. Weir, University of Iowa School of Dentistry, Iowa City, Iowa.)

ture so that there is adequate structure to retain a crown. These composites can be light-cured, self-cured, or dual-cured. They often contain pigments that colorize them so that they can be easily differentiated from natural tooth structure (Figure 6-5). Dentin-colored core materials are used when all-ceramic crowns are to be used. Amalgam would create an esthetically unacceptable dark discoloration under the all-ceramic crown as light passes through the porcelain and reflects off the amalgam. Core composites are strong and can be bonded to tooth structure to minimize bacterial leakage.

CLINICAL TIP　Not all light-cured bonding agents are compatible with chemical-cured composites, so follow manufacturer's recommendations when selecting a bonding agent for the core material.

Provisional Restorative Composites　Composites for provisional restorations are used in place of acrylic resins for the construction of provisional onlays, crowns, and bridges. They are more expensive than the acrylic resins, but they wear less and shrink less, and release less heat as they cure. They can be repaired easily with flowable composites to add to contact areas and margins. They are more brittle than the acrylic resins and tend to break more easily with longer-span bridges (see Chapter 14).

TABLE 6-1
Four Classification Methods for Composites

Classification Method				
1. Filler amount (volume %)	Sealant 0-10	Microfill 20-30	Anterior hybrid 40	Posterior hybrid 70
2. Particle size (μm)	Macro 40	Midi 4	Small 0.1-1	Micro 0.04-0.1
3. Matrix composition	Bis-GMA	Urethane dimethacrylate		
4. Polymerization method	Self-cured	Light-cured	Dual-cured	

Adapted from Marshall GW, Marshall SJ: Dental composites. In *Biomaterials science for restorative dentistry (teaching syllabus),* San Francisco, 2000, University of California.

PHYSICAL PROPERTIES OF COMPOSITES

Important physical properties of composites include biocompatibility, strength, wear, polymerization shrinkage, thermal conductivity, coefficient of thermal expansion, water sorption, elastic modulus, and radiopacity.

Biocompatibility   Newly placed composite resins can release chemicals that, in deep cavity preparations, could pass through the dentinal tubules into the pulp, causing an inflammatory reaction. When the tubules are sealed by dentin bonding agents or protected with a base, there is no problem. Polished composites are well tolerated by surrounding soft tissues. They are not known to cause any systemic disorder. A very few individuals may be allergic to one or more of the components of the material, and for these individuals another restorative material must be chosen.

Strength   Composites with larger filler particles are stronger in both tension (pulling) and compression (bearing) than microfilled composites.

Wear   Composites wear faster than amalgams. Recent improvements have made the latest generation of composites more wear resistant than early composites, and they are beginning to approach the wear rate of amalgams. Filler content has an effect on the wear rate. Composites with a lower volume of filler (microfills and flowables) wear faster than more heavily filled materials.

Polymerization Shrinkage   Polymerization shrinkage refers to the shrinkage that occurs when the composite is cured (polymerized). The matrix, when cured, usually shrinks away from the cavity walls. It was once thought that light-cured composites shrink toward the light, and a great effort was made to correctly place the light probe in order to draw the material toward the cavity wall to minimize leakage at the margins. More recent research indicates that the material does not shrink toward the light. Chemical-cured composites cure toward the center of the bulk of the material, and light-cured materials have this tendency but are also influenced by the cavity shape and size with minimal influence by the location of the light. Placing the restoration in small incremental layers and curing each layer can help minimize the effect of polymerization shrinkage. Some postinsertion sensitivity can be attributed to this shrinkage as it pulls composite away from the cavity walls and allows leakage of fluids and bacteria into the dentinal tubules. Shrinking composite that is well bonded to cavity walls can also put tension on the cusps of the tooth, causing discomfort when the patient bites down. The greater the resin content of the composite, the greater the shrinkage. Therefore microfills and flowables shrink more than hybrids and packables.

Another method of managing the shrinkage in the cavity is to do an indirect restoration (one that is prepared and cured outside of the mouth). The shrinkage occurs in the restoration before it is placed in the tooth; then the restoration is cemented in place with a thin layer of a low-viscosity composite cement such as that used to cement veneers. This thin layer of cement will have minimal shrinkage.

Thermal Conductivity   Composite resin has a thermal conductivity close to that of natural tooth structure and much lower than that of metal. It is therefore a biologically protective material for the dental pulp.

Coefficient of Thermal Expansion   Ideally the coefficient of thermal expansion (CTE) of the filling material would be the same as the tooth structure. In the case of composite, the CTE is greater and will have a greater change in dimension than will the adjacent tooth structure. This can result in debonding and leakage of the restoration. The greater the filler content, the lower the CTE. The microfilled composites and the flowable composites have a higher CTE than do the packable or hybrid varieties.

Elastic Modulus   The elastic modulus (also referred to as Young's modulus), or stiffness of composite, is determined by the amount of the filler. The greater the volume of the filler, the stiffer and more wear resistant the restoration. This is an important consideration for the selection of the type of composite. For example, an occlusal restoration on a posterior tooth must have a greater wear resistance than does a class V gingival restoration. In fact, the stiffer material is probably contraindicated at the gingival margins because it does not have the flexibility needed in that area. Microfilled and flowable composites have fewer particles and more resin. They deform more readily under function and therefore can break more easily. Microfills are generally used in non–stress-bearing restorations.

Water Sorption   The resin matrix absorbs water from the oral cavity over time. The greater the resin content, the more water is absorbed. Therefore microfills and flowables tend to have greater water sorption. The water softens the resin matrix and leads to a gradual degradation of the material.

Radiopacity   Metals such as lithium, barium, or strontium are added to the filler to make the restoration more opaque when viewed on a radiograph. However, the older composite materials did not have this additive and might appear radiolucent on the radiograph. Clinical observation of the teeth will confirm the presence of a restoration in those cases. Some present-day microfilled composites are also radiolucent. Quartz is not radiopaque, but it is sometimes used as a filler for composites used in the anterior part of the mouth, because it has good optical properties that can enhance the color match to the tooth. It allows light to transmit through the restoration more readily and to pick up coloration from the surrounding tooth structure, making for a better color match. See Table 6-2 for a ranting of the physical properties of the composite resin types relative to each other.

CLINICAL HANDLING OF COMPOSITES

Uses of Composite Resins   Composites are used in all classes of restorations, from class I through class VI. Although previously used mostly for class III and class V esthetic restorations, these materials are very popular for posterior as well as anterior restorations. Composite materials are also used for provisional restorations (see Chapter 14), core buildups, fiber-reinforced posts, and laboratory-fabricated onlays and bridges.

Selection of Materials   Several criteria can be used for the selection of composite resins for restorations. When used in the anterior part of the mouth in non–stress-bearing areas, selection is usually based on the ability of the material to match the color of the teeth and to achieve a high polish. Microfills and microhybrids are well suited for this purpose. When incisal edges or other stress-bearing areas are being restored, hybrids or microhybrids should be considered because they are stronger than microfills. In the stress-bearing areas of the posterior

TABLE 6-2

Composite Resins Ranked Relative to Each Other

Composite	Polymerization Shrinkage	Flexural Strength	Compressive Strength	Stiffness	Polishability	Wear Resistance
Macrofills	Low	High	High	High	Low	Moderate
Microfills	Moderate	Moderate	Moderate	Moderate	High	Moderate
Hybrids	Low	High	High	High	Moderate	High
Packables	Low	High	High	High	Moderate	High
Flowables	High	Low	Low	Low	High	Low

part of the mouth, hybrids and microhybrids are usually chosen for their strength, wear resistance, and polishability. Flowable composites should not be used in areas subjected to stress or abrasion because they are relatively weak and wear more rapidly. Macrofills generally are not used much since the hybrids have been developed, because they do not polish well and leave a rough surface.

Shade Guides Many manufacturers include a shade guide with color tabs that can be used to help in shade selection. Sometimes these color tabs are not an exact match to the composites they represent. Therefore it is a good practice to apply and cure a small quantity (in a thickness comparable to the finished restoration) of the composite selected onto the clean, moist tooth before the tooth is isolated and dried under rubber dam or cotton roll isolation. Some

practitioners prefer to make their own custom shade guides directly from the composite material because these will be more accurate representations of the true composite colors. The color tab should be moist, held adjacent to the tooth to be restored, and viewed under different lighting conditions (Figure 6-6) (see Shade Taking, later in this chapter).

Occasionally, a good color match is not possible with the composite as it is supplied. In this situation it may be necessary to mix a couple of different colors together to achieve the desired color match or to add special color modifiers (specially pigmented composites that contain more resin and less filler). In some circumstances the color of badly discolored teeth cannot be matched with composite resin.

Shelf Life The shelf life of composites varies with the type of resin used and the manufacturer. In

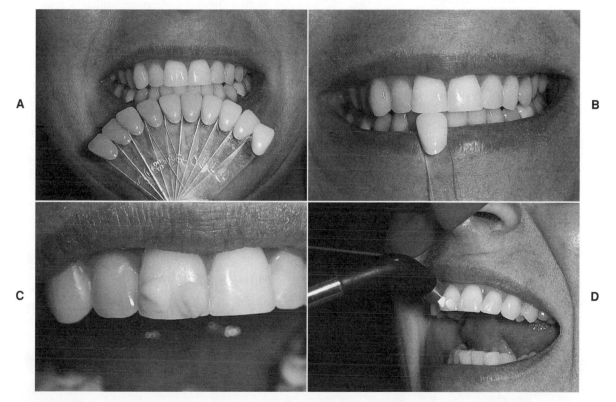

FIGURE 6-6 ■ Shade selection for composites. **A,** Hold shade guide up to the teeth and look for the shade that is the closest match. **B,** Hold that shade tab next to the tooth to be restored to confirm the match. **C,** If unsure of an exact match, place a small amount of composite in the two closest shades on the tooth. **D,** Light-cure the composite so that its final shade can be compared with the tooth. Select the closest match. Occasionally, a couple of shades will need to be mixed together to get a good match.

general, avoiding heat and light can extend the shelf life. Manufacturers usually recommend refrigerating the material. The average shelf life is 2 to 3 years if stored properly.

Dispensing and Cross-contamination Light-cured composites are supplied in compules or syringes. All of these containers are opaque so that the material is not affected by light. Some offices prefer single-use (unidose) items such as composite compules (small containers of composite resin that fit into a delivery gun) that can be disposed of after the procedure so that infection-control procedures are easier and risk of contamination is minimized. Reusable syringes require careful handling to ensure that they are not contaminated during the procedure. The delivery tip on syringes of flowable composites should be disposed of in a sharps container after use, and the syringes should be recapped and sprayed with disinfectant. Composite in screw-type syringes should be dispensed after the shade is selected and covered in a light-protected container until used. Chemical-cured composites come in jars or screw-type tubes (Figure 6-7).

Matrix Strips/Bands For class III and IV anterior restorations, a clear plastic (Mylar) matrix strip is used to contain and shape the composite. For class II restorations, metal matrix bands or precontoured plastic matrix strips that help shape the contact area are used. Metal matrix bands are either circumferential bands (fit all the way around the tooth as for mesiocclusodistal-type cavities) or sectional bands (fit only on one proximal surface at a time as with mesiocclusal or distocclusal cavities). The curing light is placed from the occlusal with metal bands for initial curing, then placed from the facial and lingual after the matrix band is removed. Clear matrix forms for class V cavities are also available for light-cured composites. For rebuilding large portions of the tooth, appropriately sized and trimmed clear crown forms can be filled with composite, pressed into place, and cured with the light-curing unit.

A wedge may be placed to seal the gingival margin or separate teeth to make up for the thickness of the matrix band. When the band is removed, a contact will be established with the adjacent tooth. Wedges can be wooden or transparent plastic to help transmit light to the gingival margin. If a wooden wedge is used, the gingival portion of the composite should be light-cured after the wedge is removed, because it may have prevented the light from curing this area with the initial light-curing. Any of these matrices can be used with chemical-cured composites as well.

Incremental Placement For most moderately sized or large cavity preparations, the composite resin should be placed in small increments about 2 mm thick. The benefits of this are twofold. First, it minimizes polymerization shrinkage; second, it permits light from the curing unit to adequately penetrate and thoroughly cure each increment. Thicker increments are more difficult for the light to cure

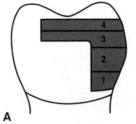

FIGURE 6-7 ■ Dispensing systems for composites. In sequence from *upper left* to *lower center,* composite may be supplied in jars or compules and delivered by a gun, syringes, or screw-type tubes.

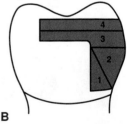

Incremental placement of composite in a Class II cavity preparation

Horizontal layers in box form   Diagonal layers in box form

A   B

FIGURE 6-8 ■ Incremental placement of composite to minimize polymerization shrinkage and ensure complete cure of composite. **A,** Increments placed horizontally. **B,** Increments placed diagonally.

through the entire thickness and therefore require longer curing times (Figure 6-8).

Resin-to-Resin Bonding   Etched enamel and dentin is infiltrated with resin bonding agents to form the resin-rich hybrid layer. The initial increment of composite resin will chemically bond to the resin bonding agent on the enamel and dentin. Each additional increment will bond to the previously placed increment of composite as long as good isolation is maintained and no contaminants are introduced. When resins polymerize there is a thin layer of unpolymerized resin on the surface, because contact with oxygen in the air inhibits the cure. This

"air-inhibited" layer looks shiny and feels slippery. This unset layer facilitates chemical bonding with the next layer of composite and will set when the layer placed over it is cured. The completed restoration comprises a series of layers of resin-based materials that are all chemically bonded to each other and micromechanically bonded to the tooth structure (Figure 6-9). In most cases, the thin-air–inhibited layer is removed during finishing and polishing. It may have an unpleasant taste and should be wiped off with gauze before the patient leaves if finishing and polishing are not required (as with pit and fissure sealants).

Contaminants   Newly etched dentin is kept moist for "wet" dentin bonding. However, after dentin bonding any form of moisture (water, saliva, gingival fluid from the sulcus or blood) should be kept away from the tooth until the restoration is completed. Contamination requires removal of the contaminant and reetching for 10 to 15 seconds. Alcohol should not be used to wet the composite placement instrument to keep the composite from sticking because it weakens the composite. Instead, a little of the bonding agent or other unfilled resin can be used to prevent sticking. Liners, bases, or temporary cements containing eugenol should not be used because eugenol inhibits the set of resins.

Light-curing   For light-cured composites the light probe should be held as close as possible to the composite without actually touching it. In many offices the light probe and handle are covered with a disposable barrier such as a clear plastic cover. The light probe may be further away from the composite than ideal in some locations, such as the first composite increment placed on the gingival floor of a class II preparation. In some circumstances the light probe may be positioned to cure through enamel overlying the composite. For class II and III cavities the light may be positioned alternately from the lingual and facial (after the occlusal in the case of class II).

Typical curing times for thin layers are 20 to 40 seconds. Thicker increments, darker composites, or composites located further than ideal from the light probe should be cured for longer times (at least 60 seconds). Areas of composite that lie just outside of the borders of the light probe should be cured separately. Newer high-speed or variable-intensity light units should use the curing times recommended by the manufacturers.

**Section of tooth with
bonded composite restoration**

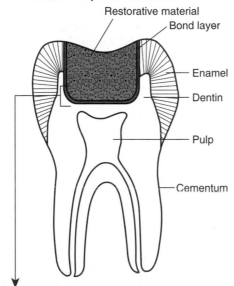

**Micro illustration of area of bond with restorative
material and dentin tubules in hybrid layer**

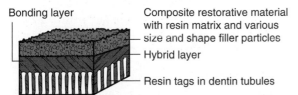

FIGURE 6-9 ■ Section of tooth with bonded composite restoration. Thin layer of bonding agent is micromechanically attached to the etched enamel and dentin and is chemically bonded to the composite resin.

Finishing and Polishing (see Chapter 9)   Excess composite can be removed with multifluted carbide finishing burs, fine and ultrafine diamonds, and sandpaper disks. Small excesses at the gingival margin or interproximal can be removed with special composite knives, a scapel blade, needle-shaped burs or diamonds, or abrasive strips.

Polishing of composites can be achieved by using successively finer sandpaper disks and interproximal finishing strips; by rubber polishing points, cups, and disks impregnated with abrasives; and by polishing pastes.

Surface Sealers   Some clinicians prefer to add an unfilled resin to the surface of the composite after finishing and polishing. This surface sealer is thought to reseal margins that might have been opened by polymerization shrinkage and to fill in any surface porosities created by small voids or air pockets in the composite that were uncovered by finishing. Usually, the surface of the composite is rinsed and dried thoroughly; it and the surrounding enamel are etched for 15 seconds; and then a thin layer of the unfilled resin is applied and thinned further with a gentle stream of air and light-cured for 20 seconds. Thick layers might interfere with the occlusion. Interproximal contacts should be flossed to ensure that resin has not been trapped.

LIGHT CURING UNITS

Many standard curing units use a halogen light bulb as the light source. The light delivery tip or probe is usually attached to the unit by a flexible fiber bundle. The probes are often glass or glass encased in metal. Some are a type of plastic. Some delivery tips are in the configuration of a wand and others in the shape of a gun. A few units have the capability of being used remotely rather than being plugged into an electrical outlet because they have rechargeable batteries and can be detached from the base unit. For infection control purposes, the wand or gun should be covered with a disposable cover and uncontaminated gloves should be worn when using the unit (see Chapter 4, Figure 4-10).

High-intensity light units are available that greatly reduce the curing times needed. Plasma arc curing (PAC) units and argon laser units can cure materials in less than 10 seconds. Rapid curing greatly speeds up the procedure because the conventional curing of many small increments each for 40 seconds increases the time required. Some studies suggest that rapid curing might cause a rapid shrinkage that can create stress in the tooth-to-restoration interface and produce microleakage. For this reason, new curing lights have been introduced that can be adjusted to start out with a low light intensity and gradually increase to a high intensity. Some of the light units send the light out in pulses rather than a continuous beam. This gradual curing is thought to relieve the stress and reduce microleakage associated with polymerization shrinkage.

Precautions

1. *Inadequate light output.* It is important to check the light-curing units frequently (monthly) because the light bulbs will deteriorate over time and not produce an adequate cure. Additionally, the light probes can darken with application of surface disinfectants or sterilization or become scratched and not transmit light as well. If composite or bonding agent has come in contact with the light tip and hardened on it, it will impede the light output. Light output can be measured by commercially available radiometers (light meters); some light units have a built-in light meter for periodic testing. If these are not available, a rough assessment of light output can be made by taking a sample of composite and placing it in a 4 mm length of drinking straw and light-curing it on one end for 40 seconds. The surface of the composite away from the light can be tested with a sharp explorer to see if the surface is hard.
2. *Premature set of composite.* The operatory light can cause an initial surface set of the surface of many composites. Once this has happened the composite can no longer be manipulated, but it is not cured through the depth of the material. The operatory light should be moved further from the composite or temporarily turned away from the field, so that the direct light is not shining in the patient's mouth.
3. *Eye protection.* The operator is cautioned to use a light-shielding protective device to protect the eyes of the patient and the staff (see Chapter 4, Figure 4-10). The patient could also be given protective eyewear that filters the light. The intense blue light has the potential to cause damage to the retina with direct exposure.

> **CAUTION**
> *Do not look directly at the light when curing*
> *materials. Use a light shield to protect the eyes.*
> *Have the patient close his or her eyes, or*
> *provide filtering eyewear.*

4. *Heat generation.* The curing light generates a certain amount of heat as it is applied to the tooth, and composite resins release heat (exothermic reaction) when they polymerize. The combination of the two heat sources has the potential to elevate the temperature of the pulp in deep cavities that have only 1 mm or less of dentin over the pulp. This increase in pulpal temperature has the potential to cause an inflammatory reaction in the pulp and even death of the pulp.

GLASS IONOMERS

Glass ionomers are self-cured, tooth-colored, fluoride-releasing restorative materials that bond to tooth structure without an additional bonding agent. Several materials have been developed in this class and are classified for use in dentistry as luting (cementation) agents (see Chapter 10) for crowns, onlays, and inlays; restorative materials; liners and bases for cavity preparations; and core buildup materials. They are supplied as a liquid composed of an aqueous solution containing copolymers of polyacrylic acid and a powder composed of an acid-soluble calcium fluoroaluminosilicate glass. An acid-base reaction occurs when the powder and liquid are mixed and fluoride is released. The powder and liquid can be measured and mixed at chairside or can come as premeasured powder or liquid capsules that are mixed in a triturator and delivered with a gun-type applicator. They are manufactured in a variety of shades.

Physical Properties   Glass ionomers have some highly desirable characteristics, as well as some drawbacks:

1. *Biocompatibility.* Glass ionomers are tolerated well by surrounding soft tissues and are considered kind to the pulp.
2. *Bond to tooth structure.* They can bond to enamel and dentin through a chemical ion exchange mechanism that allows the material to bind with the calcium ions in the tooth. Because they set

gradually and shrink very little, they do not generate the great internal stresses that composite resins do when they set rapidly. Therefore glass ionomers maintain their seal to the tooth better.
3. *Fluoride release.* They release an initial high level of fluoride that helps in the control of secondary caries. They can absorb fluoride and rerelease it, thereby acting as a fluoride reservoir. The fluoride has some antibacterial properties and is thought to suppress bacteria associated with tooth decay, especially *mutans* types of streptococci.
4. *Solubility.* Their less desirable properties include their sensitivity to moisture during the first 24 hours after placement. They are highly soluble during this time and must be covered with a protective varnish. They also are prone to crack or craze (develop numerous shallow cracks on their surface) if dried too much during the first 24 hours. Therefore they should not be finished until they have completely set after 24 hours.
5. *Thermal expansion.* They have a thermal expansion similar to tooth structure.
6. *Thermal protection.* They are good insulators against temperature extremes.
7. *Compressive and tensile strength.* They have a moderately high compressive strength but are weaker in tension and therefore should not be used in stress-bearing areas such as occlusal surfaces and incisal edges.
8. *Wear resistance.* Glass ionomers wear faster than composite resins. Their surface gets rougher over time. They cannot be polished to as smooth a surface as composites.
9. *Radiopacity.* They are more radiopaque than dentin.
10. *Color.* Glass ionomers are more opaque than composites. Translucency and the number of colors available have improved over the years.

Clinical Uses

Luting Cements (see Chapter 10)   Glass ionomer luting cements were very popular because they are pulpally kind, bond to tooth structure, release fluoride, and have a low film thickness so crowns can be seated easily. Their use has decreased since the introduction of hybrid ionomer cements and resin cements that have better physical properties (stronger and less soluble).

Restorative Materials   Glass ionomer restoratives are used in non–stress-bearing areas because they are weak in tensile strength and are not as wear resistant as composites. They are used for restoration of root caries because they bond to the root better than composites and release fluoride to resist recurrent caries. They are useful for restoration of noncarious cervical lesions because they can be placed conservatively without the need for cutting a lot of mechanical retention in the tooth to retain the restoration as with amalgam. They can be used in anterior class III cavities when color match is not an issue. Encapsulated materials are desirable because powder/liquid ratios are improved and mixing is consistent. They can also be dispensed directly into the cavity from the capsules, which have a dispensing tip attached (Figure 6-10). Some restoratives called *cermets* have metal particles added to improve the physical properties (i.e., abrasion resistance and compressive strength). Cermets are used in locations where esthetics is not a concern and as core buildup materials where the bulk of the subsequent crown will be supported by tooth structure. As with composite resins, glass ionomer restoratives require good isolation. Two to three minutes after mixing, the material undergoes an initial gelation whereby the material cannot be manipulated but has not completely hardened. Over the next minute or so, the material hardens but continues to undergo chemical setting reactions for several hours. Only gross excess of material should be removed, and the material should be covered with a varnish to protect it from moisture until the final set has occurred at least 24 hours later. Finishing can be done after 24 hours. Core buildup cements can be reduced as part of the crown preparation approximately 8 minutes after the initial set, because they will be subsequently covered by a provisional and then a final crown.

Liners and Bases Glass ionomer liners are materials used to cover the dentin for pulpal protection from temperature changes, from chemicals within other restorative materials, or from acid etchants. They have a low powder content and are applied in thin layers that are relatively weak. Glass ionomer bases are used to rebuild missing dentin within the cavity preparation and are usually much thicker layers than liners. They have a higher powder content and stronger physical properties.

Lamination or "Sandwich" Technique Occasionally glass ionomer is used in combination with another restorative material to gain the best properties of each material. The most common situation where this lamination technique is used is within the proximal box of a deep composite cavity preparation where the gingival floor is located on the root. Glass ionomer can obtain a better seal to the root than composite and additionally will release fluoride into the surrounding root surface to resist secondary decay. Glass ionomer is placed in the proximal box on the gingival floor as the initial layer, and composite resin is used to complete the restoration (Figure 6-11).

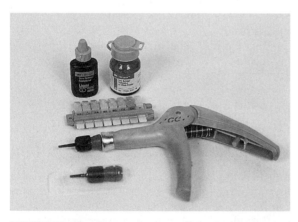

FIGURE 6-10 ■ Delivery systems for glass ionomers (regular and resin-modified). Glass ionomer may be supplied as powder and liquid in containers or in capsules. The encapsulated material is mixed in a triturator and delivered by a gun dispenser.

**Sandwich technique
in a Class II cavity preparation**

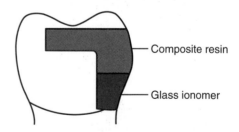

Composite resin

Glass ionomer

Glass ionomer (GI) is "sandwiched" between the tooth and composite. GI seals better on the root while composite is more wear resistant and esthetically pleasing.

FIGURE 6-11 ■ Sandwich technique with glass ionomer "sandwiched" between the tooth and another restorative material.

HYBRID (RESIN-MODIFIED) IONOMERS

To improve on the physical properties of the glass ionomers, resin mostly in the form of hydroxyethyl methacrylate (HEMA) has been added. These materials are called **hybrid (resin-modified) glass ionomers.** They have some properties of composites and many of the properties of glass ionomers. The resin makes them stronger, more polishable, and more wear resistant. The resin also protects the material from exposure to moisture once the resin has polymerized. This makes them less soluble and gives them an early strength. They release fluoride, act as a fluoride reservoir, and have a thermal expansion similar to tooth structure. The hybrid ionomers are available as light-cured materials. Some of these materials also have a chemical cure of the resin in the absence of light, as well as the acid-base reaction of the glass ionomer cement. They are used for the same applications as glass ionomers. They are popular for use in primary teeth for most classes of cavity preparation because the teeth are usually exfoliated before excessive wear can become a problem.

COMPOMERS

The **compomers** are essentially composite resins that have been modified with polyacid. The resin component contains polycarboxylic acid and methacrylates together. This provides methacrylate groups for cross-linking as with composites and carboxyl groups for the acid-base reaction as with glass ionomers. Light-activation chemicals are included, and the fillers are glasses as in composites along with some fluoride-containing glasses. The release of the fluoride, however, is not the same as for the glass ionomers, because the resin binds these fillers together as soon as the light activation starts the curing process. The fluoride release, if it occurs at all, is delayed for some months and does not seem to be at all comparable to the self-cured or light-cured glass ionomers. Likewise, there is little or no recharging of the compomer with fluoride as with glass ionomers. Some compomers have fluoride-releasing monomers added to enhance the level of fluoride release, but it is still much less than with glass ionomers.

The setting reaction in compomers occurs in two phases. Phase one is similar to that of the light-activated composite resins and forms a resin network encompassing the fillers. This causes the material to harden in the cavity preparation. Phase two reaction occurs more slowly as an acid-base reaction proceeds over a span of a month or so. These materials do not bond to tooth structure through ion exchange as glass ionomers do. Acid etching and primer or adhesive are indicated during the placement of the compomers. The bonding agents will reduce the chances of fluoride leaching from the material into the dentin. Research indicates that they have about the same cervical margin adaptation as composite resins. They can be used in most situations where a microfilled composite would be used.

Table 6-3 compares the properties of the direct esthetic restorative materials.

Indirect-Placement Esthetic Restorative Materials

Indirect-placement esthetic materials are materials that are prepared outside of the mouth on replicas of

---

TABLE 6-3

Comparison of Properties of Direct Esthetic Restorative Materials

Material	Color Match	Bonding Agent Needed	Fluoride Release	Wear Rate	Polishability	Compressive Strength	Flexural Strength
Glass ionomer	Low	No	High	High	Low	Low	Low
Hybrid ionomer	Medium	No	Medium	Medium	Low	Medium	Medium
Compomer	High	Yes	Low	Medium	High	Medium	Medium
Microfill composite	High	Yes	Low	Medium	High	Medium	Medium
Hybrid composite	High	Yes	Low	Low	Medium-high	High	High

Adapted from Craig RG, Powers JM, Wataha JC: *Dental materials: properties and manipulation,* ed 7, St Louis, 2000, Mosby.

the prepared teeth and then fitted and cemented to the teeth. They include inlays, onlays, or veneers of porcelain or composite resin; porcelain-bonded-to-metal crowns; all-ceramic crowns; and crowns with composite resin facings.

PORCELAIN

Porcelain is in the class of dental materials known as *ceramics.* Porcelain is a very hard esthetic material that has been used for tooth-colored restorations for many years. The porcelain restoration has wide acceptance because of its excellent esthetic appearance, biocompatibility, low wear rate, and stain resistance. The major drawbacks of porcelain are its potential to fracture, its wear of opposing tooth structure, and the difficulty in repolishing it after adjusting it. Although it is very strong in compression, it is brittle and weak when placed in tension (pulling). What is more important is its *transverse strength* (a combination of compressive and tensile strength), which is a better indicator of its resistance to fracture. The transverse strength of dental porcelain is in the range of 50 to 450 MPa (mega-Pascals). The traverse strength varies with the type of porcelain used. When porcelain restorations are placed in parts of the mouth where they are under heavy loading, they are at greater risk for fracture. Many patients are willing to accept the risk of porcelain fracture in order to obtain the esthetic appearance they desire.

Porcelain is manufactured from fine crystalline powders of alumina, feldspar, and silica mixed with a flux of sodium or lithium carbonate. As the powder is heated to certain critical temperatures, the powders fuse together to form a type of glass. Within this glass, leucite crystals are formed from feldspar. Leucite increases the hardness of the porcelain and its fusing temperatures. The porcelain is manufactured in a variety of colors that are produced from the addition of metal oxides to create the different colors (shades) that will match the teeth. The laboratory technician selects powders based on the shade prescription provided by the dentist. The technician mixes each powder with distilled water to form a paste and "stacks," or forms the mix to the shape of the tooth, using layers of different colors of porcelain to replicate the tooth. An absorbent material such as gauze, felt, or tissue paper removes excess water. Then the porcelain shape is placed in an oven that

Diagram of longitudinal section through (A) All-ceramic crown (B) Porcelain-bonded-to-metal crown

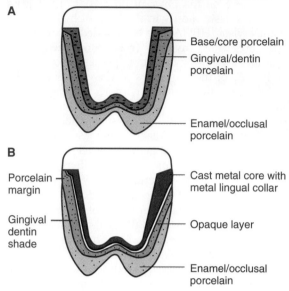

FIGURE 6-12 ■ Section through an all-ceramic crown and a porcelain-bonded-to-metal (PBM) crown showing the layers of porcelain and the metal substructure of the PBM crown.

heats the material to a temperature at which the powder crystals fuse together into a noncrystalline material. Surface defects and flaws produced during porcelain stacking and firing can lower the strength of the final restoration. Porcelains are classified according to their fusing temperature as *high fusing* (2360° to 2500° F [1288° to 1371° C]), *medium fusing* (2000° F to 2300° F [1093° to 1260° C]), and *low fusing* (1600° to 1950° F [871° to 1066° C]). Most dental restorations are made with the low-fusing porcelain. The high-fusing porcelain is used for the manufacture of denture teeth, and medium-fusing porcelain is used for the all-ceramic restorations (Figure 6-12).

It is important for the clinician to identify the junction of the tooth and the margins of any of these ceramic restorations when removing excess cement or when doing scaling or root-planing procedures. The scaler may cause chipping of the margins if the clinician is not careful. However, properly fabricated and adjusted ceramic restorations should present minimal problems for the clinician doing these procedures. If there is a significant overhang or catching of the margins, the assistant or hygienist should alert the dentist, who may correct them or prescribe replacements.

PORCELAIN-METAL RESTORATIONS

The most commonly used restorations in fixed (crown and bridge) prosthodontics are combinations of porcelain and metal. The main advantage of this combination of materials is derived from the strength given to the restoration by the bond between a metal internal core and the esthetic external porcelain covering. Low-fusing porcelain is used for the bonding of porcelain to metal, which occurs through an oxide on the metal surface. These restorations are referred to as porcelain-fused-to-metal (PFM) or porcelain-bonded-to-metal (PBM) restorations. The metals that are used as the core for the PBM/PFM crowns are specially made so that an oxide layer will be formed as the metal is heated during bonding with the porcelain. They are classified as high noble (precious), noble (semiprecious), or base (nonprecious) metal alloys based on the presence and amount of gold, palladium, and other valuable metals (see Chapter 8). The metal in the area where the porcelain is to be bonded is usually relatively thin, approximately 0.3 to 0.5 mm thick. Before the prescribed colors of porcelain are placed on the metal core, an opaque coating of porcelain is placed over the metal to keep the dark color of the metal oxides from showing through the more translucent porcelain. The porcelain is heated (or fired) in an oven at temperatures that cause the porcelain crystals to fuse together (called *sintering*). A layer of dentin-colored porcelain is placed in the cervical half of the restoration and fired. Then an incisal porcelain is added and fired followed by a thin layer of glazing porcelain that produces a glassy smooth surface. The incisal porcelain is more translucent than the dentin porcelain so that it can take on the appearance of enamel (see Figure 6-12). Occasionally, special porcelain stains are used on the surface to help in matching the natural tooth color and characteristics such as discolorations or fine crack lines in enamel.

Most porcelain failures are from problems related to the chemical bond between the porcelain and the metal oxides. The oxide layer may be too thick or inadequate in quantity and quality, leading to the formation of cracks at or near the interface of the porcelain and metal. These cracks propagate (spread) over time as the porcelain is loaded by chewing or bruxing, and eventually the porcelain fractures.

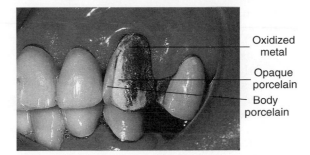

FIGURE 6-13 ■ Porcelain failure with PBM crown. The metal is exposed, as well as a portion of the opaque layer of porcelain used to prevent metal from showing through the more translucent outer layers of porcelain.

However, the coefficient of thermal expansion of the porcelain and the metal must be compatible. The best arrangement is for the porcelain to have slightly less thermal expansion than the metal. This will keep it from cracking at the metal-porcelain interface and reduce the chance of failure (Figure 6-13). When porcelain failures do occur, there are materials that can be used to repair the PBM restorations, but they are not as good as the original bonded porcelain (see Chapter 5). The alternative is to do expensive replacements of the entire crown or bridge.

The porcelain surface, once it has been fused under temperature, is very hard and smooth. When porcelain or PBM restorations are delivered, the proximal contacts or occlusal surfaces often must be adjusted. These restorations could be returned to the laboratory to be reglazed (refired at porcelain fusing temperatures to form a glassy surface) before cementing. Because this is seldom practical, a variety of abrasives have been developed for polishing the porcelain surface after adjustment (see Chapter 9).

ALL-CERAMIC RESTORATIONS

All-ceramic restorations have been available for almost 100 years. They were made with the low-fusing "stacked" porcelains and used in areas of the mouth that demanded esthetic treatment, yet were not under high stress. When used for crowns they were called *porcelain jackets* and were used mainly on maxillary incisors. New ceramic materials have been developed that are stronger and, when used in conjunction with resin bonding to tooth structure, have found wider application, including use in the posterior region of the mouth. However, the fracture rate for all-ceramic crowns in the posterior part of the mouth is still higher than for PBM crowns. The newer low-fusing porcelains are less abrasive to opposing tooth structure and can be repolished easier after adjustments. There are three techniques to form the newer all-ceramic crowns: (1) Molten ceramic material is injected into a mold and pressed over a die of the preparation, and then surface coloration (called *stain*) is added to the porcelain to develop the proper shade. (2) A castable ceramic is cast into a mold developed from a wax pattern that was burned out in an oven (lost wax technique as for gold crowns is discussed in Chapter 15), and then heat-treated in an oven. (3) A strong core porcelain acts as the foundation and conventional "stacked" porcelains are added to enhance the esthetics.

All-ceramic crowns have a more lifelike appearance (sometimes called *vitality*) than porcelain-bonded-to-metal crowns, because they do not have an opaque layer to hide metal. Porcelains appear vital (similar to natural teeth) because they are fluorescent. That is, they emit light in the visible wave spectrum when ultraviolet light hits them. They are also opalescent because they take on a bluish tinge when light reflects off them and an orange-yellow tinge when light passes through them.

COMPUTER-AIDED DESIGN/COMPUTER-AIDED MANUFACTURE (CAD/CAM) PORCELAIN RESTORATIONS

Advances in technology have made it possible for porcelain restorations (usually inlays, onlays, and veneers) to be made in the office or the laboratory starting with a solid block of ceramic material. An optical scanner is used to capture the image of the tooth preparation directly from the tooth or from a replica (die) of the tooth and store it in a computer. The restoration is fabricated by means of a milling machine that shapes the ceramic block into the restoration as instructed by the computer program. The advantage of this type of porcelain restoration is that it can be fabricated in hours and delivered the same day (the traditional laboratory "fired" method takes several days). The disadvantage is that these restorations do not fit as precisely and thus have margins that have large resin cement lines that can potentially wear down, leak, and irritate gingival tissues. As the technology improves, higher-quality restorations and a greater variety of restorations will likely become available.

VENEERS

Veneers are thin layers of esthetic materials that are bonded to the fronts of teeth, mostly anteriors and premolars, to lighten the color of teeth, to cover stains or defects, to close diastemas, or to reshape crooked teeth so that they look as though they are in proper alignment. Indirect porcelain veneers are made in the laboratory of traditional or newer low-fusing porcelains. They are bonded at a subsequent appointment with resin cements (Figure 6-14).

INDIRECT COMPOSITES

In addition to their use for direct application to teeth for restorations or veneers, composites can also be used indirectly. That is, a composite restoration is made on a replica (die) of an inlay, onlay, or veneer preparation. It is tried in the mouth, adjusted, and bonded into place with a resin cement and bonding agent. Indirect materials were developed to try to eliminate the problems associated with polymerization shrinkage, such as marginal leakage, posttreatment sensitivity, and recurrent caries, and to reduce the wear seen with direct composites.

Laboratory-Processed Composites An impression of the preparation, opposing cast, and bite registration and a prescription with the proper shade are sent to the laboratory for construction of the restoration. There are several advantages to having the restoration constructed in the laboratory. The technician can process the composite material under heat and pressure. This creates a restoration that is denser, polymerizes more completely, and is tougher. The polymerization shrinkage occurs outside of the mouth, and then the restoration is cemented with a thin layer of resin cement. The shrinkage from the thin layer of resin cement is much less than that which would have occurred with a composite that is cured in the tooth. Therefore there is less stress created internally on the composite and the walls of the cavity preparation. Microleakage should be reduced. Three different types of materials can be used:

1. Conventional composites
2. Fiber-reinforced composite that contain a fiber mesh composed of carbon Kevlar (similar to the material used in bullet-proof vests), glass fibers, or polyethylene for improved strength
3. Particle-reinforced composite that is heavily filled (70% to 80% by weight) with particles of submi-

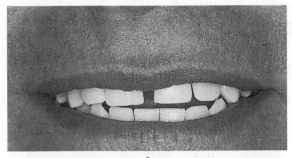

A

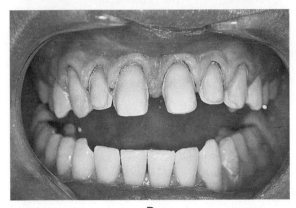

B

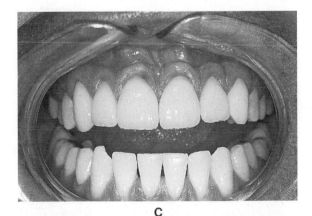

C

FIGURE 6-14 ■ Placement of porcelain veneers to correct large diastema. (Refer also to Color Plate 2 at the beginning of the book.) **A,** Pretreatment photograph showing large midline diastema. **B,** Maxillary anterior teeth prepared for veneers. Retraction cord is in place. **C,** After cementation of veneers with a resin cement.

(Courtesy Dr. Cary Behle and Dentsply Corp.)

cron-size ceramic filler for improved wear, polishability, and strength

Indirect Chairside Technique   An impression is made of the prepared tooth with alginate. Immediately, a fast-setting die stone or a polyvinyl siloxane die material is injected into the impression. The resulting die is used to make the restoration with light-cured composite material at the chairside. The composite restoration is seated into the preparation and adjusted. It is removed from the mouth and polished on the die. Then it is cemented with a resin cement in the same manner as the laboratory-processed composite inlays (Figure 6-15).

CLINICAL TIP   Ultrasonic scalers, if improperly applied, can chip and craze margins of esthetic materials. Acidulated fluorides can etch porcelain surfaces.

Shade Taking

HUE, CHROMA, AND VALUE

When teeth are viewed for shade taking, three characteristics should be taken into consideration: hue, chroma, and value. *Hue* is the color of the tooth and may include mixtures of colors, such as yellow-brown. *Chroma* is the amount or intensity of color present; for example, a bold yellow has more chroma than a pastel yellow. *Value* is the amount of lightness or darkness of the tooth (some describe it as the grayness of the tooth). A tooth with low value is darker and one with high value is brighter.

INVOLVING THE DENTAL ASSISTANT AND PATIENT

The dentist often relies on the chairside assistant to help obtain a good color match for restorations with porcelain or composite. Three pairs of eyes (doctor, assistant, and patient) are usually better than one. Involving the patients in shade taking helps determine if their expectations can be met. Matching shades can be very difficult, because many teeth do not match the standard shade guides. In general, the shade should be taken before preparation of the tooth and before a rubber dam is placed. The color of the rubber dam can interfere with accurate matching, and teeth dry out and become lighter when under the dam or if isolated with cotton rolls. For best shade matching the teeth should be clean, free of stain, and moist.

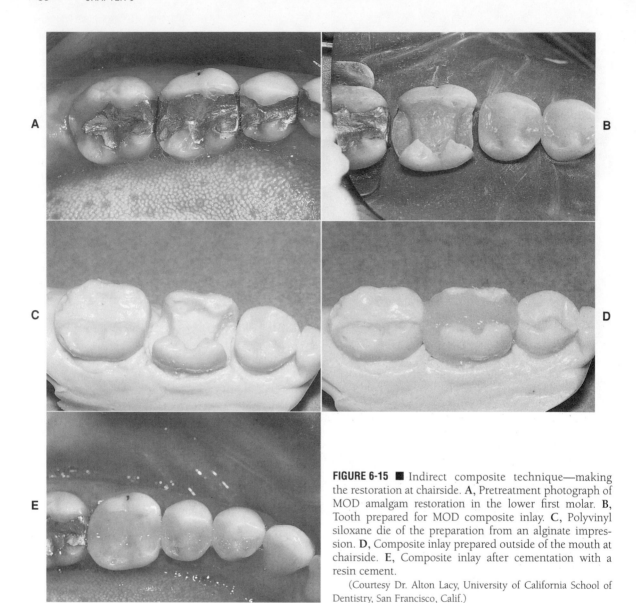

FIGURE 6-15 ■ Indirect composite technique—making the restoration at chairside. **A,** Pretreatment photograph of MOD amalgam restoration in the lower first molar. **B,** Tooth prepared for MOD composite inlay. **C,** Polyvinyl siloxane die of the preparation from an alginate impression. **D,** Composite inlay prepared outside of the mouth at chairside. **E,** Composite inlay after cementation with a resin cement.

(Courtesy Dr. Alton Lacy, University of California School of Dentistry, San Francisco, Calif.)

CLINICAL TIP A good use of time is to take the shade after the injection of local anesthetic while you are waiting for the patient to get numb.

LIGHTING FOR SHADE TAKING

The lighting in which the shade is viewed is very important. Shade matching should be done in two different types of light, because the perception of shade may vary in different lights, a phenomenon called *metamerism*. Most dental offices have fluorescent or incandescent lights (or both). Fluorescent lights emit more blue light, and incandescent lights emit more yellow light. Some dentists install color-corrected light bulbs to help in shade taking. A natural north light is considered a good light for shade taking. However, early morning and late after-

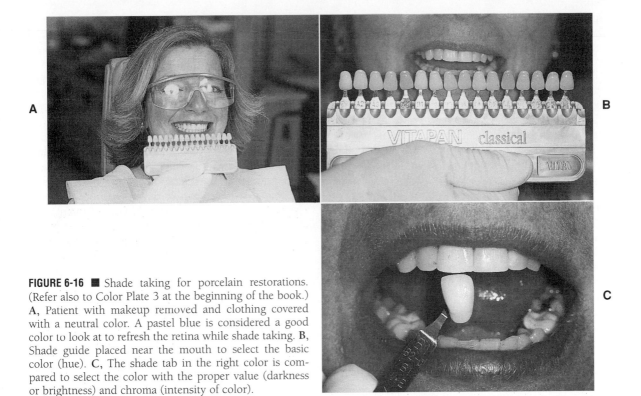

FIGURE 6-16 ■ Shade taking for porcelain restorations. (Refer also to Color Plate 3 at the beginning of the book.) **A,** Patient with makeup removed and clothing covered with a neutral color. A pastel blue is considered a good color to look at to refresh the retina while shade taking. **B,** Shade guide placed near the mouth to select the basic color (hue). **C,** The shade tab in the right color is compared to select the color with the proper value (darkness or brightness) and chroma (intensity of color).

noon natural light contains more yellow and orange light and less green and blue. If possible, the shade should also be taken in the type of lighting that the patient is in most often. The bright light from the dental unit will tend to increase the perceived brightness of the shade and decrease the color intensity.

MATCHING THE SHADE

A neutral background is important so that the colors do not distract the eye and alter the perceived shade. A pastel-blue patient bib is a good color for shade taking. Female patients should be requested to remove lipstick and colorful makeup because these colors may influence the shade. Colorful clothes should be covered. The shade guide is placed near the patient's teeth and the basic color (hue) is chosen. If the color intensity is low it may be more difficult to determine the color. In this case the cervical area of a tooth with a more intense color, such as a maxillary canine, should be used to help pick the initial color. Next, shade tabs from that color

should be moistened and individually held adjacent to the teeth to be matched. The patient, dentist, and assistant should view the tabs and rank them as to the closest match for color intensity (chroma) and lightness or darkness (value). It is often necessary to take separate shades for the cervical portion of the tooth, for the occlusal surfaces of posterior teeth, and for the incisals of anterior teeth (Figure 6-16).

CHARACTERIZING THE SHADE

In addition to the shade, the surface luster and texture should be noted. As a person ages, the surface of the teeth gets smoother from wear and reflects light differently than highly textured teeth. Textured teeth tend to scatter light. *Luster* is the degree to which the surface appears shiny and reflects light. The laboratory technician can add surface glazes to porcelain to create a shiny surface and can add texture to scatter light. The amount of translucency of the enamel and its location (e.g., incisal edge) should be communicated to the laboratory also. Teeth may have opaque white spots or lines, stained cracks, wear facets, and other characteristics that should be conveyed to the laboratory if the patient is trying to match existing teeth (this process is called *characterization*). Often it is helpful to the technician if a photograph of the teeth is included. If photography is used, the shade tab should be included in the picture, because some photographs will be a little more red or blue than the actual color. The bright operatory light should not be used to illuminate the patient's mouth. The shade tab should be in the same plane as the tooth to be matched so that it will be in the same focus as the teeth. That is, it should not be in front of the teeth or outside of the mouth and will have the same illumination as the teeth when flash photography is used. Occasionally, some teeth are not a close match to the shade tabs and require that the technician see the teeth so that he or she can custom blend different shades of porcelain to match the color. The patient may be sent to the laboratory, or the technician may come to the operatory for this "custom" shade taking.

SUMMARY

A wide variety of tooth-colored esthetic materials are available to the dental team to use to restore a patient's dentition. Patients demand high-quality restorations with a close match to their existing teeth, or in some cases they demand restorations that produce a lighter, youthful smile. It is important that all members of the dental team understand the handling characteristics, physical properties, and potential shortcomings of these materials. Before working in the patient's mouth it is wise to review the dental charting section of the patient's record or perform a brief oral inspection to detect the presence of esthetic restorations. Drying the teeth with the air syringe can help reveal some of the materials because they may have a different luster than the enamel or margins may be more readily visible once the saliva has been removed. The selection and use of proper polishing and scaling devices is an important consideration for the hygienist and the chairside assistant when working around these restorations. Ultrasonic scalers have the potential to chip or craze the margins of all-ceramic or composite restorations. When applying topical fluoride, it is important to keep in mind that the surfaces of these esthetic restorations can be affected by the use of acidulated fluoride solutions and gels. The use of these products can dull the surface of the restoration and change the esthetic effect of the original restoration, making for an unhappy patient. Neutral sodium fluoride products can be use as an alternative. Certain abrasives used for coronal polishing can also adversely affect the surface luster of composites and porcelain. The radiographic appearance may be different with each of the various esthetic restorative materials. As new esthetic materials are adopted in the practice, it is important to become familiar with their handling characteristics, physical properties, uses, and precautions.

CHAPTER REVIEW

Select the one correct response for each of the following multiple-choice questions:

1. **In order for a composite to have greater wear resistance, it needs**
   a. To have larger filler particles
   b. A higher polish
   c. To have a higher filler content
   d. To be light cured

2. **Composite resins are often classified according to their**
   a. Strength
   b. Polishability
   c. Resin content
   d. Filler particle size

3. **The shortcomings of flowable composites as compared with hybrid composites include all of the following EXCEPT one. Which one is this EXCEPTION?**
   a. They are weaker.
   b. They wear faster.
   c. They shrink more when polymerized.
   d. They are more difficult to polish.

4. **The purpose of a silane coupling agent for composite resins is**
   a. To improve the bond between the filler particles and the resin matrix
   b. To help the composite retain the color
   c. To reduce the oxygen-inhibited layer
   d. To help the various layer stick together

5. **The curing light requires repair**
   a. If it causes a slower set of a dark-color composite
   b. If it has not been tested
   c. If a 2-mm thick piece of composite does not cure through the bottom at the recommended exposure time
   d. If the light appears blue

6. **The polymerization shrinkage of a composite**
   a. Is cause for alarm
   b. Is greater than 10% of the volume
   c. Can be minimized by placing and curing a series of small increments
   d. Has no effect on the final restoration

7. **All composite restorative materials appear the same on radiographs of the teeth.**
   a. True
   b. False

8. **One of the advantages of glass ionomer is**
   a. The ability to finish it immediately
   b. That it has a higher strength than composite because of the glass fillers
   c. That because it contains water, it does not need to have a dry field for insertion into a cavity
   d. That it has been shown to release fluoride

9. **Hybrid (resin-modified) glass ionomers have all of the following advantages over conventional glass ionomers EXCEPT one. Which one is this EXCEPTION?**
   a. Stronger
   b. Less sensitive to moisture when set
   c. Can be finished the same appointment
   d. Contain quartz fillers like some composites

10. **Compomer restorative materials**
    a. Release as much fluoride as glass ionomer materials
    b. Are only self-cure resins
    c. Are closer to composite resins in their makeup than to glass ionomers
    d. Are like glass ionomers in that they do not require a separate bonding agent

11. **Porcelain restorations have**
    a. Great stain resistance
    b. Low wear resistance
    c. No disadvantages
    d. Easy reparability

12. **Porcelain bonds to metal by which one of the following mechanisms?**
    a. Micromechanical retention such as resin to etched enamel
    b. Penetrates the surface of the metal
    c. Fuses to oxides on the surface of the metal
    d. Shrinks when it is fired and locks itself onto the metal

13. **The main advantage of all-ceramic crowns over porcelain-bonded-to-metal crowns is**
    a. Their superior esthetics
    b. Their strength
    c. Their ease of cementation
    d. The ease of taking shades

CASE-BASED DISCUSSION TOPICS

◉ A 24-year-old aspiring actress comes to the dental office seeking replacement of occlusal amalgams in her mandibular molars, because they are visible when she talks and sings. She does not grind her teeth. *From among the esthetic materials discussed in this chapter, which ones have properties that would make them suitable for use in this situation? Which ones are more suitable for anterior class III cavities?*

◉ A 75-year-old retired plumber who is taking medication to control his blood pressure is found on examination to have a dry mouth and numerous root caries. *Which types of direct-placement esthetic materials discussed in this chapter would have the greatest advantage for restoring root caries? Why? How do these materials bond to tooth structure?*

◉ A 43-year-old nurse comes to the office complaining of tooth sensitivity to air, cold, and sweets. Examination reveals several deep class V toothbrush abrasion lesions. No dental caries is present. *Considering that resistance to wear is an important physical property, are flowable composites suitable materials? Why or why not? What other materials could be used successfully in this situation?*

◉ A 57-year-old secretary comes to the dental office for a periodic examination and prophylaxis. She has maxillary anterior composite veneers and all-ceramic crowns on her mandibular incisors. *Describe the factors that might contribute to fracture of the porcelain restorations. What must the dental hygienist and dental assistant be concerned about when treating patients who have esthetic composite and porcelain restorations present in their mouths?*

◉ An active 80-year-old woman comes to the dental office for preparation of her maxillary anterior and premolar teeth for porcelain veneers. She wants to lighten her teeth but wants to keep the same color (hue). She is wearing brightly colored clothing and makeup. *What steps can the dental assistant or hygienist perform to help in the initial shade taking? Under what lighting conditions should the shade be taken?*

REFERENCES

Albers HF: Composite classification, resin bonding, polymer chemistry. In *Tooth-colored restoratives,* ed 8, Santa Rosa, CA, 1996, Alto Books.

Baum L, Phillips R, Lund M: The metal-ceramic restoration. In *Textbook of operative dentistry,* ed 3, Philadelphia, 1995, WB Saunders.

Bird D, Robinson D: Restorative materials and dental cements, restorative and cosmetic dentistry. In *Torres and Ehrlich modern dental assisting,* ed 6, Philadelphia, 1996, WB Saunders.

Craig RG, Powers JM, Wataha JC: Direct esthetic restorative materials and dental porcelain. In *Dental materials: properties and manipulation,* ed 7, Philadelphia, 2000, Mosby.

Donly KJ, Segura A, Weffel JS: Evaluating the effects of fluoride-releasing dental materials, *J Am Dent Assoc* 130:819, 1999.

Gladwin M, Bagby M: Direct polymeric restorative materials. In *Clinical aspects of dental materials,* Philadelphia, 2000, Lippincott Williams & Wilkins.

Marshall GW, Marshall SJ, Bane SC: Restorative dental materials: scanning electron microscopy and x-ray microanalysis, *Scanning Microscopy* 2(4):2007, 1998.

Mount GJ, Hume WR: Glass-ionomer materials, composite resins, and rigid materials used in tooth restoration. In *Preservation and restoration of tooth structure,* Philadelphia, 1998, Mosby.

Neisler L, Kamins D: Prospectives from the dental laboratory: shade tab photography. In *Contemporary esthetics and restorative practice,* Jamesburg, NJ, Sept 1999, Dental Learning Systems.

Phillips RW, Moore KB: Dental ceramics. In *Elements of dental materials for dental hygienists and dental assistants,* ed 5, Philadelphia, 1994, WB Saunders.

Rosenstiel SF, Land MF, Fujimoto J: Color science and shade selection. In *Contemporary fixed prosthodontics,* Philadelphia, 1988, Mosby.

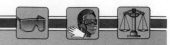

PROCEDURE 6-1 (see p. 324 for competency sheet)

Placement of Class II Composite Resin Restoration

EQUIPMENT/SUPPLIES (Figure 6-17)

- Rubber dam setup
- Curing light and light shield
- Composite placement instruments
- Light-cured hybrid composite resin
- Bonding agent and finishing glaze
- Mixing wells or Dappen dish
- Finishing burs, diamonds, disks
- Articulating paper in paper forceps
- Local and topical anesthesia setup
- High-volume evacuator tip
- High- and low-speed handpieces
- Shade guide
- Etchant and applicator
- Matrix system and wedges
- Polishing points, cups, paste

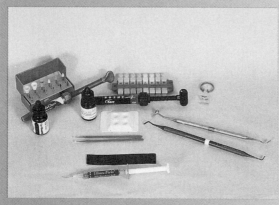

FIGURE 6-17

PROCEDURE STEPS

1 Apply topical anesthetic. Local anesthetic is administered.

2 Take composite shade. Hold shade guide close to the patient's mouth and select two or three shade tabs that are close to the patient's tooth color. Moisten and check each tab individually against the tooth under room light (and natural light, if possible) (Figure 6-18). Verify shade by taking a small amount of

composite in the closest shade and light-curing it on the tooth for 20 seconds.

NOTE: Shade is taken before applying the rubber dam, because the color of the dam might interfere with taking an accurate shade and the teeth might dry out under the dam and appear lighter. Lipstick should be removed, and brightly colored clothing should be covered with a pale blue or gray patient bib to prevent the colors from influencing the perceived shade.

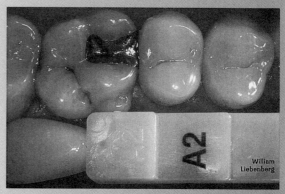

FIGURE 6-18
(Courtesy Dr. William Liebenberg)

3 Apply the rubber dam.

NOTE: Cotton roll isolation can be used, but rubber dam provides a more reliable isolation. Moisture from the breath can affect the bond adversely.

4 Rinse and dry cavity prepared by dentist.

5 Apply sectional matrix, wedge, and a spring ring or stick compound (Figure 6-19).

NOTE: A Tofflemire matrix can be used, but it is much more difficult to obtain a tight contact when both mesial and distal interproximal spaces have matrix band in them at the same time. The wedge helps close the matrix band at the gingival margin to prevent overhang of composite, and it helps separate the teeth to make up for the thickness of the matrix band so that firm contact with the adjacent tooth can be established. The spring ring helps adapt the matrix against the facial and lingual surfaces of the tooth and helps separate the teeth slightly. Stick compound could be used instead to hold the band against the facial and lingual surfaces, but it does not have the benefit of separation of the teeth.

Continued on following page

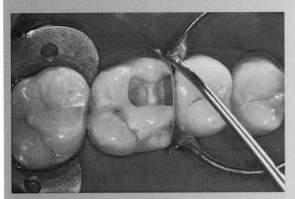

FIGURE 6-19
(Courtesy Dr. William Liebenberg)

6 Apply etchant to enamel first for 10 to 20 seconds, and then apply it to dentin for 10 seconds (Figure 6-20).

NOTE: Etching dentin for more than 10 seconds will overetch it and contribute to a weaker bond strength and postoperative sensitivity by opening the tubules excessively.

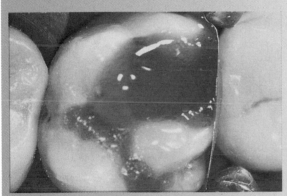

FIGURE 6-20
(Courtesy Dr. William Liebenberg)

7 Rinse thoroughly and dry lightly so that the dentin remains slightly moist (glistening but no pooling of water).

NOTE: Drying the dentin will cause collapse of the collagen fibrils and interference with penetration of the dentin primer into the tubules and etched dentin surface (see Chapter 5).

8 Apply dentin primer/bonding agent with a brush applicator as directed by the manufacturer (dentist's choice of one- or two-bottle materials) and thin with a gentle stream of air (Figure 6-21).

NOTE: See Chapter 5 for one-bottle and two-bottle dentin primers and bonding agents. When the dentin primer and bonding agent are applied in separate steps, the dentin primer is usually light-cured for 10 to 20 seconds before placement of the bonding resin. Some dentists prefer to use a base or liner on the dentin before acid etching.

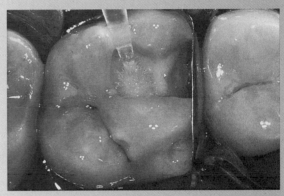

FIGURE 6-21
(Courtesy Dr. William Liebenberg)

9 Dry gently and light-cure for 20 seconds.

NOTE: Drying at this step removes water and volatile solvents from the resin.

10 Apply composite resin in small increments starting with the proximal box (Figure 6-22). Each increment should be no more that 2 mm thick and light-cured for 20 to 40 seconds.

NOTE: Small increments are used to minimize the effects of polymerization shrinkage. Dark or opaque shades are more difficult for the light to penetrate and require longer curing times. Newer curing lights may have an initial low setting that ramps up to a high intensity to minimize shrinkage and stress within the material. Some very high intensity curing lights require less curing time. Manufacturer's recommendations should be followed.

Continued on following page

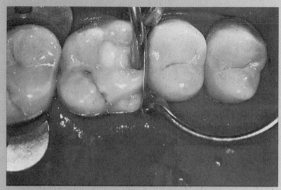

FIGURE 6-22
(Courtesy Dr. William Liebenberg)

11 Remove spring ring, wedge, and matrix band after the cavity preparation is slightly overfilled with composite and cured thoroughly. Contour occlusal surface and remove excess material with finishing diamonds and burs. Disks and interproximal finishing strips are used on the proximal surfaces (Figure 6-23).

NOTE: The composite in the proximal box should be cured again from the facial and lingual after removal of the matrix and wedge because these materials may have partially blocked light transmission to the floor of the box, causing an incomplete cure of the composite.

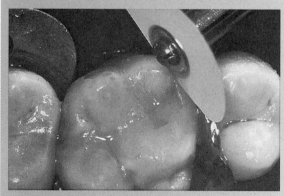

FIGURE 6-23
(Courtesy Dr. William Liebenberg)

12 Remove rubber dam. Check occlusal contacts with articulating paper and adjust.

NOTE: A high restoration can cause a sore tooth by stressing the periodontal ligament or a tooth that is temperature sensitive.

13 Polish surfaces with polishing points and cups at low speed. A polishing paste can be used to produce a highly polished surface (Figure 6-24).

NOTE: Some dentists prefer to apply a finishing glaze to the composite. A finishing glaze is an unfilled resin that bonds to the composite resin. Its purpose is to reseal the margins if polymerization shrinkage has caused composite to pull away from the enamel margin, and it fills in any small voids in the surface that contribute to wear and staining. To use the glaze the tooth is isolated with cotton rolls, and the composite and adjacent enamel are etched for 10 seconds, rinsed, and dried. A brush is used to apply a very thin layer so as not to interfere with the occlusion. It is light cured for 20 seconds.

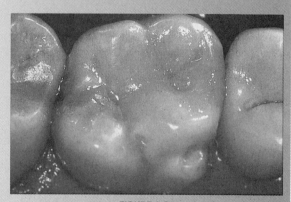

FIGURE 6-24
(Courtesy Dr. William Liebenberg)

PREVENTIVE AND BLEACHING MATERIALS

CHAPTER OUTLINE

Fluoride
Topical versus systemic effects
Protection against erosion
Bacteria inhibition
Fluoride and antibacterial rinses for
    control of dental caries
Methods of delivery
Safety

Pit and Fissure Sealants
Purpose
Indications
Composition
Working time
Color and wear
Placement
Effectiveness

Desensitizing Agents
Causes of tooth sensitivity
Function
Categories and components

Mouth Guards and Splints
Sports mouth guards
Night guards (bruxism mouth guards)
Maintenance

Teeth Bleaching
How bleaching works
Types of stains
In-office bleaching
Home bleaching
Over-the-counter products
Role of the dental assistant or hygienist
Potential side effects
Restorative considerations
Contraindications
Re-treatment

Summary

Chapter Review

Case-Based Discussion Topics

References

Procedures
Applying topical fluoride
Applying dental sealants
In-office bleaching
Clinical procedures for home bleaching
Fabrication of custom bleaching trays
Fabrication of a sports mouth protector

OBJECTIVES

On completion of this chapter the student will be able to:

1. Describe the use of fluoride in prevention.
2. Explain how fluoride protects teeth from caries.
3. Discuss the various methods for fluoride delivery.
4. Explain the benefit of using an antibacterial rinse in conjunction with fluoride.
5. Describe the antibacterial effects of chlorhexidine.
6. Apply topical fluoride gel correctly.
7. Discuss the use of sealants for prevention of pit and fissure caries.
8. Describe the composition of sealants.
9. Recite the steps for applying sealants.
10. Apply pit and fissure sealants correctly.
11. Recite causes for tooth sensitivity.

12. List the various materials used for treating sensitive teeth.
13. Explain how desensitizing agents work.
14. Describe the uses of mouth guards.
15. List the materials for the fabrication of mouth guards.
16. Fabricate a sports mouth guard.
17. Describe the methods used to bleach teeth.
18. Discuss the similarities and differences among the materials used to bleach teeth.
19. Explain the differences between professionally supervised home bleaching and over-the-counter systems.
20. Apply high-strength bleach on prepared teeth.
21. Fabricate custom trays for home bleaching.

KEY TERMS

Prevention/preventive aids—Chemicals, devices, or procedures that reduce or eliminate disease or tooth destruction in the oral cavity.

Fluoride—Naturally occurring chemical that helps protect tooth structure from dental caries.

Fluorosis—Enamel abnormality caused by consumption of excessive levels of fluoride.

Demineralization—Action that removes mineral from the tooth, usually caused by acids.

Dental caries—A process whereby bacteria in plaque metabolize carbohydrates and produce acids that remove mineral from teeth and permit bacteria to invade.

Fluorapatite—Tooth mineral that results when fluoride is incorporated into the tooth.

Cariogenic—Substances or microorganisms that promote dental caries.

Erosion—Loss of tooth mineral caused by acids not from bacterial metabolism.

Antibacterial mouth rinse—Liquid used to rinse the oral cavity to reduce mouth odor, prevent dental caries, or suppress bacteria associated with periodontal disease.

Substantivity—Property of a material to have a prolonged therapeutic effect after its initial use.

Over-the-counter (OTC)—Available in retail or drug stores without a doctor's prescription.

Sealant—A protective resin that is bonded to enamel to protect pits and fissures from dental caries.

Desensitizing agent—A chemical that seals open dentinal tubules in order to reduce tooth sensitivity to air, sweets, and temperature changes.

Mouth guard—A hard or pliable resin that protects teeth from trauma during sports activities or from teeth grinding.

Custom-made—Made specifically to fit one individual.

Bleaching—A cosmetic process that uses chemicals to remove discolorations from teeth or to lighten them.

Extrinsic stains—Stains occurring on the tooth surface.

Intrinsic stains—Stains that are incorporated into the tooth structure, usually during the tooth's development.

*Patients often ask dental assistants and hygienists about the prescription or over-the-counter (nonprescription) agents the dentist has recommended for the prevention of tooth decay and periodontal disease and for tooth whitening. In addition, the dental assistant or hygienist is often asked by the dentist to dispense, apply, or fabricate devices to deliver these **prevention/preventive aids**. Therefore it is essential that all members of the dental team are familiar with the mechanism of action and application of these products. This chapter presents information on fluorides, antibacterial mouth rinses, sealants, desensitizing agents, mouth guards, and tooth bleaching materials.*

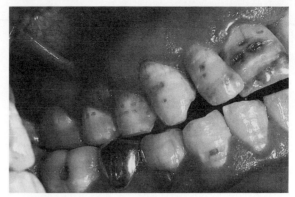

FIGURE 7-1 ■ Fluorosis. Note enamel defects (mottling) and discolorations.

(Courtesy Dr. Steve Eakle, University of California, San Francisco.)

Fluoride

Fluoride is a naturally occurring mineral found in many forms in the modern world. It may be found in well water, in food that has absorbed fluoride from the soil, and as an additive in many dental products that we buy over the counter or that are prescribed by dentists and physicians. The accepted optimal level of fluoride in the drinking water is in the range of 0.7 to 1.0 parts per million (ppm). Consumption of excess fluoride during formation of the teeth may lead to a condition known as **fluorosis.** Severe fluorosis can cause brown staining and pitting of the enamel surface, called *mottled enamel* (Figure 7-1). Mild or moderate fluorosis may create cosmetic concerns for some people by causing opaque white spots or bands on the teeth. Fluorosis is usually caused by the concentration of fluoride in the water being too high, but it may also be caused by excess fluoride toothpaste swallowed by the child or by other iatrogenic (doctor-induced) factors such as overly prescribed fluoride drops. Some cultures consume beverages such as tea that are high in fluoride and that, when consumed during tooth development along with other natural or supplemented fluorides, can contribute to fluorosis.

TOPICAL VERSUS SYSTEMIC EFFECTS

The enamel and dentin of the tooth are composed of tiny mineral crystals (hydroxyapatite) within a protein/lipid matrix. Tiny gaps or pores between these millions of crystals are filled with protein,

lipid, and water. It is in these matrix gaps that small molecules such as lactic acid and ions such as hydrogen, calcium, and phosphate are allowed to pass. There is a constant interchange of mineral ions between the tooth surface and the saliva. Usually, the minerals entering the surface balance the minerals coming out of the tooth surface. The tooth crystals are not pure hydroxyapatite but contain carbonate, which makes them much more soluble in acid. When bacteria in the plaque on the tooth surface metabolize cooked starches or sugars, they produce acids. The acids remove more mineral (**demineralization**) than the amount of mineral coming into the tooth from the saliva. When these acid attacks are repeated over time, the surface becomes more porous and allows bacteria to enter the tooth. This is the start of the caries process.

For years it has been thought that fluoride incorporated into the teeth at the time of development was the main reason for the lowering of the **dental caries** (tooth decay) rates seen in areas of water fluoridation. However, work by Featherstone and others (1990) has shown that fluoride's greatest anti-caries benefit is gained from topical application. Research has shown that the solubility of the tooth mineral with fluoride incorporated at the time of development is not much different than that formed without systemic fluoride and is insufficient to have a measurable effect on its acid solubility. However, fluoride in the saliva surrounding the tooth is incorporated into the surface of enamel crystals during **remineralization** (replacing minerals lost from the tooth surface) to form a surface veneer containing **fluorapatite** with a much lower solubility than the original carbonated tooth mineral. The pH (a measure of acidity) at which tooth mineral dissolves is 5.5 (7.0 is neutral pH—neither acid nor base). However, when the mineral is converted to fluorapatite, the pH at which it dissolves is lowered to 4.5 (a lower number indicates that it is more acidic; e.g., stomach acid has a pH of less than 1.0). Therefore fluoride makes it more difficult for the acids produced by **cariogenic** (decay-causing) bacteria in plaque to demineralize tooth structure and cause dental caries. There is evidence that fluoride from drinking water, toothpastes, mouth rinses, and some foods remains in the saliva for several hours and has a prolonged topical effect.

PROTECTION AGAINST EROSION

Highly acidic foods and beverages such as citrus fruits, sodas, and wine can contribute to loss of tooth mineral that is called **erosion** (Figure 7-2). Erosion differs from caries in that bacteria are not involved and most of the mineral loss is at the surface. It is important to maintain a well-balanced diet to minimize excess acidic foods. Some medical conditions also cause erosion of the teeth by causing stomach acid to enter the mouth. Examples are acid reflux (burping up stomach acid) and bulimia (chronic forced vomiting to control weight gain after binge

eating). By making the tooth structure less soluble in acids, fluoride provides some degree of protection against erosion.

BACTERIA INHIBITION

Fluoride interferes with the essential enzyme activity of the bacteria. Although the fluoride ion has been shown not to cross the bacterial cell wall, it can travel through it in the form of hydrofluoric acid (HF). As the decay-causing bacteria produce acids during the metabolism of sugars and cooked starch, some of the fluoride present in the plaque fluid combines with the hydrogen ion of the acid to become HF and rapidly diffuses into the cell. Once in the alkaline cytoplasm of the cell, the HF separates into the fluoride ion and the hydrogen ion again. These ions disrupt the enzyme activities essential to the functioning of the bacteria and cause their death.

FLUORIDE AND ANTIBACTERIAL RINSES FOR CONTROL OF DENTAL CARIES

Studies have shown that fluoride alone is not as effective in managing dental caries as when it is used in conjunction with an **antibacterial mouth rinse.** Therapeutic mouth rinses help suppress bacteria associated with dental caries but are not meant to be substitutes for daily mechanical plaque removal.

Chlorhexidine gluconate is a bis-bisguanide that is effective against a broad spectrum of microorganisms. In several European countries it is used at a concentration of 0.2%, but in the United States the maximum concentration allowed by the Food and Drug Administration (FDA) is 0.12%. It is a prescription mouth rinse that is available commercially through several companies. The most common trade names are Peridex, Periogard, and Oris CHX. It is one of the most effective agents for reduction of plaque (55%) and gingivitis (45%). Patients typically rinse with it for 30 to 60 seconds twice a day after brushing and flossing. It is usually not used continuously because the bacteria may build up resistance to it. It is often used for a 2- or 3-week period, then not used for 2 months before repeating the sequence.

Chlorhexidine kills bacteria by binding strongly to the bacterial cell membrane, causing it to leak and lose its intracellular components. It binds very strongly on many sites in the oral cavity, including

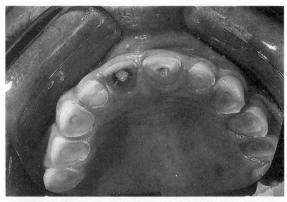

FIGURE 7-2 ■ Erosion from stomach acid. Note severe loss of enamel and dentin from the teeth due to chronic vomiting.

(Courtesy Dr. Steve Eakle, University of California, San Francisco.)

the mucous membranes and plaque, and is released slowly, giving it a prolonged effect (called **substantivity**). The antibacterial effect from a single dose is greatest for several hours after use, but it may last for as long as 5 days. It is used in the management of many bacteria associated with periodontal disease and also is effective in suppressing *mutans*-type streptococcus associated with dental caries.

The side effects associated with this product are the formation of a brown stain on the teeth and tongue; on glass ionomer, compomer, and composite restorations; and on artificial teeth. It has a bitter taste and may affect the taste of some foods. Staining seems to be more rapid in some individuals. Diet and brushing habits are thought to play an important role in how rapidly staining occurs. Some flavoring agents have been introduced to offset the bitter taste. More frequent professional teeth cleaning and polishing is usually necessary for patients who use these compounds routinely.

The longest-used mouth rinse agents are the phenolic compounds also called *essential oils*. The best-known product is Listerine, which has received the American Dental Association (ADA) Seal of Acceptance. It is a combination of phenol-related essential oils (thymol, eucolyptol, and menthol) mixed in methylsalicylate in a 26.9% hydroalcoholic vehicle. The antibacterial action of these compounds is a result of their alteration of the bacterial cell wall. It has not been shown to be an effective anticaries rinse, but clinical studies have shown reduction of plaque scores by about 25% and gingivitis by 30% with use of these compounds. In some patients these compounds cause a burning sensation in the tissues and a bad taste. Flavoring agents have been added to try to overcome the taste problem.

METHODS OF DELIVERY

Ingested Fluorides (Systemic)   Fluoride may be obtained through the drinking water, either naturally occurring or in fluoridated water supplies. In nonfluoridated communities dentists may prescribe fluoride supplements for children in the form of tablets, drops, or lozenges. Consideration should be given to the total fluoride exposure the child receives from other sources, such as school rinse programs, toothpaste, or prepared foods with fluoride. Tablets and lozenges should be sucked to gain a topical effect. A portion of systemically ingested fluoride,

including that in drinking water, is returned to the oral cavity by way of the saliva, thereby contributing to a topical effect.

In-Office Fluoride Applications (Topical)   Children with newly erupted permanent teeth or children and adults at high risk for caries are good candidates for professionally applied fluorides. The dental hygienist is most often the professional applying the fluoride in conjunction with a dental prophylaxis. In some states properly trained dental assistants can also play this important role. The most commonly used fluorides come in the form of topical gels or foams that are applied for 4 minutes in disposable trays. Some manufacturers market topical fluorides that they suggest need only be applied for 1 minute. The 1-minute application delivers approximately 85% of the fluoride that a 4-minute application delivers, but it has the advantage that it is in the mouth for a much shorter time. This can be particularly beneficial with small children who have active tongues and profuse salivary flow, and it is helpful with patients who tend to gag easily. When used one to two times a year, topical fluoride treatments have been shown to produce 20% to 26% caries reduction. Acidulated phosphate fluoride (APF) is most often used with children, because it contains 12,300 ppm fluoride and has good uptake in the enamel. Two percent neutral sodium fluoride (NaF) contains 9000 ppm fluoride and is used more often with adults because the acid in APF tends to etch the surface of restorations made of porcelain, composite resin, glass ionomer, or compomer. Fluoride varnishes are available as 5.0% sodium fluoride and are applied directly to the surfaces of the teeth. They remain on the teeth for 1 to 3 days if the patient brushes gently. They are particularly useful for direct application to early dental caries that can remineralize (Figure 7-3).

Self-Applied Topical Gels   Self-applied fluoride gels are recommended for individuals who are at moderate-to-high risk for dental caries. They are also used for orthodontic patients to prevent caries and decalcification around brackets and bands that causes permanent white spots and lines on the enamel. These white spots are unsightly and represent the early stages of the caries process. Elderly patients who take medications that dry up their salivary flow are at high risk for root caries and can receive benefit from gels used at home. Self-applied

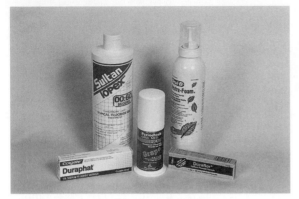

FIGURE 7-3 ■ In-office fluoride products include foams, gels, and varnishes.

gels are available by prescription as 1.1% neutral sodium fluoride (5000 ppm fluoride) or 0.4% stannous fluoride (900 ppm fluoride). Stannous fluoride may cause some staining of the surfaces of the teeth, and it delivers less fluoride ion to the teeth. These gels can either be brushed on the teeth or applied in custom fluoride trays. Four minutes of use in a custom tray is much more effective than 1 minute of brushing with the gel because the saliva quickly dilutes the gel and removes it from contact with the teeth. The custom trays, however, involve some additional expense for the time required to make impressions, pour casts, and construct the trays. Children under 6 years of age should not use these gels, because they tend to swallow too much of the gel. In place of a brush-on gel, some manufacturers have made a prescription toothpaste containing 1.1% neutral sodium fluoride. The idea is that it will aid compliance because the patient will not have to brush the teeth first and then brush again with a gel. The patient can brush once with the paste containing the stronger fluoride.

Over-the-Counter Fluoride Rinses Over-the-counter (OTC) fluoride rinses have been demonstrated to provide a 28% caries reduction when used in a daily rinse program. Rinses are available as 0.05% sodium fluoride (225 ppm fluoride). Patients typically are instructed to rinse for 30 to 60 seconds, spit out the excess, and not to eat or drink anything for at least 30 minutes. It is often used just before bedtime so that a residue of fluoride can remain in the saliva during sleep. Prescription rinses contain 0.2% sodium fluoride or 0.63% stannous fluoride (Figure 7-4).

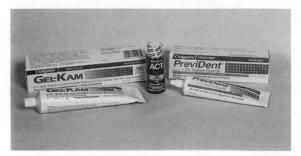

FIGURE 7-4 ■ Common home-use fluoride products

Fluoride-Containing Toothpaste Studies with Crest toothpaste conducted in the 1950s first established the caries-preventive capability of fluoride in toothpaste. Many studies conducted since then have shown sodium monofluorophosphate (MFP) and sodium fluoride to be more effective and chemically stable than stannous fluoride. The fluoride content of most toothpastes is about 1000 ppm. Children under 6 years of age should be supervised when brushing and should only be given a pea-size amount of toothpaste once a day. They tend to swallow the paste and run the risk of mild fluorosis of the permanent teeth if they consume too much.

Fluoride-Containing Prophylaxis Pastes Prophylaxis pastes contain pumice as an abrasive to remove surface stains and plaque from the teeth. In the process they remove a small amount of the fluoride-rich enamel surface. By incorporating fluoride in the paste, it is thought that some of the lost fluoride can be regained. The most common fluoride additive is 1.23% APF. These pastes have not received the ADA Seal as effective for caries prevention, because studies have not shown them to be effective for this purpose.

SAFETY

All fluorides should be used as directed and kept well away from small children for safety reasons. The lethal dose for a child weighing 20 pounds is approximately 700 to 1500 mg of sodium fluoride, or about 300 fluoride tablets. Acute symptoms could arise with a lesser dose. If it is determined that a child has consumed an excessive amount of fluoride, vomiting should be induced and milk of magnesia should be given to tie up the fluoride. Cow's milk could be given to slow the absorption from the stomach. The most common reaction seen in the dental office or shortly after leaving the office when a child has swallowed fluoride gel is nausea and vomiting. The fluoride irritates the stomach. (See Procedure 7-1 at the end of this chapter for the clinical technique for in-office topical fluoride application. Table 7-1 lists common in-office and home-use fluoride products.)

Pit and Fissure Sealants

PURPOSE

Sealants are unfilled or lightly filled resins that are used to seal the noncarious pits and fissures of deciduous and permanent teeth (see Chapter 6). The purpose of a sealant is to prevent dental caries in

TABLE 7-1
Common In-Office and Home-Use Fluoride Products

Use	Product	Fluoride Content (ppm)	Common Brands	Frequency of Use	Precautions
In-office treatment	1.23% APF gel or foam	12,300	Minute-Foam and Minute-Gel (Oral-B) Nupro APF Gel (Dentsply) Care 4 (Sultan Chemists) Denti-Care Topical Fluoride (Medicom) Fluoridex Foam (Discus Dental)	Twice a year	Gastrointestinal upset, vomiting if swallowed; may etch esthetic restorations; not for children under age 3
	2.0% NaF	9,000	Neutra-foam (Oral-B) NuproNeutral (Dentsply) Denti-Care Topical Foam or Gel (Medicom)	Twice a year	Gastrointestinal upset, vomiting if swallowed; not for children under age 3
Prescription home use	1.1% NaF gel or toothpaste	5,000	Prevident (Colgate) NeutraCare (Oral-B) Denti-Care gel (Medicom) Fluoridex gel (Discus Dental)	Daily	Not for children under age 6
	0.4% SnF_2 gel	900	Gel-Kam (Colgate) Stop (Oral-B) Denti-Care gel (Medicom) Perio Plus (Discus Dental)	Daily	May cause surface staining of teeth; not for children under age 6
	0.2% NaF rinse	900	Fluorinse (Oral-B) PreviDent Dental Rinse (Colgate)	Weekly	Not for children under age 6
Over-the-counter home use	0.05% NaF rinse	250	ACT (Johnson & Johnson) Fluorigard (Colgate)	Daily	Not for children under age 6
	Toothpaste 0.24% NaF	1,100	Numerous brands and manufacturers	Daily	Not for children under age 6
	Toothpaste 0.8% MFP	1,000	Numerous brands and manufacturers	Daily	Use pea-size amount with children under 6

the pits and fissures. The widespread use of fluoride has caused a dramatic reduction in dental caries in children. Although the overall caries rate has dropped, the greatest benefit from fluorides has been on smooth enamel surfaces. The location of the majority of caries (about 88%) in children is in pits and fissures. The nature of the shape of the pits and fissures makes them vulnerable to dental caries. Pits and fissures are often deep, narrow channels in the enamel surface that can extend close to the denti-noenamel junction (Figure 7-5). They collect bacteria and food debris that cannot be removed by toothbrushing, so dental caries can occur readily in these locations. Sealants provide a conservative means of protecting pit and fissures by preventing bacteria and food products from entering them. Caries is often difficult to detect in its early stages in pits and fissures. If caries is inadvertently sealed in the pits and fissures, the caries process stops because the bacteria are cut off from their nutrients. When a sealant is placed early before decay has penetrated the enamel, it is a highly effective preventive restorative material. However, if a sealant leaks because it is not properly placed, caries can occur beneath it.

INDICATIONS

Not all teeth require sealants. Teeth indicated for sealants are those with deep pits and fissures. Teeth not needing sealants are those with enamel that is well coalesced (fused) so that pits and fissures are shallow or nonexistent. Sealants are targeted for young children so that susceptible pits and fissures are protected before they have the chance to decay. Sealants are used mostly on deciduous molars and permanent molars and premolars. However, some maxillary central and lateral incisors may have deep pits that could be protected by sealants.

COMPOSITION

Sealants are chemically similar to composite resins. Their resin component is based on a dimethacrylate monomer that is either bisphenol A-glycidyl methacrylate (bis-GMA) or urethane dimethacrylate (UDMA). Polymerization of the resin occurs either solely by chemical reaction (self-cure) or by light activation (light-cure). The self-cure is by the conventional peroxide-amine system that requires the mixing of two components. The light-cured sealants are one-component systems that use blue light to polymerize them. The vast majority of sealants in use today are light-cured. Many manufacturers add filler particles to the sealants to make them more wear resistant. Sealants are not as heavily filled as most composites, because they would be too viscous to flow into the narrow fissures. Some of the filler particles used in sealants may be radiopaque and allow the sealants to be seen on x-rays. Many of the sealants, however, are radiolucent (see Chapter 6).

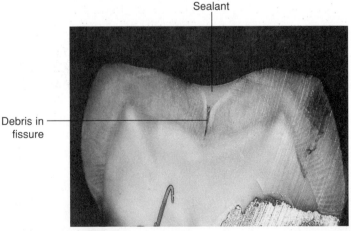

FIGURE 7-5 ■ Section of tooth showing long, narrow fissure containing debris.
(Courtesy Dr. Steve Eakle, University of California, San Francisco.)

WORKING TIME

The self-cured sealant polymerizes to final set within approximately 2 minutes from the start of mixing of the two components, one with the initiator and the other with the accelerator. An experienced operator can apply the material to one or two quadrants of posterior teeth with one mix of material, so it has the advantage of being applied faster than the light-cured material on a comparable number of teeth. The light-cured material requires a 20-second application of light on each tooth to polymerize the sealant. The light-cured material has the advantages of not requiring mixing, which often incorporates bubbles into the material, and allowing the operator to place and cure the material when the operator is ready.

COLOR AND WEAR

Manufacturers provide sealants in a variety of colors. Sealants may be clear, amber, tooth colored, or opaque white. Patients usually prefer the clear or tooth-colored sealants, but it is easier for the dental team to identify the presence of the sealant at the time of placement and at subsequent examination visits if it contrasts with the tooth color. Sealants are subject to wear from the occlusion. Sealants that contain no organic filler particles will wear faster than those that have filler particles added. Some clinicians use flowable composites as sealants, because they are more heavily filled and therefore are more resistant to wear while at the same time having adequate flow to enter the fissures. Sealants seldom flow to the bottom of long, narrow fissures because of the presence of debris and trapped air. Some clinicians prefer to open the fissures with a small-diameter bur or diamond to look for decay, remove debris, and allow better penetration of the sealant. Wear does not create much of a problem as long as the fissure remains sealed. If part of the fissure is uncovered, repair is recommended.

PLACEMENT

The technique of placement of sealants requires attention to detail (see Procedure 7-2 at the end of this chapter). The technique has many steps in common with the placement of other bonded restorations (see Chapters 5 and 6). The surface must first be cleaned with pumice to remove any surface debris that would interfere with acid etching or bonding. Retention of the sealant is obtained by etching the enamel with 37% phosphoric acid to roughen it and open pores in the enamel for penetration of the resin sealant. After etching, rinsing, and drying of the enamel, isolation of the field is *very* important. The sealant is applied to the pits and fissures and surrounding enamel and cured. Any moisture on the tooth could result in a failure of the sealant. Moisture could come from saliva, an air/water syringe that leaks water into the air, or even moisture from the patient's breath. Failure may be seen as an immediate loss of the sealant, complete or partial loss of the sealant seen at subsequent visits, or retained sealants that are leaking and could result in dental caries beneath the sealant. Maxillary and mandibular second molars are the teeth that most frequently lose sealants, probably because they are the ones for which it is difficult to maintain isolation when a rubber dam is not used. The dental hygienist plays an important role in the maintenance of sealants by carefully checking them at hygiene visits. In many states dental hygienists and dental assistants can be licensed to place sealants. State practice act guidelines must be followed as to the oral health care providers permitted to place sealants.

EFFECTIVENESS

Carefully placed sealants are very effective at preventing decay in the pits and fissures. Simonsen (1991) followed sealants for 15 years after placement found them to be highly effective. In that study sealants were placed on permanent posterior teeth, then followed with periodic examinations. If sealants were completely or partially lost, they were not replaced or repaired. (In dental practice lost sealants would be replaced.) At the end of 15 years, more than 68% of teeth were caries free compared with 17% in a control group. A much greater reduction in caries could have been obtained by replacement of lost sealants.

Desensitizing Agents

Many patients experience sensitivity in their teeth to cold foods or beverages, sweets, or cold air. Professionally applied or OTC materials applied to the teeth by the patient to reduce or eliminate the sensitivity are called **desensitizing agents**. Dental hygienists and assistants will be called on to apply certain types of desensitizing agents or to explain to the patients the causes of the sensitivity.

CAUSES OF TOOTH SENSITIVITY

Teeth may become sensitive when there are dentinal tubules exposed to the oral cavity. When some stimulus causes the fluid within the tubules to move, sensitive nerve endings located at the junction of the pulp and the dentin are deformed, causing them to fire and produce a quick, localized sharp pain (hydrodynamic theory of dentin sensitivity). Temperature, usually cold, and sugars and acidic foods are common offenders. Causes for the exposed dentin include roots abraded by improper toothbrushing (see Chapter 9, Figure 9-6), loss of enamel and dentin from dietary acids (erosion), loss of tooth structure in the cervical part of the tooth by abfraction (grinding of the teeth can cause bending of the teeth at the microscopic level with breaking away of enamel and dentin in the cervical area), and scaling and root planing procedures. If the dentinal tubules become plugged, the sensitivity stops. Acidic foods and beverages, toothbrushing, or scaling and root-planing procedures can remove the plugs and create sensitivity again. Desensitizing agents have been developed to treat sensitivity (Figure 7-6). Other causes of sensitivity include a cracked tooth or a leaking restoration. In the latter two cases, desensitizing agents are not the treatment of choice and corrective restorations are indicated.

FUNCTION

Many desensitizing agents work by closing the open ends of the dentin tubules to reduce the fluid movement. This may be by a chemical or mechanical blocking process. Some materials actually create a bond with the dentin or mineralize the openings of the exposed tubules (Figure 7-7). Some desensitizing agents, potassium nitrate in particular, work by passing through the dentinal tubules to the pulp and acting directly on the nerve. This produces a soothing effect on the pulp. Desensitizing agents are used in several different ways. They may be used at the time of placement of a restoration, after a prophylaxis or scaling and root planing procedure, or for teeth with gingival recession and exposed root surfaces that are hypersensitive to touch or temperature. One of the side effects of teeth bleaching can be tooth and gum sensitivity during the bleaching process. Some bleaching products contain chemicals such as potassium nitrate or fluoride that are claimed to reduce or eliminate the sensitivity during bleaching.

> ### COMMON CAUSES OF ROOT SENSITIVITY
>
> - Root caries
> - Toothbrush abrasion
> - Erosion by acids
> - Abfraction associated with bruxism
> - Scaling and root planing
> - Leaking restoration on the root

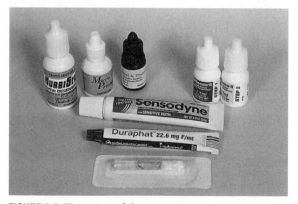

FIGURE 7-6 ■ Variety of desensitizing agents.

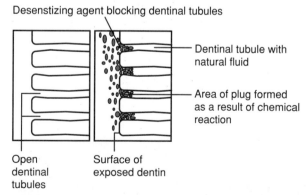

FIGURE 7-7 ■ Illustration of a desensitizing agent that forms a precipitate that occludes the dentinal tubules.

CATEGORIES AND COMPONENTS

A variety of desensitizing agents are available. They may be categorized as toothpastes, fluoride gels and varnishes, inorganic salt solutions, and resin primers and bonding agents (Table 7-2). Desensitizing toothpastes usually require repeated use over several days or weeks to achieve some relief. Fluorides also may take a while before results are seen. Some of the inorganic salts that precipitate into the open dentinal tubules and seal their openings will have immediate results; others may take repeated applications. The resin desensitizing agents will have immediate results if all of the open tubules are sealed. A reduced level of sensitivity may remain if some of the tubules are still open. Desensitizing systems using bonding resins may require etching of the surface first, sometimes creating additional temporary sensitivity, particularly with rinsing and application of air. However, some

TABLE 7-2

Desensitizing Agents

Product Category	Product Name	Manufacturer	Active Ingredient
Toothpastes	Sensodyne	Block Drug	Strontium chloride
	Sensodyne F	Block Drug	Potassium nitrate
	Sensitive Maximum Strength	Colgate	Potassium nitrate
	Sensitive toothpaste with fluoride	Oral B	Potassium nitrate and sodium fluoride
	Thermodent	Lee Pharmaceuticals	Strontium chloride
Fluoride gel/varnish	Gel-Kam	Colgate	0.4% stannous fluoride
	Prevident	Colgate	1.1% sodium fluoride
	Dentin Block	Colgate	Sodium, stannous, and strontium fluorides
	Duraphat	Colgate	5% sodium fluoride varnish
	Duraflor	Pharmascience	5% sodium fluoride varnish
	Fluor Protector	Vivadent	Fluoride varnish compound
Inorganic salts	Protect	Butler	Potassium oxalate
	Sensodyne Sealant	Block Drug	Ferric oxalate
	D/Sense 2	Centrix	Two solutions each containing two salts
	UltraEZ	Ultradent	3% potassium nitrate plus 0.11% sodium fluoride
	Desensitize	DenMat	5% potassium nitrate
	Relief	Discus Dental	Potassium nitrate
Resin agents	Hurriseal	Beutlich	HEMA, 0.5% sodium fluoride, benzakonium chloride
	Microprime	Danville Materials	HEMA, 0.5% sodium fluoride, benzakonium chloride
	Gluma Desensitizer	Kulzer	5% gluteraldehyde 35% HEMA
	Gluma Comfort Bond and Desensitizer	Kulzer	GLUMA 4-META resin
	Pain-Free	Parkell	Poly (methyl MA co-parastyrenesulfonic acid
	Clearfil SE Bond	J. Morita	Phosphate monomers with acid (self-etching)
	All-Bond DS	BISCO	NTG-GMA and BPDM primers
	Seal & Protect	Caulk/Dentsply	Prime&Bond NT with 7% filler

HEMA, Hydroxyethyl methacrylate; *GLUMA,* glutaraldehyde and HEMA; *4-META,* methacryloxyethyl trimellitate anhydride; *NTG,* N-toluene glycine; *GMA,* glycidil methadrylate; *BPDM,* biphenyl dimethacrylate.

self-etching dentin primers are available that do not require rinsing after etching (see Chapter 5). The duration of relief varies greatly, from a few days to close to 1 year. None of these agents provides permanent relief. The duration of relief can be prolonged if the original cause of the sensitivity is eliminated. That is, the poor toothbrushing habit, the acidic diet, or the teeth grinding must be curtailed, or the desensitizing agent will be removed and the tubules reopened. The dental hygienist must provide the patient with one of the desensitizing agents following scaling and root planing if the patient has a history of sensitivity. Chronically sensitive root surfaces may require restoration with glass ionomers, compomers, or composites to provide definitive relief.

Mouth Guards and Splints

The purpose of **mouth guards** and splints is to protect the teeth and their supporting structures. The widespread use of mouth guards in school sports prevents thousands of injuries each year. Most states mandate, and the Centers for Disease Control and Prevention recommends, that participants in school contact sports wear mouth guards (also called mouth protectors). Most professional and amateur adult athletes wear them, too.

Mouth guards are also recommended for patients who are bruxers (grind their teeth). Dental offices can provide valuable preventive measures for their patients by offering mouth guards. Dental assistants and hygienists can play an active role in recommending mouth guards, making impressions for their construction and even constructing them in the office laboratory.

SPORTS MOUTH GUARDS

Mouth guards for sports can be purchased over the counter or can be **custom-made** in the dental office or commercial dental laboratory. The OTC guards are of two types. One type is a stock guard that comes in several sizes. These generally are thick and poor fitting and may be somewhat uncomfortable to wear. They are not adapted to the patient's bite. The second type is constructed of a flexible thermoplastic material (softens when heated) that is in a horseshoe shape. The material is softened in boiling water, placed in the mouth while still moldable, hand adapted to the

teeth and arch, and then adapted to the bite by closing the teeth into the guard. Excess material is cut away with heavy-duty scissors. These are often difficult for inexperienced individuals to adapt properly and may have a poor fit. Professionally made guards are custom-fit to casts made of the patient's mouth. A thermoplastic material is heated and vacuum adapted to the cast. Because the fit is excellent and the bite is comfortable, compliance with its use is much better than the OTC guards. (See Procedure 7-6 at the end of this chapter.)

NIGHT GUARDS (BRUXISM MOUTH GUARDS)

Many patients who grind their teeth do so mostly at night while they are sleeping. Because the guard is worn at night, it has become known as a night guard. The guard does not stop the grinding habit, but it prevents wear of the incisal and occlusal surfaces, chipping of enamel, and even fracture of cusps. When used for treatment of temporomandibular dysfunction (TMD), the guards are frequently referred to as splints.

Two main types of materials are used: (1) hard acrylic (methylmethacrylate resin and monomer) and (2) thermoplastic sheets of polyethylene material. The guards made from thermoplastic sheets may be fabricated in the dental office by the assistant, hygienist, or dentist or sent to a commercial dental laboratory.

MAINTENANCE

The hygienist and assistant should instruct the patient in the proper home care of the guard. The guard should be cleaned daily. When it is removed from the mouth it should be rinsed thoroughly to remove saliva, then brushed with a toothbrush or denture brush and liquid soap. After final rinsing, excess water should be shaken off and the guard stored in a rigid container that is left open so that the guard can air-dry. If it is sealed in a container while it is still moist, it may promote the growth of bacteria and mold. A rigid container prevents the guard from being distorted by other articles inadvertently placed on top of it. Staining is common with all types of guards. Contact with amalgam restorations will cause a dark gray stain over time in the area of contact. Solutions containing alcohol or bleach should not be used because they will degrade the material. Commercially available soaks for orthodontic retainers or dentures are useful to freshen the guard.

Teeth Bleaching

A desire by patients for brighter, whiter smiles has caused an explosion in the demand for cosmetic services. Teeth **bleaching** has become an active part of many dental practices. Patients request it to make their teeth whiter. The dental hygienist or dental assistant, depending on the state dental practice act, can perform many of the bleaching procedures. Bleaching can be done as an in-office procedure or as a home procedure supervised by the dentist. Controlled research and case studies indicate that bleaching with peroxide products is safe and effective. Some bleaching products are available that do not contain peroxide.

HOW BLEACHING WORKS

Teeth bleaching occurs when the hydrogen peroxide or nonperoxide bleaching material passes through the enamel to the dentin and oxidizes pigments in the dentin, resulting in a lighter color. This process is accelerated by the use of low-intensity heat or high-intensity light, such as a conventional composite curing light, a laser, or a high-intensity plasma arc light. Some manufacturers have suggested that acid etching before the application of the bleach chemical may enhance penetration of the bleach. Research has shown that this does not improve the bleaching, and it can contribute to additional complications. It may necessitate polishing the enamel before the dismissal of the patient because of the surface roughness it creates. Depending on the manufacturer, the main ingredients of bleaching products are hydrogen peroxide, carbamide peroxide, or urea peroxide or a non hydrogen peroxide system that contains sodium chloride, oxygen, and natrium fluoride. Some products also contain additives such as potassium nitrate and fluoride to help reduce sensitivity.

TYPES OF STAINS

Teeth may be discolored by **extrinsic stains** on the tooth surface, **intrinsic stains** incorporated internally into the tooth structure (often when the tooth is developing), or a combination of both (Table 7-3). Some extrinsic stains can be removed, all or in part, by hand or ultrasonic scaling and coronal polishing (Figures 7-8 and 7-9). Some stains have penetrated the enamel surface and cannot be polished or scaled

TABLE 7-3 ▨

Causes and Colors of Extrinsic and Intrinsic Discoloration

Cause	Color
Extrinsic Stain	
Poor oral hygiene	Yellow, brown, green, black
Coffee, tea, foods	Brown to black
Tobacco products	Yellow-brown to black
Intrinsic Stain	
MEDICATIONS DURING TOOTH DEVELOPMENT	
Tetracycline	Brown, gray, black bands
Fluoride	White, brown spots or bands
MEDICATIONS AFTER TOOTH DEVELOPMENT	
Minocycline (tetracycline-type drug)	Brown, gray
DISEASES/CONDITIONS DURING TOOTH DEVELOPMENT	
Conditions such as purpura (a blood disorder)	Red, brown, purple
Trauma	Blue, black, brown
PULPAL CHANGES	
Pulp canal obliteration	Yellow
Pulp necrosis with hemorrhage	Gray, black
Pulp necrosis without hemorrhage	Yellow, gray-brown
OTHER CAUSES IN NONVITAL TEETH	
Trauma during pulp extirpation	Gray, black
Tissue remnants in the pulp chamber	Brown, gray, black
Restorative dental materials	Brown, gray, black
Endodontic materials	Gray, black
Combination Intrinsic/Extrinsic Stains	
Fluorosis	White, brown
Aging	Yellow

Adapted with permission from *Contemporary Esthetics and Restorative Practice*. Hayward VB: Current status and recommendations of dentist-prescribed, at home tooth whitening, *Contemp Esthet Rest Pract* 3(suppl):2-9, 1999.

away. These may require bleaching to remove them. In general, discolorations that are yellow-brown in color are easier to bleach than are blue-gray and

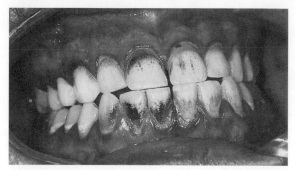

FIGURE 7-8 ■ Extrinsic stain on the teeth. Greenish stain as a result of accumulation of plaque, pellicle, food debris, and pigment-producing bacteria. (See also Color Plate 4 at the beginning of the book.)

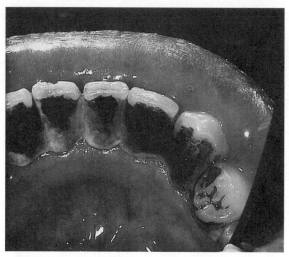

FIGURE 7-9 ■ Extrinsic stain on the teeth. Dark brown and black stains as a result of poor oral hygiene and heavy use of tobacco (smoking). (See also Color Plate 5 at the beginning of the book.)

black colors. The latter stains are often caused during tooth development by chemicals or drugs, such as tetracycline. As a consequence, they are incorporated deep within the dentin and are also in the enamel. Externally applied, vital bleaching usually takes much longer to lighten these stains. Stains associated with endodontically treated teeth may require internal bleaching. Some stains are resistant to bleaching, and repeated attempts may not achieve the result the patient desires.

IN-OFFICE BLEACHING

Bleaching of Vital Teeth Bleaching is done in the dental office for both vital and nonvital teeth. Bleaching involves the use of various strengths of hydrogen peroxide solutions and gels. For years bleaching was done by means of a liquid of 35% hydrogen peroxide and the application of a heating lamp. This can be effective for single-tooth bleaching, but it is a time-consuming process and is technique sensitive. If any of the liquid contacts the soft tissues it can cause a chemical burn that can be painful. One product (Hi-Lite, Shofu Dental Corp.) uses a powder and liquid system that can be applied in the office as a light-cure or chemical-cure procedure. This product contains 35% hydrogen peroxide liquid and a powder containing manganese sulfate as a light activator and ferrous sulfate for a chemical activator. After the powder and liquid are mixed, it is a translucent green color that changes to an opaque white after the oxygenation reaction is completed. The use of a curing light accelerates the process by a factor of 3. This is a better system than the use of the 35% hydrogen peroxide solution alone, but it must be carefully administered in the office or tissue burns can occur. The procedure may require more than one visit to achieve the desired whitening result.

The high-concentration gel of 35% carbamide peroxide is more controllable than the liquid hydrogen peroxide and seems to be more effective. All of these high-concentration products require the use of the dental dam and an additional gingival protection with petroleum jelly or the paint-on light-cured dental dam materials (Opal Dam, UltraDent). When a bleaching procedure is going to be done, it is best to record the starting shade of the patient's teeth before beginning the bleaching procedure. (See Procedure 7-3 at the end of this chapter.)

In-office "power bleaching" (use of a strong bleach activated by high-intensity light) has become a popular procedure, because it can be completed in one visit and there is no need to rely on patient compliance as with the home-use systems. Many patients simply do not want to spend the time to bleach at home for several hours a day over a period of 2 or more weeks. When used with a curing light, plasma arc light, or laser light, the "power bleach" in-office system can be done in as little as 45 minutes to 1 hour. Recently materials have been developed that do not require the use of a high-intensity light. Some patients may need a longer bleaching time or additional visits depending on the type of discoloration. The gels or paste systems each have indicators that change color when the oxygenating cycle is complete. Applications are repeated until the desired whiteness is achieved or the patient begins to develop sensitivity. The bleaching materials should be stored in the refrigerator to prolong their limited shelf life.

It is important to remember that teeth dehydrate when they are isolated by the rubber dam for a period of time and appear whiter than they will be after they have rehydrated several hours later. Dehydration of the teeth can also contribute to an increase in sensitivity during the procedure.

Bleaching of Nonvital Teeth   When the pulp of a tooth dies, the necrotic breakdown products of the pulpal tissue or hemoglobin from blood in the pulp escapes into the surrounding dentinal tubules. Chemicals from these tissues (e.g., iron sulfide from hemoglobin) cause staining of the dentin (Figure 7-10). Bleaching of nonvital teeth in the dental office typically involves removing the restoration from the endodontic access cavity (the hole through which the root canal therapy was performed) and bleaching internally through this access. The tooth is isolated with a rubber dam to prevent bleaching solutions from contacting and burning soft tissues. A 30% hydrogen peroxide solution (Superoxol) is placed in the pulp chamber on a saturated cotton pellet. A hot instrument is plunged into the cotton several times to activate the peroxide. An alternative approach is the "walking bleach" technique, in which a commercially prepared bleaching gel or paste made in the office from sodium peroxyborate monohydrate (Amosan) and 30% hydrogen peroxide is sealed into the pulp chamber with a temporary restoration. With the paste, both products release oxygen that helps bleach the tooth. When the patient returns in 2 to 5 days, the bleaching material is removed, and a composite or an amalgam restoration is placed. All of the internal bleaching procedures require that a seal be established at the base of the endodontic access preparation just coronal to the level of the gingival attachment to the tooth. This is to prevent bleach from leaking out through open dentinal tubules or accessory canals into the periodontal ligament. There have been cases of external root resorption that were caused by the bleach activating an inflammatory reaction in the periodontal tissues. External root resorption is an attack on the root surface by cells and enzymes in the

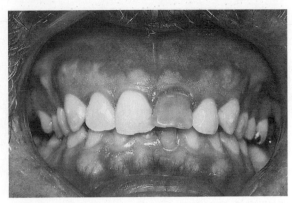

FIGURE 7-10 ■ Intrinsic stain in a maxillary central incisor as a result of trauma leading to pulpal death. Staining is due to blood products entering the dentinal tubules. (See also Color Plate 6 at the beginning of the book.)

periodontal tissues. It can actually eat a hole through the root, and the patient may lose the tooth.

HOME BLEACHING

Home bleaching (also called night guard bleaching) is a popular and cost-effective means of bleaching. The chemical that is used in most home bleaching systems is 10% to 16% carbamide peroxide at a pH near neutral in a viscous gel. Carbamide peroxide is made up of two components, urea and hydrogen peroxide, and is mixed into a gel of either propylene glycol or glycerin or both. Carbopol is added as a thickener, and flavoring agents are also added. Nonperoxide gels are also available and claim not to cause tooth sensitivity or gingival irritation, as peroxide products may do with some patients. The gel is placed in a custom-formed soft, thin plastic tray and worn by the patient for periods as short as 30 minutes twice daily or as long as overnight. Trays may or may not have spaces, called reservoirs, built into them to hold the bleaching material (see Procedure 7-5 at the end of this chapter). Most offices use reservoirs, but some studies suggest that they may not be needed. The length of treatment varies for each patient depending on his or her discoloration and sensitivity. The usual period is 2 weeks, but discolorations such as those from tetracycline may take several weeks or months (Figure 7-11). Not all stains can be removed or lightened with bleaching. The home bleaching process is as effective as the in-office process and is sometimes used as a follow-up to the

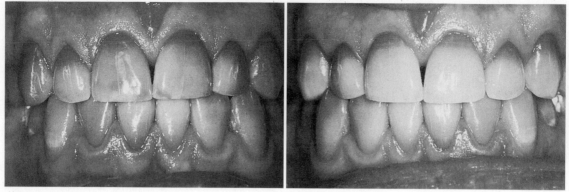

FIGURE 7-11 ■ Intrinsic stain. Teeth with tetracycline stains (**A**) before and (**B**) after home bleaching. (See also Color Plate 7 at the beginning of the book.)
(Courtesy UltraDent Products, Inc.)

in-office procedure that "jump-starts" the bleaching process. The recommended time for follow-up visits is every 2 to 3 weeks, and the procedure is performed with supervision by the dentist.

OVER-THE-COUNTER PRODUCTS

A recently introduced product for home bleaching (Crest Whitestrips, Procter & Gamble) does not require the construction of bleaching trays. The material consists of clear, flexible strips that are adapted over the teeth and worn for 30 minutes at a time twice a day. The shorter treatment time may be beneficial for patients who developed sensitivity with longer treatment times when using trays. The strips deliver 5.3% hydrogen peroxide to the teeth. The strips are thin and do not interfere with speech. Early indications are that they are just as effective as bleaching with custom trays at a considerable reduction in cost. The strips cover only the anterior six teeth in each arch, so patients who want to bleach additional teeth may need to resort to night guard bleaching.

Several tray bleaching systems are sold directly to the public by manufacturers. The trays in these systems are either preformed stock trays or thermoplastic trays that are heated in boiling water and adapted to the teeth. These trays are often poorly fitting and are not properly trimmed to prevent excess material from contacting the gingiva. Additionally, there is no professional evaluation before bleaching to ensure that decay and leaking restorations are repaired, nor is there professional supervision during bleaching. Individuals with pre-

existing sensitive teeth will probably worsen their condition. The bleach in these systems is usually 10% carbamide peroxide.

ROLE OF THE DENTAL ASSISTANT OR HYGIENIST

The dental assistant and hygienist can play an important role in the delivery of bleaching services to the patients. In addition to chairside assisting for in-office bleaching, assistants and hygienists can be active oral health providers for home bleaching. They can perform several important clinical procedures (see Procedure 7-4 at the end of this chapter), as well as fabrication of the bleaching trays. It is important that the patient is fully informed of the pros and cons of bleaching. The assistant or hygienist can obtain the informed consent from the patient. Additionally, she or he can provide the patient with instructions for proper use of the bleach and care of the trays.

POTENTIAL SIDE EFFECTS

Tooth sensitivity, usually short term, can occur from the bleaching process and can be managed by shortening the bleaching time each day, as well as using fluoride, potassium nitrate, or other desensitizing agents as an adjunct as previously described. Other possible side effects include irritation of the gingiva, mucosa, and throat from excess bleaching material coming out of the trays. If patients wear the bleaching trays overnight, they may experience some soreness of the muscles of mastication and temporomandibular

HOME BLEACHING INSTRUCTIONS GIVEN IN THE DENTAL OFFICE

At the Bleaching Sessions
1. Brush and floss.
2. Place small amount of bleaching gel in the front of each tooth section of the tray. Do not overload because excess gel may irritate mouth tissues and throat.
3. Place tray over the teeth and seat it gently. Remove excess gel with toothbrush or clean finger.
4. Wear tray for the time prescribed by the dentist.
5. At end of bleaching session remove tray, rinse mouth with water, and use toothbrush to remove residual gel.
6. Clean tray under running water with toothbrush. Liquid soap may be used. Shake off water. Place in storage container with the lid open to allow tray to air-dry.

Additional Information
1. Store bleaching gel in cool dry location out of direct sunlight.
2. Bleaching is not recommended while pregnant or nursing.
3. Avoid coffee, tea, red wine, cola drinks, berries, and tobacco because they can cause staining of teeth.
4. Bleaching results usually last 1 to 3 years. Gradual restaining may necessitate occasional rebleaching.
5. Keep bleaching trays so you only need to buy additional bleach for rebleaching.
6. If tooth sensitivity or other problems develop, call the office for advice.

joints if the trays cause them to clench or grind or slightly displace the condyles (heads of the mandible) from the joints.

RESTORATIVE CONSIDERATIONS

Before starting the bleaching process, cavities should be filled and leaking restorations should be replaced to prevent excessive penetration of bleach through the dentinal tubules that might irritate the pulp and cause sensitivity. Bleaching may be done as a pre-restorative procedure to whiten the teeth before composite bonding procedures, veneers, or porcelain crowns. However, research has shown that bonding to newly bleached surfaces will be weaker than if the teeth are allowed to restabilize. Patients need to be informed that the color of existing restorations will not lighten with bleaching. So if they have restorations in visible areas of the mouth that match the teeth before bleaching, they will appear darker after bleaching because the surrounding tooth structure will be lighter. Some patients have bleached their teeth so much that the shades found in regular composite kits may not be light enough to match the color of the bleached teeth. Several manufacturers have now developed composite shades for bleached teeth. Some bleaching gels that are mildly acidic have caused slight roughness of the surface of some composites, compomers, or glass ionomers. During the bleaching process, patients should also be advised to limit their intake of foods and beverages that can stain the teeth, including coffee, tea, red wine, and berries or their juices. Smoking can also contribute to staining of the teeth.

CLINICAL TIP A period of at least 2 weeks is needed after bleaching to allow the color of the teeth to stabilize before placing esthetic restorations. Also, the bond to newly bleached surfaces is weaker than if the teeth are allowed to stabilize.

CONTRAINDICATIONS

Bleaching is not for everyone. Patients who are allergic to components of the bleaching materials or the tray material should not attempt bleaching. Patients with extremely sensitive teeth should also avoid the procedure. Patients who have several tooth-colored restorations in the anterior part of the mouth and who do not want to replace these restorations should think twice about bleaching. Patients with unrealistic expectations about what bleaching can do should be discouraged from bleaching.

RE-TREATMENT

Both in-office and home bleaching will fade with time and may require re-treatment to maintain the whiteness. Typically, patients may find that in 1 to 3 years they will want to do some additional bleaching. With in-office bleaching this often means that patients will have to pay the full bleaching fee again. With home bleaching patients need only purchase additional bleach if they keep their custom bleaching trays.

SUMMARY

Conservative dentistry mandates that the allied oral health practitioner be familiar with and use the various preventive materials available. By performing caries risk assessment and using topical applications of fluoride, as well as fluoride and antibacterial rinses, early caries can be arrested and tooth structure can often be remineralized. Sealants placed to protect pits and fissures of teeth are recognized as being effective in the prevention of tooth decay. Desensitizing agents are more important now than

ever before because people are retaining their teeth longer and as a result are subject to the factors that produce root sensitivity. These agents provide relief to patients whose teeth have gingival recession and exposed dentin that subjects them to chronic or episodic pain. Likewise, the use of mouth guards not only helps those patients with TMD problems, but also is effective in the prevention of excessive tooth wear and fracture.

Bleaching of teeth for cosmetic reasons is a recent and popular aspect of cosmetic dentistry. Because patients are realizing the benefits of these procedures and products, the allied oral health practitioner must be knowledgeable of the products and their application techniques. To be effective in providing bleaching services and advice to patients, clinicians must be knowledgeable about in-office, prescribed home-use, and OTC products, including their indications and contraindications and potential side effects.

CHAPTER REVIEW

Select the one correct response for each of the following multiple-choice questions:

1. **High levels of fluoride can be found as naturally occurring in which one of the following?**
   a. Coffee
   b. Tea
   c. Raw seafood
   d. Beans

2. **When tooth enamel first begins to demineralize, what is one of the corrective measures to stimulate remineralization?**
   a. Stop eating foods with proteins and amino acids
   b. Use a daily rinse containing fluoride
   c. Brush with baking soda and salt
   d. Check the labels on the food packages to determine whether they contain fluoride

3. **When enamel is remineralized with fluoride,**
   a. It is a different color
   b. The fluoride contains a poison that kills all bacteria associated with dental caries
   c. The resultant remineralized crystal is more resistant to acids
   d. All of the calcium is replaced

4. **Fluorosis is always considered to be**
   a. Destructive to the tooth
   b. Very unsightly
   c. A sign that the person has ingested more that the optimum amount of fluoride
   d. A sign that the person will need to have bleaching and restorations

5. **Nightly home fluoride treatment with 1.1% sodium fluoride as a brush-on gel or in custom trays is indicated for**
   a. Children under 6 years of age
   b. Adolescents with one or two pit and fissure caries
   c. Middle-age women going through menopause
   d. Elderly patients taking medications that cause dry mouth

6. **Sealant material is**
   a. Indicated for *all* permanent molars
   b. Used for protection of smooth surface caries
   c. An unfilled or lightly filled resin
   d. Never in need of replacement once it is placed

7. **When placing a dental sealant, the technique**
   a. Is exactly the same as bonding to dentin
   b. Requires the field to be kept dry
   c. Can be done by dental hygienists and assistants in all states
   d. Always requires the use of a curing light

8. **The main purpose of most desensitizing agents**
   a. Is to close the openings of the enamel rods to prevent temperature and osmotic changes in the enamel fluids
   b. Is to help the dental hygienist keep the patient comfortable during the dental prophylaxis procedure
   c. Is to plug the openings of the exposed dentinal tubules
   d. When added to toothpaste, is to improve the taste and keep it from burning the gingiva

9. **When a mouth guard is prescribed by the dentist, fabrication can be done by**
   a. The dental assistant   c. The laboratory technician
   b. The dental hygienist   d. All of the above

10. **The main purpose of a mouth guard is**
    a. To help protect the teeth and supporting structures during contact sports
    b. To use as a tray for placing fluoride on the teeth
    c. To use as a bleaching tray
    d. To keep teeth in alignment after orthodontic treatment

11. **Custom-made mouth guards and splints may be made of**
    a. A plastic material softened by boiling
    b. Thermoplastic sheets of resilient plastic or hard processed acrylic resin
    c. Composite resin
    d. Tray acrylic

12. **Bleaching of teeth**
    a. Can cause them to become soft   c. Is very predictable
    b. Affects only extrinsic stains   d. Can cause sensitivity of the teeth

13. **Bleaching of teeth works**
    a. By removing surface stains
    b. By penetrating both enamel and dentin and oxidizing the stain
    c. By sealing surface porosities so that stain cannot enter the tooth surface
    d. By creating a white coating on the surface of the enamel

14. **In-office bleaching**
    a. Is superior in results to home bleaching
    b. Produces equivalent results to home bleaching but is faster
    c. Does not cause tooth sensitivity
    d. Has no effect if the bleach contacts the gingiva

CASE-BASED DISCUSSION TOPICS

◉ A 14-year-old female high school student with no restorations comes to the dental office with poor oral hygiene and early caries in the fissures of her mandibular first molars. An analysis of her diet reveals frequent consumption of sodas and between-meal snacking on sugary foods. *Discuss preventive measures that should be recommended for this young woman and the rationale for their use.*

◉ A 75-year-old retired plumber who takes medication for hypertension comes to the dental office with moderate marginal gingivitis, root caries, and a complaint of dry mouth. *Discuss which of the antibacterial rinses this man should use. Discuss the type of fluoride regimen he should be using. Explain the rationale for each of these recommendations.*

◉ A 35-year-old housewife has been using an over-the-counter bleaching system with trays adapted to the teeth after boiling the material in water. She has been wearing the trays while she sleeps. She comes to the dental office complaining of sensitivity in her teeth, inflamed and painful gingivae, and sore jaw muscles. *Discuss possible causes for each of her complaints and make recommendations to treat the problems and prevent their recurrence.*

◉ A 56-year-old business executive comes to the dental office for her annual examination and cleaning. Her chief complaint is that her front teeth are chipping on the incisal edges. She also notes sensitivity to cold, sweets, and air on the roots of her maxillary premolars in areas of gingival recession. Questioning reveals that she grinds her teeth. She also loves lemons and uses lemon juice frequently in cooking and on her salads. *Discuss the etiology of her complaints and preventive and therapeutic measures that should be recommended for her.*

REFERENCES

Azuma Y et al: Pharmacological studies on the anti-inflammatory action of phenolic compounds, *J Dent Res* 65:53, 1986.

Baum L, Phillips RW, Lund MR: Prevention of dental disease. In *Textbook of operative dentistry,* ed 3, Philadelphia, 1995, WB Saunders.

Bird D, Robinson D: Preventive, restorative and cosmetic dentistry. In *Torres and Ehrlich modern dental assisting,* ed 6, Philadelphia, 1999, WB Saunders.

Featherstone JD: Prevention and reversal of dental caries: role of low-level fluoride, *Community Dent Oral Epidemiol* 27:31, 1999.

Featherstone JD et al: Dependence of in vitro demineralization and remineralization of dental enamel on fluoride concentration, *J Dent Res* 69:620, 1990.

Gladwin MA, Bagby MD: Tooth bleaching; oral appliances. In *Clinical aspects of dental materials,* Philadelphia, 2000, Lippincott Williams & Wilkins.

Haywood VB: Current status and recommendations for dentist-prescribed, at-home tooth whitening, *Contemp Esthet Rest Pract* 3(1):2, 1999.

Kugel G: Effective tooth bleaching in 5 days: using a combined in-office and at-home bleaching system, *Compendium* 18(4):378, 1997.

Leinfelder K: Ask the expert: anything new in pit and fissure sealants? *J Am Dent Assoc* 130:533, 1999.

Magid KS: In-office power bleaching with a plasma arc curing light, *Contemp Esthet Rest Pract* 3(8):14, 1999.

Mandel JD: Chemotherapeutic agents for controlling plaque and gingivitis, *J Clin Periodontol* 15(8):488, 1988.

Simonsen RJ: Retention and effectiveness of dental sealant after 15 years, *J Am Dent Assoc* 122:34, 1991.

Ten Case JM, Featherstone JDB: Mechanistic aspects of the interactions between fluoride and dental enamel, *Crit Rev Oral Biol* 2:283, 1991.

Warren JJ: Fluorosis of the primary dentition: what does it mean for the permanent teeth? *J Am Dent Assoc* 130:347, 1999.

PROCEDURE 7-1 (see p. 325 for competency sheet)

Applying Topical Fluoride

EQUIPMENT/SUPPLIES (Figure 7-12)

- Disposable trays of various sizes
- Topical fluoride foam or gel
- Air-water syringe
- Watch or timer
- Cotton rolls
- Saliva ejector
- High-volume evacuation (HVE) tip

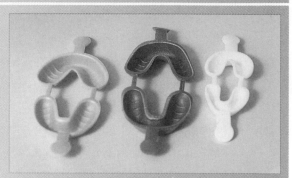

FIGURE 7-13

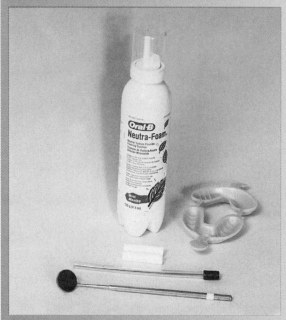

FIGURE 7-12

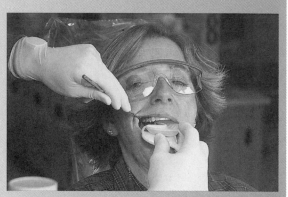

FIGURE 7-14

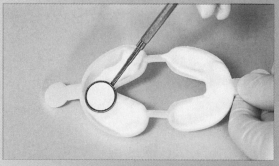

FIGURE 7-15

PROCEDURE STEPS

1 Select appropriate disposable tray for the size of the patient's mouth (Figures 7-13 and 7-14).

2 Examine the patient for the presence of calculus. If present, perform scaling procedure before proceeding.

NOTE: Do not polish teeth with premanufactured prophylaxis paste. This reduces the absorption of the fluoride.

3 Seat the patient upright.

NOTE: This reduces the amount of the gel going down the patient's throat.

4 Load trays with fluoride (Figure 7-15). Do not overfill, because that will cause excess fluoride to run into the patient's mouth.

NOTE: Follow appropriate guidelines for the age of the patient.

Continued on following page

PROCEDURE 7-1 (Continued)

5 Place trays in the patient's mouth. Place cotton rolls between the trays and have the patient close on the cotton rolls to keep the trays in place.

6 Place the saliva ejector in the mouth either on the cheek side or between the trays in the space created by the cotton rolls (Figure 7-16).

NOTE: The taste of the gel and the presence of the trays will greatly increase the flow of saliva.

7 Time the fluoride application.

8 Remove the trays after appropriate time. Remove excess gel/foam and saliva from the patient's mouth with HVE.

9 Instruct the patient not to rinse, eat, or drink for 30 minutes.

NOTE: Fluoride circulating in the saliva will continue to have a topical effect for a few hours after treatment.

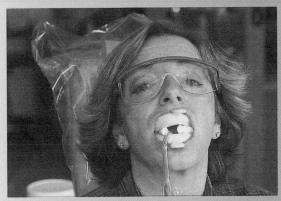

FIGURE 7-16

PROCEDURE 7-2 (see p. 326 for competency sheet)

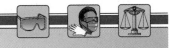

Applying Dental Sealants

EQUIPMENT/SUPPLIES (Figure 7-17)

- Basic examination setup
- Prophy setup: slow-speed handpiece with prophy angle, prophy cup, or bristle brush
- HVE, saliva ejector tips, and air-water syringe tip
- Dental dam setup (check for latex allergy); alternative isolation: cotton rolls and holder
- Flour of pumice or special prophy paste without fluoride or oils
- Dappen dish for pumice and mixing well for sealant, if supplied in bulk
- Curing light if using light-cure sealant and light shield
- Sealant material: self-cure or light-cure
- Etching solution/gel: 35% phosphoric acid
- Applicator brush or tips (some sealant materials have an applicator)

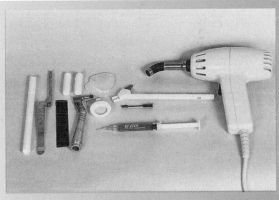

FIGURE 7-17

- Articulating paper, dental floss
- Bullet-shaped finishing bur or polishing stone

Continued on following page

PROCEDURE 7-2 (Continued)

PROCEDURE STEPS

1 Place dental dam or cotton rolls and saliva ejector to isolate teeth to be sealed.

NOTE: Moisture contamination with saliva or water can cause a lost or leaking sealant.

2 Clean the surfaces of the teeth to be sealed with pumice or oil/fluoride-free paste (Figure 7-18).

3 Use three-way syringe and HVE to rinse and dry teeth thoroughly. Remove any retained polishing paste (Figure 7-19).

NOTE: Some dentists prefer to clean out the fissures with a small round or needle-shaped bur or diamond rotary instrument. This allows them to inspect the fissures for the presence of caries.

4 Place etchant on enamel to be sealed for 20 to 30 seconds (Figure 7-20).

NOTE: Some teeth need longer etching times, such as primary teeth and teeth with fluorosis.

5 Rinse with water for 10 to 15 seconds.

6 If using cotton rolls, carefully replace them or dry them out with the HVE.

NOTE: Be certain that saliva does not contaminate the freshly etched surfaces or the enamel will need to be reetched for 15 seconds.

7 Dry the teeth thoroughly.

NOTE: Properly etched enamel should appear frosty (Figure 7-21). If not adequately etched, reetch for an additional 30 seconds. The fissures in Figure 7-21 were opened minimally with a small bur before etching.

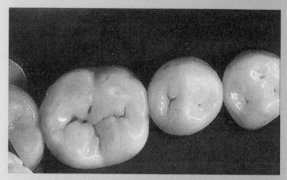

FIGURE 7-19

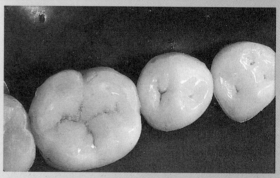

FIGURE 7-20

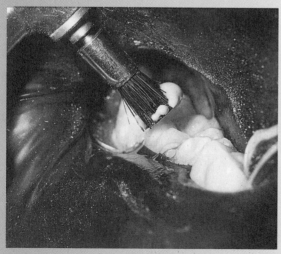

FIGURE 7-18

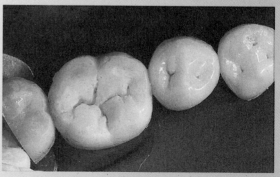

FIGURE 7-21

Continued on following page

8 Apply sealant according to the manufacturer's instructions.

NOTE: Sealant should be gently worked into the pits and fissures to displace trapped air. It should cover the entire fissure but should not overfill the groove pattern because that will probably interfere with the occlusion.

9 Cure appropriately for the required length of time (self-cure or light-cure) (Figure 7-22).

NOTE: If light-curing, each area under the light probe should be cured for at least 20 seconds.

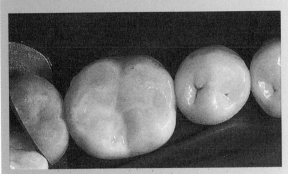

FIGURE 7-22

10 Check with explorer to ensure that all fissures and pits are covered, no holes in the material exist, and sealant is well retained. Apply more material, if needed.

11 Remove dental dam or cotton rolls and thoroughly rinse.

12 Check occlusion with articulating paper and adjust sealant where needed.

NOTE: Follow state laws as to which health care practitioners are allowed to do adjustment.

13 Check contact areas with floss.

NOTE: Excess material may have blocked these areas.

14 Check retention at each subsequent visit.

NOTE: Sealants should be checked for partial or complete loss. Make sure fissures are still covered. With retained sealants, check periphery for staining that may indicate leakage. Extensive decay can occur under leaking sealants if not detected early. Replace lost or leaking sealants.

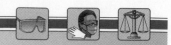

PROCEDURE 7-3 (see p. 327 for competency sheet)

In-Office Bleaching

EQUIPMENT/SUPPLIES (Figure 7-23)

- Basic examination setup
- Prophy setup: low-speed handpiece with prophy angle, prophy cup, flour of pumice
- Tooth shade guide
- Dental dam setup (check for latex allergy)
- Tissue-protective material (petroleum jelly or manufacturer's coating or foam)
- High-strength bleaching material (varies with manufacturer)
- High-intensity light, curing light, laser, or heat source (depending on bleach type)
- Appropriately tinted safety lenses or light shield
- Timer or watch
- Three-way syringe and HVE with disposable tips
- Waxed dental floss, 2 × 2 gauze
- Optional: extraoral or intraoral camera for taking photograph

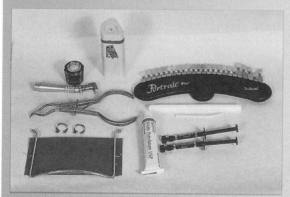

FIGURE 7-23

PROCEDURE STEPS

1 Clean teeth with flour of pumice or nonfluoride/oil polishing paste.

2 Take starting shade and record. Photograph may also be taken, if desired.

3 Place tissue protection on gingiva and interdental papillae according to manufacturer's directions.

NOTE: Gingiva is often coated with petroleum jelly or other protective layer under the dental dam in case the dam leaks.

4 Place dental dam isolating teeth to be bleached (Figure 7-24).

NOTE: Holes must be appropriate size and spacing to prevent leakage. Invert edge of dam around each tooth to form a seal so bleach will not contact gingiva.

5 Place waxed floss around each tooth and tuck dam tightly at the cervical margin.

6 Place high-strength bleach as provided by the manufacturer (usually 35% hydrogen peroxide) and follow specific directions as to time and light/heat source application (Figures 7-25 and 7-26). Be aware of developing tooth or gum sensitivity during the procedure. Respond accordingly.

NOTE: Tooth sensitivity may be due to overheating the tooth, previously exposed root areas, or penetration of strong bleach into vital dentin. Gum sensitivity may be caused by a chemical burn from the bleach. Mild sensitivity usually goes away in a few days. Severe burns to the gingiva or mucosa can be painful and cause tissue necrosis that may take weeks to heal. Mild burns with surface whitening of the gingiva heal quickly.

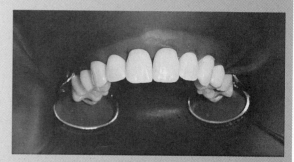

FIGURE 7-24

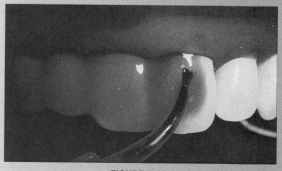

FIGURE 7-25

Continued on following page

PROCEDURE 7-3 (Continued)

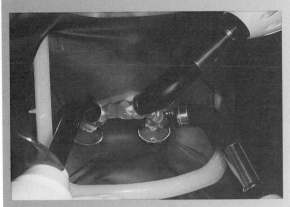

FIGURE 7-26

7 Rinse off bleach, wipe clean with 2 × 2 gauze, and examine for shade. Repeat application of bleach as needed to achieve desired shade.

NOTE: Teeth appear whiter with the dental dam in place because of the contrast in color and the dehydration that occurs under the dam. True color appears after teeth are rehydrated with saliva. Color stability is achieved 2 weeks after bleaching.

8 Further appointments may be needed to achieve tooth whiteness goal.

NOTE: Desired results cannot always be achieved. Some stains are more resistant to bleaching.

PROCEDURE 7-4 (see p. 328 for competency sheet)

Clinical Procedures for Home Bleaching

EQUIPMENT/SUPPLIES (Figure 7-27)

- Basic setup for examination
- Rubber mixing bowl and spatula
- Alginate, measures for water and powder
- Dental plaster or stone
- Alginate impression trays
- Tooth shade guide and camera (optional)
- Home bleaching kit and instructions

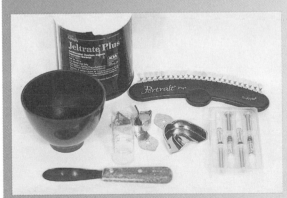

FIGURE 7-27

PROCEDURE STEPS

First Appointment

1 Dentist examines teeth and arches for type of discoloration and oral conditions that might influence the success of bleaching. Potential areas of concern are corrected or planned for correction.

NOTE: Dental caries, sensitive teeth, and leaking restorations may need correction before bleaching to prevent further sensitivity or pulpal problems.

2 Discuss pros and cons of bleaching. Obtain informed consent.

NOTE: A signed informed consent form signifies that the patient fully understands what is involved, has had his or her questions answered, and agrees to the treatment.

3 Record patient's tooth shade (Figure 7-28; see also Color Plate 8 at the beginning of the book). Take photographs with shade tab next to teeth, if desired.

NOTE: Many manufacturers include a shade card that can be used to match the initial shade and later to compare it with the bleached shade at future visits.

Continued on following page

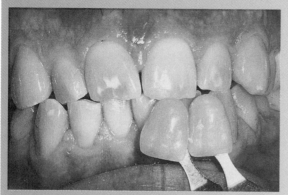

FIGURE 7-28
(Courtesy Ultradent Products, Inc.)

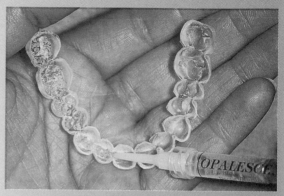

FIGURE 7-29
(Courtesy Ultradent Products, Inc.)

4 Select impression trays of the correct size and make alginate impressions.

5 Rinse impressions, spray with disinfectant or immerse in suitable disinfectant for 15 minutes, wrap in wet paper towel, and seal in zippered plastic bag.

6 Pour impressions in dental stone. (Block out tongue and palatal area with wet paper towel to make trimming casts easier when making trays.) Trays are fabricated in the office (see Procedure 7-5) or sent to a commercial laboratory.

Second Appointment

7 Try in trays for fit and comfort.

8 Demonstrate loading of trays with gel, tray insertion, and removal of excess gel (Figures 7-29, 7-30, and 7-31).

9 Demonstrate cleaning of trays after bleaching session.

10 Give verbal and written instructions. Review possible side effects. Dispense home bleaching kit.

NOTE: Written instructions are important because patients forget what has been told to them.

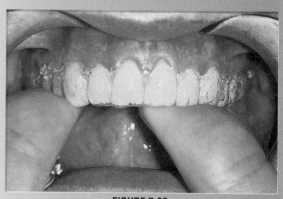

FIGURE 7-30
(Courtesy Ultradent Products, Inc.)

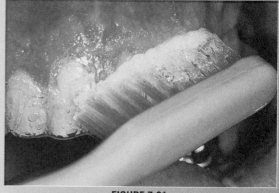

FIGURE 7-31
(Courtesy Ultradent Products, Inc.)

Continued on following page

PROCEDURE 7-4 (Continued)

11 Schedule follow-up appointment in 2 to 3 weeks following initial delivery. Take and record tooth shade at each subsequent visit (Figure 7-32; see also Color Plate 9 at the beginning of the book). Procedure continues until desired shade is achieved.

NOTE: Bleaching will not change the color of existing tooth-colored restorations (composite, glass ionomer, compomer, or porcelain). The patient must understand that these restorations will appear darker than the surrounding bleached teeth and may need to be replaced to achieve the desired cosmetic result. Not all stains respond to bleaching, and patients may not achieve desired results. Cosmetic restorative procedures are done after bleaching has stabilized for a period of 2 weeks or more.

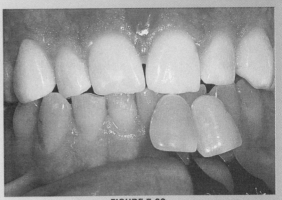

FIGURE 7-32

(Courtesy Ultradent Products, Inc.)

PROCEDURE 7-5 (see p. 329 for competency sheet)

Fabrication of Custom Bleaching Trays

EQUIPMENT/SUPPLIES (Figure 7-33)

- Casts (models) of patient's dentition
- Bleach reservoir material: light-cured block-out resin or adhesive reservoir strips
- Vacuum former
- Two sheets of 6 × 6 inch by 0.02- or 0.035-inch-thick vinyl tray material
- Fine-tipped scissors for trimming the trays

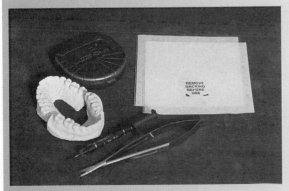

FIGURE 7-33

PROCEDURE STEPS

1 Trim casts to eliminate much of the facial peripheral border. If the maxillary cast has a palatal area, drill a hole in the deepest part of the palate or grind away most of the palatal area (Figure 7-34).

NOTE: Ledges or concave areas on the casts that trap air when the molten tray material is lowered over the casts will prevent good adaptation of the tray to the cast and result in a poorly fitting tray that leaks bleaching gel into the patient's mouth. Before pouring stone into the alginate impressions, block out the tongue and palate areas with a wad of wet paper towel. This will save time trimming stone away from these areas later.

2 Allow casts to dry, then apply reservoir material to the facial surfaces of the teeth (on the cast) to be bleached in one of the two following ways:

a. Light-cured block-out resin is applied to the facial surfaces of the teeth to be bleached in a thin layer about 1 mm thick. It should extend 1 mm short of the gingival crest and the interproximal embrasures. Resin on each tooth

Continued on following page

PROCEDURE 7-5 (Continued)

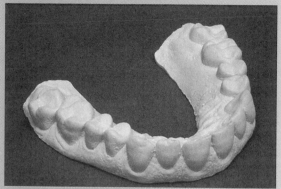

FIGURE 7-34
(Courtesy Ultradent Products, Inc.)

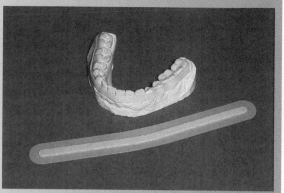

FIGURE 7-35B

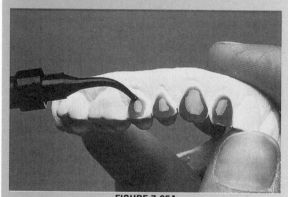

FIGURE 7-35A
(Courtesy Ultradent Products, Inc.)

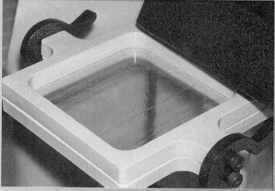

FIGURE 7-36

should be cured for 10 seconds with a curing light, or the entire cast can be placed in a Triad light-curing unit for 1 minute (Figure 7-35, *A*).

NOTE: The reservoir is left short of the gingival crest so the tray will seal in that area and prevent bleach from contacting the gingiva.

b. As an alternative to block-out resin, plastic adhesive reservoir strips can be applied to the teeth. Cut a reservoir adhesive strip (3M Corp.) to the appropriate length to extend over the facial surfaces of the teeth to be bleached. Remove the plastic backing and press the adhesive strip firmly on the dry cast (Figure 7-35, *B*).

NOTE: The cast must be very dry or the adhesive strip will not stick. The plastic reservoir strip becomes attached to the inside of the bleaching tray when the vinyl is softened and adapted over the cast.

3 Clamp a sheet of vinyl tray material in the frame of the vacuum-forming unit (Figure 7-36). Raise the frame until it is just below the heating element. Turn on the heating element.

4 Place one cast in the center of the platform (it contains many holes) of the vacuum former.

5 When the vinyl material has heated and sagged an inch or more (Figure 7-37), lower the frame to the platform and turn on the vacuum. The molten material will be pulled down tightly over the cast.

NOTE: If a pocket of air is trapped under the vinyl, push it out by adapting the tray to the cast by hand with a wet paper towel while the material is still soft and the vacuum is on.

Continued on following page

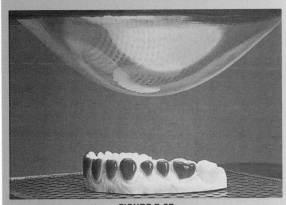

FIGURE 7-37
(Courtesy Ultradent Products, Inc.)

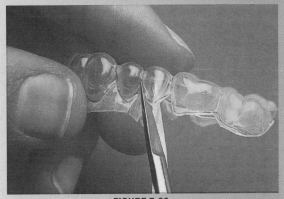

FIGURE 7-38
(Courtesy Ultradent Products, Inc.)

6 Allow tray material to cool for at least 1 minute before removing from the frame. Place under cold running water to cool thoroughly.

7 Trim excess material away from the cast with scissors. Remove cast from the tray.

8 Use fine scissors to trim tray so that it extends over the teeth just to the gingival crest (Figure 7-38). It should have a scalloped appearance as it traces the outline of the gingival crest (Figure 7-39).

NOTE: If tray extends over the gingiva on the facial surfaces, bleach can contact the gingiva and irritate it.

9 Repeat process for the other cast.

10 Wash trays with soap and water. Spray trays with surface disinfectant and store until delivery in zippered plastic bag marked with patient's name.

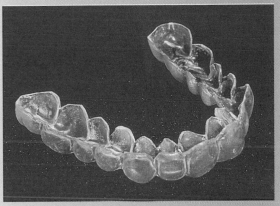

FIGURE 7-39
(Courtesy Ultradent Products, Inc.)

PROCEDURE 7-6 (see p. 330 for competency sheet)

Fabrication of a Sports Mouth Protector

EQUIPMENT/SUPPLIES (Figure 7-40)

- Trimmed casts (study models)
- Vinyl mouth guard material—one sheet 6 × 6 inches, 0.15 inch thick
- Vacuum former unit
- Heavy-duty scissors
- Straight-line hinge articulator
- Petroleum jelly
- Alcohol torch
- Disinfectant spray and zippered plastic bag

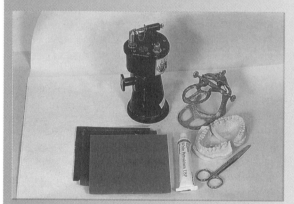

FIGURE 7-40

PROCEDURE STEPS

1 Inspect casts (study models) and remove any blebs of dental stone on the teeth.

NOTE: These blebs (bumps) of stone represent trapped air bubbles in the impression. Painting alginate on the occlusal surfaces of the teeth and in the palate just before inserting the loaded tray will help minimize trapped air in the impression.

2 Trim casts in a horseshoe shape so that the central portion representing the tongue and palate areas is mostly removed.

NOTE: To save time trimming the casts, these areas can be blocked out with a piece of wet, crumpled paper towel when the impressions are poured.

3 Insert a sheet of vinyl mouth guard material in the frame of the vacuum former and clamp it in place. Lift clamping frame up to heating element and turn on the heat to soften the material.

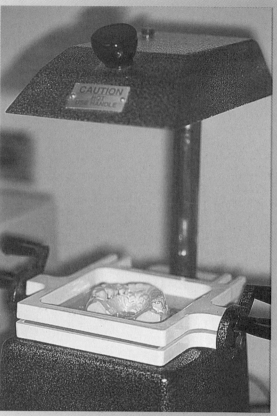

FIGURE 7-41

NOTE: The vinyl sheets come in a variety of colors that are appealing to young athletes or can be clear.

4 Place the maxillary cast on the platform and center it under the sheet of material.

5 Lower the frame when the sheet of material has softened and sags an inch or more. Turn on the vacuum when the molten tray material covers the cast. Leave the vacuum on for at least 30 seconds to allow the molten material to adapt to the cast (Figure 7-41).

NOTE: With some machines the vacuum activates automatically when the frame is lowered. If air is trapped between the cast and the vinyl, use a wet paper towel to quickly press the vinyl against the cast while the vacuum is still on to force the air out and closely adapt the vinyl to the cast.

Continued on following page

6 Remove the vinyl and the cast from the clamping frame and allow the vinyl to cool.

NOTE: Hold it under cold water to cool it rapidly.

7 Trim excess material from the cast. Carefully remove cast from the vinyl.

NOTE: Removing excess vinyl at the sides of the cast will help free the cast more easily.

8 Place the maxillary and mandibular casts together in their proper bite relationship (centric occlusion) and mount them on the articulator using fast-set plaster (Figure 7-42).

NOTE: For patients whose bite relationship is not clear, a separate bite registration should be taken at the time of the alginate impressions.

9 Trim vinyl away using heavy-duty scissors until the guard extends about 3/8 inch onto the palatal and facial gingiva of the cast.

NOTE: The guard is extended over the gingiva to give added protection but is kept short of the depth of the vestibule so it will not irritate the tissues when the athlete bites on the guard.

10 Place the guard on the maxillary cast and check to see that the guard material is not too thick in the molar area (Figure 7-43). The mandibular cast should close evenly onto the guard and not prop the bite open.

11 Correct the bite. If the guard hits the mandibular molars first, apply a thin coat of petroleum jelly to the occlusal surfaces of the mandibular cast, soften the vinyl in both right and left molar areas with an alcohol torch, and close the casts together into the softened vinyl

(Figure 7-44). Repeat this process by heating the vinyl in the molar, premolar, and cuspid areas until the mandibular teeth touch the guard evenly in the posterior and anterior.

NOTE: A guard corrected in this manner will allow the athlete to close comfortably and not be in a strained jaw position.

12 Round out with an acrylic bur in the laboratory handpiece the indentations in the guard caused by the mandibular cast. Next, create smooth borders and occlusal surface by flaming with an alcohol torch to soften the material, then lightly rubbing the surface of the vinyl with a gloved finger coated with petroleum jelly.

NOTE: Be careful not to overheat the vinyl. Just soften the surface by lightly flaming it. If it is too hot, it could cause a burn to the finger. Overheating the vinyl can cause it to burn.

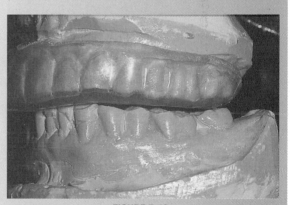

FIGURE 7-43

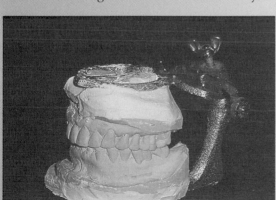

FIGURE 7-42

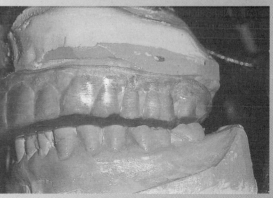

FIGURE 7-44

Continued on following page

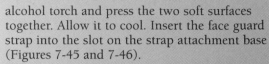

PROCEDURE 7-6 (Continued)

13 A commercially purchased strap can be added to the anterior part of the guard for those sports in which a face guard is used. The strap allows the athelete to remove the guard from the mouth while not in activity and have it attached to the face guard and ready to reinsert when needed. While still on the cast, heat the vinyl guard on the facial surface and heat the back surface of the strap attachment base with an alcohol torch and press the two soft surfaces together. Allow it to cool. Insert the face guard strap into the slot on the strap attachment base (Figures 7-45 and 7-46).

14 Wash the guard with liquid soap and water. Rinse thoroughly and spray it with a disinfectant. Store it until the delivery appointment in a zippered plastic bag marked with the patient's name.

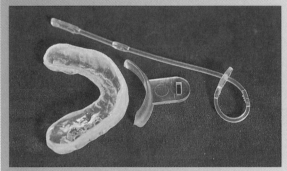

FIGURE 7-45

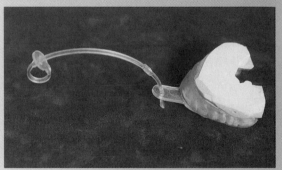

FIGURE 7-46

8 METALS IN DENTISTRY

OBJECTIVES

On completion of this chapter the student will be able to:

1. Discuss the safety of amalgam as a restorative material.
2. List the main components in dental amalgam.
3. Describe the advantages of high-copper amalgams over low-copper amalgams.
4. Describe the role of the gamma-2 phase on corrosion of the amalgam.
5. Describe the particle shapes in lathe-cut, admix, and spherical alloys and discuss their effect on the condensation resistance of the freshly mixed amalgam.
6. Define *creep, corrosion,* and *tarnish.*

7. Discuss the effect of mixing time on the strength and manipulation of amalgam.
8. Describe the advantages and disadvantages of bonded amalgam restorations.
9. Discuss mercury hygiene in the dental office.
10. Describe the differences among the types of gold alloy used for dental restorations.
11. Define *karat* and *fineness*.
12. Differentiate among high noble, noble, and base metal alloys.
13. Describe the characteristics needed for porcelain bonding alloys.
14. Describe the characteristics of metals used for casting partial denture frameworks.
15. Describe the biocompatibility problems associated with some alloys.
16. Explain how solders are used.
17. List metals used for solders.
18. Describe how wrought metal alloys differ from casting alloys.
19. Describe the uses of wrought wire.
20. Describe the metals used for orthodontic brackets and how they bond to teeth.
21. Explain the use of the different types of metal wire for orthodontic arch wire.
22. Describe the basic types of implants in use today.
23. Describe the different types of metals used for dental implants.
24. Explain osseointegration of an implant.
25. Discuss the clinical care of dental implant fixtures.
26. Explain the rationale for use of plastic instruments for cleaning implants and when metal instruments can be used.
27. List the home care aids for implants and explain how they are used.
28. Explain the purpose of a post.
29. List the various classifications of posts.
30. Describe the types of materials used for preformed posts.

KEY TERMS

Alloy—A mixture of two or more metals.

Amalgamation—Reaction that occurs when silver-based alloy is mixed with mercury.

Dental amalgam—Restorative material composed of silver-based alloy mixed with mercury.

Lathe-cut alloy—Irregular-shaped particles formed by shaving fine particles from an alloy ingot.

Spherical alloy—Alloy particles produced as small spheres.

Admixed alloy—Mixture of lathe-cut and spherical alloys.

Gamma-2 phase—A chemical reaction between tin in the silver-based alloy and mercury that causes corrosion in the amalgam.

Tarnish—Oxidation affecting a thin layer of a metal at its surface. Not as destructive as corrosion.

Corrosion—Oxidation from interaction of two dissimilar metals in the presence of a solution containing electrolytes (such as saliva). It results in breakdown of the amalgam.

Creep—Gradual change in the shape of a restoration caused by compression from occlusion or adjacent teeth.

Triturator (amalgamator)—Mechanical device used to mix the silver-based alloy particles with mercury to produce amalgam.

Noble alloy—Alloy composed of metals that do not corrode readily.

High noble alloy—Alloy containing at least 60% noble metals, 40% of which must be gold.

Base metal alloy—Alloy composed of nonnoble metals. Corrodes more readily.

Precious metal—Classification of metal based on its high cost.

Porcelain bonding alloys—Special casting alloys manufactured for their compatibility with porcelain that has been bonded to it at high temperature.

Solder—An alloy used to join two metals together or repair cast metal restorations.

Wrought metal alloy—An alloy that has been mechanically changed into another form to improve its properties.

Yield strength—Amount of stress at which a substance deforms.

Anneal—To modify physical properties of a metal by heating it.

Gauge—A measure of the thickness of a wire; the lower the gauge, the thicker the wire (e.g., 8 gauge is thicker than 16 gauge).

Subperiosteal implant—Implant placed on top of the bone and under the periosteum.

Transosteal implant—Implant that penetrates entirely through the bone.

Endosseous (endosteal) implant—Implant placed into the bone.

Osseointegration—Bone growing into intimate contact with an implant.

Post—A metal or nonmetal dowel placed within the root canal to retain a core buildup.

Active post—Post that engages the root canal surface like a screw.

Passive post—Post that sits in the prepared canal space but does not engage the root surface.

Custom post—A post cast to fit precisely in the root canal space; usually has the core attached.

Preformed post—Factory-made post supplied in several sizes.

Historically and currently, the most widely used material in restorative and corrective dentistry is metal. The dental clinician is in contact with and involved in the manipulation of metal dental materials in various ways every day. It is essential that the clinician have an understanding of the characteristics of the various metal materials in order to correctly manipulate and care for them and to be able to answer questions by patients relative to a particular material that will be used for their treatment.

Dental Amalgam

Dental amalgam has been used for the restoration of teeth successfully for over 165 years in the United States. Approximately 50 million amalgam restorations are placed each year. Although composite resins are being used with increasing frequency for posterior restorations, amalgam is still the primary direct-placement material used in this region of the mouth. A survey conducted in 1995 reported that approximately 76% of dentists used amalgam as the main restorative material for posterior teeth with approximal caries. There is still no other direct restorative material that has the durability, ease of handling, and good physical characteristics of amalgam. The safety of amalgam has been called into question in recent years, but a study conducted by the National Institutes of Health (NIH) in 1991–1993 concluded that amalgam is safe for human use. Less than 0.01% of people have an adverse reaction to components of the amalgam. However, a combination of concerns by patients about its safety and its lack of esthetics has caused many patients to request tooth-colored restorative materials. Insurance carriers have seen a reduction in the use of amalgam for posterior restorations by approximately 35% in the last decade.

ALLOY VERSUS AMALGAM

An **alloy** is a mixture of two or more metals. The alloy used to produce dental amalgam is predominantly composed of silver but also contains copper and tin. A variety of other metals, such as palladium, indium, or zinc, may be added in much smaller quantities to produce specific properties in the alloy. When the silver-based alloy is mixed with mercury, a liquid metal, the reaction that occurs is called **amalgamation** and the material that is produced is called **dental amalgam.**

SILVER-BASED AMALGAM ALLOY PARTICLES

Silver-based amalgam alloys are classed according to the shape of the particles in the powder as irregular, admixed, or spherical (Figure 8-1). Each of these particle shapes contributes certain handling characteristics to the amalgam, and to some degree the amalgam type is selected by the dentist according to these char-

acteristics. Irregular-shaped particles are formed by shaving fine particles off an ingot of the alloy by means of a lathe **(lathe-cut alloy).** The particles are sifted to separate them into fine and ultrafine particles. Spherical particles are produced by spraying molten alloy into an inert gas **(spherical alloy).** Spherical particles are formed as the atomized droplets cool. Admixed particles consist of a mixture of lathe-cut and spherical particles **(admixed alloy).**

COMPOSITION

Modern dental alloys are considered to be high copper in content (10% to 30%) compared with their predecessors, which had 2% to 4% copper by weight (Table 8-1). They generally contain 40% to 70% silver and 12% to 30% tin. They are mixed with mercury 43% to 50% by weight. Spherical alloys require less mercury to wet the particles and generally set faster than lathe-cut particles. Manufacturers may also add

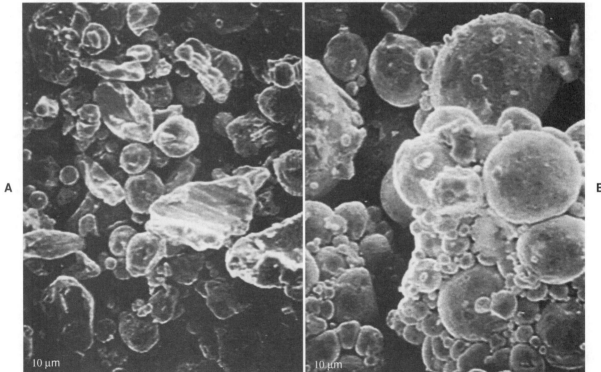

FIGURE 8-1 ■ **A,** Scanning electron micrograph (SEM) of admixed alloy showing a mixture of irregular-shaped particles and spherical particles. **B,** SEM of spherical alloy with different size spherical particles.
(Courtesy Dr. Grayson W. Marshall, University of California School of Dentistry, San Francisco, Calif.)

indium (1% to 4%), palladium (0.5%), and zinc (0.01% to 2%). Zinc may inhibit corrosion by reducing the oxidation of the other metals in the amalgam. In the high-copper amalgams it increases the clinical longevity of the restorations. In the low-copper amalgams zinc was responsible for the gradual expansion of the amalgam over time (delayed expansion) if moisture contamination was present during placement. Contact of moisture with the zinc caused the formation of hydrogen gas within the amalgam, which caused it to expand. Delayed expansion could cause the restoration to expand beyond the cavity walls and to cause cracking in the adjacent enamel. Because of this undesirable property, most alloys contain no zinc or very low levels of zinc and are called *zinc-free alloys.*

SETTING TRANSFORMATION

When the alloy in powder form is mixed with the liquid mercury, a chemical reaction occurs. The mixture has a puttylike consistency that can be packed into the cavity preparation. Over the next several minutes it gradually becomes firmer. During the first part of this firming phase, the amalgam can be carved (during the *working time,* or time available to manipulate the amalgam) to the anatomic shape of the tooth. Once it reaches its initial set it can no longer be carved and is firm but is not fully reacted. It is relatively brittle at this point, and the patient is advised not to bite on it for several hours. It takes up to 24 hours for most amalgams to gain their maximum strength. Once fully set, they are hard, strong, durable restorations.

SETTING REACTIONS

The chemical reaction that occurs when the alloy and mercury are mixed has three phases. The first phase, called the *gamma phase,* is the silver alloy phase. It is the strongest phase and has the least corrosion. The second phase is the *gamma-1 phase* consisting of mercury reacting with the silver. It is strong and corrosion resistant, although not as resistant as the gamma phase. The third phase is the **gamma-2 phase** and consists of the reaction of mercury with tin. Gamma-2 is weak and corrodes readily. Tin is used to control the rate of set of the amalgam. Both silver and tin dissolve into the liquid mercury until the solution becomes saturated with them, and they also absorb mercury. Newly formed particles begin to precipitate (crystallize) out of the mercury until there is no more mercury left to react. This process may take up to 24 hours to go to completion. The low-copper amalgams had much more corrosion because of the chemical reaction of tin and mercury (gamma-2 phase). Copper reacts with the tin to keep it from being available for the gamma-2 phase. High-copper amalgams do not have a gamma-2 phase and are superior in their clinical performance.

TARNISH

Tarnish is an oxidation that attacks the surface of the amalgam and extends slightly below the surface. It comes from contact with oxygen, chlorides, and sulfides in the mouth. It causes a dark, dull appearance, but it is not very destructive to the amalgam. The rougher the surface, the more it tends to tarnish.

TABLE 8-1

Main Components of Amalgam Alloy

Component	Function	Other Effects	High-Cu Alloy (%)	Low-Cu Alloy (%)
Silver (Ag)	Strength Corrosion	Setting expansion	40-70	65
Tin (Sn)	Improves physical properties when compounded with Ag	Setting expansion Strength	12 30	25
Copper (Cu)	Strength Hardness Corrosion	Setting expansion Creep	10-30	5-6
Zinc (Zn)	Oxidation of other metals	Delayed expansion with moisture contamination	0-2	0-2

Metals such as palladium are sometimes added to help reduce the tarnish. Polishing of the restoration can also reduce the tarnish. Polishing of amalgams is best done after the restoration has set for a period of 24 hours or more. Some clinicians have advocated polishing fast-set amalgams in as little as 20 minutes after placement. However, amalgams polished this soon after placement usually do not achieve a high shine. High-copper amalgams have a smoother surface after carving than low-copper amalgams and tend to tarnish less. Polishing is not as critical to their longevity as with low-copper amalgams. Because of this fact, controversy exists among dental educators and clinicians as to whether high-copper amalgams need polishing if they are well carved and contoured at the time of placement. Generation of excessive heat during polishing can cause a release of mercury from the silver-mercury phase that results in a mercury-rich surface that will corrode more readily and deteriorate at the margins.

CORROSION

Corrosion can occur from a chemical reaction between the amalgam and substances in saliva or food resulting in oxidation of the amalgam. It can also occur when two dissimilar metals interact in a solution containing electrolytes (saliva is such a solution). An electric current is generated between the metals (much like a battery) in a process called *galvinism.* The result of the galvanic reaction is oxidation of one of the metals. This oxidation is responsible for the corrosion of the amalgam. Corrosion also takes place within the amalgam by interaction of its metal components. It weakens the amalgam over time, can stain surrounding tooth structure as corrosion products enter the dentinal tubules, and can lead to deterioration of the margins (Figure 8-2). The high copper content of newer alloys eliminates the formation of the gamma-2 reaction product that caused the weakening of the amalgam. High-copper alloys have virtually replaced low-copper alloys, because the amalgams they produce are more durable with less deterioration at the margins (better marginal integrity), less corrosion, and higher strength.

Clinically, a galvanic reaction may occur when a newly placed amalgam contacts another metal restoration such as a gold crown. The patient feels a mild electric shock and may experience a metallic

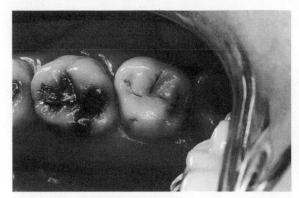

FIGURE 8-2 ■ Amalgam restoration showing surface tarnish, margin deterioration, and corrosion. Tooth has darkened as corrosion products from the amalgam have penetrated the dentinal tubules.

taste. This problem may persist until the amalgam completes its setting reactions, until enough oxides build up on one of the metals to stop the electric current, or until the offending restoration is replaced with a nonconducting restoration such as composite or with a restoration of a metal similar to the one next to it. Corrosion, however, can occur within an amalgam without the patient ever being aware of the process.

CREEP

Creep in dental amalgams refers to the gradual change in shape of the restoration from compression by the opposing dentition during chewing or by pressure from adjacent teeth. It was a phenomenon associated with the gamma-2 phase seen with low-copper alloys and resulted in deterioration of the margins. High-copper alloys exhibit far less creep and have superior marginal integrity.

DIMENSIONAL CHANGE

Ideally, the dimensions of a newly placed amalgam should not change. If it contracts excessively, it will open gaps at the margins and contribute to leakage of fluids and bacteria and cause sensitivity. If it expands excessively, it can put pressure on the cusps and cause pain with biting pressure or could result in fracture of the cusps. Some expansion and contraction occur during the setting reaction of the amalgam. It is the net effect of these two processes that is important. The composition of the alloy particles, the ratio of the mercury-to-alloy powder by weight, and salivary/moisture contamination are other factors that contribute to dimensional changes.

STRENGTH

Amalgam is among the strongest of the directly placed restorative materials. It has the ability to resist the strong forces of the bite repeatedly over many years when it is properly placed. Amalgams are stronger in compression (approximately 400 to 450 MPa) than composites or glass ionomers. However, they are relatively weak in tension (about 12% of compressive strength) and shear and therefore require adequate bulk to resist breaking. If thin excesses of amalgam are left over the cavosurface margins, they will chip away over time, creating an irregular margin that tends to collect plaque and contribute to recurrent caries. Generally, high-copper amalgams have a higher early compressive strength (1 hour) than low-copper amalgams. This is advantageous because it helps resist breakage if the patient inadvertently bites on a newly placed amalgam. Some high-copper amalgams gain approximately 80% of their strength in the first 8 hours. Low- and high-copper amalgams are comparable in compressive strength once they have completely set at about 24 hours.

HANDLING CHARACTERISTICS OF HIGH-COPPER ALLOYS

High-copper alloys are mostly admix or spherical types. Spherical particles provide a greater surface area with which the mercury can react. Therefore they need approximately 10% less mercury for the amalgamation process. Freshly mixed spherical amalgam has very little resistance to condensation into the cavity preparation and feels soft compared with an admixed amalgam. Spherical amalgams do not displace a matrix band and keep it in contact with the adjacent tooth in class II preparations as well as admixed amalgams. Therefore spherical amalgams may require a bit more physical separation of the teeth with the wedge in order to establish a good contact after the matrix band has been removed. Spherical amalgams have higher 1-hour and 24-hour compressive strengths than admixed amalgams. Newly placed spherical amalgams have slightly more shrinkage than admixed amalgams. At 24 hours both admixed and spherical high-copper amalgams shrink slightly, whereas low-copper amalgams expand.

MANIPULATION OF AMALGAM

Selection of Alloy   The dentist selects the dental alloy based on personal preference for its handling characteristics. There are variations among the commercially available alloys in the working and setting times, resistance to condensation pressures, and resistance to carving pressures. High-copper alloys are used almost universally because they have superior properties to low-copper alloys. Amalgam can be used for all classes of cavity preparation in the posterior part of the mouth and in select applications in the anterior part of the mouth when it is not visible. It is also used to build up badly broken down teeth before crown preparation.

Dispensing of Alloy and Mercury   The amalgam must be handled properly from the start through the entire placement process if the restoration is to be successful. The preferred dispensing of alloy powder and mercury is in commercially prepared capsules containing factory-measured amounts of alloy and mercury separated from each other by a plastic membrane. The manufacturers set the optimum ratio of alloy and mercury for their product based on their testing of the materials for the best properties. Usually capsules are available with different quantities of materials depending on the size of the restoration. They are offered as single mix (also called spill), double mix, or more depending on the manufacturer. With large preparations, several capsules may be needed.

Trituration   The powder and mercury are mixed together in a mechanical device called a **triturator (amalgamator)**. The triturator has settings that allow adjustment in the speed and time of the mixing process. The manufacturer's recommendations should be followed for the selected material. Some capsules require activation before trituration to break the membrane and allow the powder and mercury to mix. Other capsules are self-activating in that the membrane ruptures with the forces created by the rapid movement of the triturator. A capsule is placed in the retaining arms of the triturator (see Procedure 8-1, Figure 8-18), the proper settings of time and speed are made, and the device is activated. The retaining arms move back and forth rapidly to mix the powder and mercury, much like an automatic paint mixer. A less frequently used form of alloy is a pellet that is placed into a reusable capsule with a small pestle (a rod that pulverizes the pellet into a powder during mixing in the triturator) and mercury that is added from a dispenser. This older method of mixing the amalgam has declined in use, because the capsules often leak mercury into the operatory during mixing, mixes are not as consistent, and the dispenser is a potential source of mercury spills.

> **CLINICAL TIP** Do not activate the capsule before you are ready to begin mixing it. Activating the capsule and placing it in the triturator before completing the cavity preparation will allow the alloy powder to be partially wet by the mercury. When the mix is actually triturated a few minutes later, some of the reaction will have already started. The resulting amalgam will not have optimum properties and may have reduced working time. Self-activating capsules avoid this potential problem.

Expansion, contraction, creep, and corrosion can be caused by improper manipulation, moisture contamination, overtrituration, and undertrituration. Undertriturated alloy has a dry, crumbly appearance and sets too quickly. It results in a weaker restora-

tion because the components have not totally mixed, leaving a higher level of unreacted mercury and alloy particles. On the other hand, overtriturated alloy is too wet. It also results in an amalgam that sets too quickly because of the heat produced by prolonged mixing. It results in a weaker restoration that will corrode more readily, because it forms too many reaction products (silver-mercury and copper-tin). Properly triturated alloy has a satin appearance (Figure 8-3) and produces the desired physical properties.

Placement and Condensation   After mixing, the amalgam is removed from the capsule and placed into an amalgam well or the small end of a dappen dish. The amalgam is picked up in increments from the well by an amalgam carrier and placed by either the assistant or the dentist into the cavity preparation. Amalgam condensers are used to carefully work the amalgam into all of the corners and retentive areas of the preparation using vertical and lateral condensation. Condensers should be carefully stepped around the preparation in overlapping steps to prevent voids in the material and to adapt the material closely to the walls of the preparation. High-copper spherical amalgams have less resistance to condensation pressures and require the use of larger condensers. The cavity preparation is slightly overfilled to allow enough material to carve to contours and to remove excess mercury that has been forced to the surface during the condensation

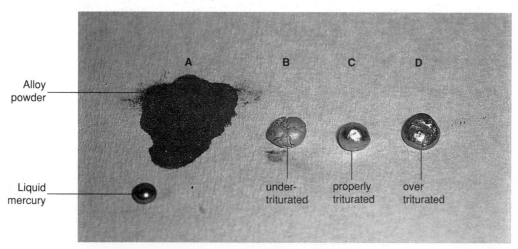

FIGURE 8-3 ■ **A,** Alloy powder and mercury. **B,** Undertriturated amalgam is dry and crumbly. **C,** Properly triturated amalgam has a satinlike appearance. **D,** Overtriturated amalgam appears too wet.

process. If excess mercury is left, physical properties will be poorer.

> **CLINICAL TIP** Amalgam should be placed as soon as it is mixed. If allowed to stand for a couple of minutes, the amalgam will be weaker because crystals that are forming will be disrupted during condensation. The amalgam will feel drier and more crumbly. Discard this mix and make a new one.

Burnishing and Carving Many clinicians prefer to burnish the amalgam before they begin carving. A large burnisher is used to further condense the amalgam with heavy pressure in faciolingual and mesiodistal directions. Burnishing before carving produces denser amalgam at the margins that enhances their longevity. With most amalgams, carving can be started with care immediately after placement. Working time varies among types of materials. Generally, spherical amalgams set faster and have more strength at an earlier time than admixed amalgams. Finishing and polishing is best done 24 hours or more after the initial placement to allow crystallization within the amalgam to go to completion (see Chapter 9).

> **CLINICAL TIP** Care should be taken when polishing amalgam not to generate heat. Heat over 140° F causes mercury to be released and weakens the surface and margins of the restoration. Do not polish dry. Use low speed and a light touch, particularly with abrasive rubber points and cups.

BONDING AMALGAM

Amalgam is retained in the cavity preparation by parallel walls or undercut walls and by its adaptation to irregularities in the tooth created during preparation. Amalgam placed in this manner simply occupies the space of the cavity preparation and is not bonded to the surrounding tooth structure. Low-copper amalgam expands slightly as it sets and forms corrosion products at the tooth/amalgam interface as it ages. The expansion and corrosion help reduce microleakage at the tooth/amalgam interface. High-copper amalgams shrink slightly during setting and form corrosion products more slowly and to a lesser degree. They tend to have more microleakage ini-

tially, which in some cases can result in transient tooth sensitivity.

More recently, many dentists have been bonding amalgams to the tooth with resin bonding agents. The cavity preparation is etched with phosphoric acid in the same manner as for composite resins. Bonding is done either with one or two bonding resins. In one technique, a bonding agent is applied to enamel and dentin first to establish a resin layer that hybridizes the dentin and seals the dentinal tubules (see Chapter 5). An adhesive resin that is chemical-cured is applied, and the amalgam is condensed directly onto the wet resin. In another technique, a single chemical-cured bonding agent is applied to the cavity preparation before the amalgam is placed. With either technique, the wet resin mechanically intermixes with the amalgam during condensation, and when the resin sets, it bonds the amalgam to the tooth. A seal is created by the resin along the margins, reducing microleakage. Research in the laboratory has shown a slight increase in the strength of the tooth from this procedure, as well as increased retention of the amalgam without undercuts in the preparation. Because healthy tooth structure does not need to be cut away to produce mechanical retention, more conservative cavity preparations can be used.

MERCURY SAFETY PROCEDURES

Mercury is toxic in high levels. Concerns about the safety of amalgam and the mercury it contains should be considered from three aspects: safety of the patient, safety of the dentist and staff, and safety of the environment. The amount of mercury that is released from a set amalgam is very small and has not been shown to be dangerous to patients. However, prudent oral health providers should limit the exposure of their patients to mercury. Mercury can enter the body through ingestion, through direct contact with the skin, and by inhalation of the vapor. When placing or removing amalgam restorations care should be taken to prevent the swallowing of amalgam particles or the inhaling of mercury vapor. The use of the rubber dam and high-volume evacuation will help minimize both.

In some dental offices, the dentists and their staff have been found to have higher levels of mercury than the population in general. Precautions should be taken in the dental office to limit the exposure to the dental team. The Occupational Safety and Health Administration (OSHA) has set an acceptable level of exposure to mercury at 0.005 mg/m^3 for a 40-hour workweek. Because excessive exposure to mercury can cause it to build up in the body faster than it is eliminated, it is prudent to practice good mercury hygiene. Most dental offices comply with mercury hygiene standards, as demonstrated by studies that have shown mercury levels in most dental offices to be far below OSHA's recommended minimum.

Several measures can be taken to minimize mercury exposure by the office staff. Heating of amalgam above 80° C causes the release of free mercury vapor. Instruments contaminated with amalgam should never be heated to this temperature in the operatory. Sterilization rooms must have adequate ventilation to disperse any mercury vapor that may come from the sterilizer during the sterilization process. Operatory floors should have surfaces that are nonporous and easy to clean. Carpets and tiled floors with seams tend to trap amalgam particles and mercury droplets and therefore are not recommended. Gloves, masks, and eye protection should be worn when working around amalgam and mercury. Use of preencapsulated alloy and mercury will minimize handling of mercury and reduce risk of mercury spills. Amalgam scrap should be stored under water in airtight containers. Operatories should be well ventilated. If staff members have concerns about mercury exposure, offices can be monitored for mercury vapor (available through private companies).

Although dental offices do not contribute as much mercury to the environment as large companies, their contribution is not insignificant. Special collection devices are available to collect amalgam particles that might escape into the wastewater. Amalgam scrap that is collected from used capsules, remnants from the amalgam well, and amalgam debris from the high-volume evacuation traps should be appropriately recycled. Commercial firms are available to provide this service.

SOURCES OF OFFICE STAFF EXPOSURE TO MERCURY

- Placing or removing amalgam
- Leaking amalgam capsules (less frequent with factory-sealed capsules)
- Mercury droplets collecting on triturator surfaces
- Sterilizing instruments contaminated with amalgam
- Improper disposal of amalgam capsules and waste
- Improper storage of amalgam scrap
- Amalgam particles in traps within the high-volume evacuation system
- Carpeted operatories or floors with tile or linoleum seams that can collect spilled mercury

---

METHODS FOR MERCURY VAPOR REDUCTION

1. Use amalgam capsules, not bulk alloy and mercury that could spill.
2. Use an amalgamator with a completely enclosed mixing arm.
3. Store amalgam scrap under water in a sealed container. Do not use x-ray fixer for amalgam scrap storage because the fixer is another source of an environmental hazard.
4. Recap used amalgam capsules and dispose of them in a sealed container.
5. Use copious water and high-volume evacuation when removing old amalgam.
6. Use rubber dam whenever possible.
7. Use facemask and shield to avoid splatter and vapors.
8. Use traps or filters (or both) in evacuation systems. Check and clean regularly.
9. Avoid the use of mechanical or ultrasonic condensers. They increase mercury vapor release.
10. Clean up spilled mercury promptly with a commercial spill kit or freshly mixed amalgam. Avoid handling with bare skin. Dispose of in a sealed container (one comes with the kit).
11. Clean instruments of any adherent amalgam before sterilization.
12. Avoid carpeted operatories. Use floor coverings that are nonabsorbent, seamless, and easy to clean.
13. Remove professional protective clothing before leaving the workplace.

MERCURY-FREE AMALGAM

A "mercury-free" metal compound was developed that had an appearance and handling characteristics similar to amalgam. It used gallium as a substitute for mercury. It turned out not to be a good alternative to amalgam because of the relatively high corrosion that occurred in the mouth and the reduced strength as compared with amalgam containing silver, copper, tin, and mercury. The expansion of the gallium-containing alloy was thought to contribute to the high number of tooth fractures seen with this material. These products are still used in some countries but not in the United States.

Casting Alloys

ALL-METAL CASTINGS

In the early 1900s Taggart developed a technique for making dental restorations from metal that was melted and cast into a mold using the lost wax technique (see Chapter 15). Pure metals are seldom used in dentistry, because they are weaker than when they are combined with other metals. Alloys used with the lost wax technique are called dental casting alloys (alloys are composed of two or more metals.) Unlike amalgam, restorations made from these alloys are not placed directly into the preparation but are made outside the mouth using the indirect technique and cemented in place (see Chapters 6 and 13). Cast-metal restorations can be classified as either intracoronal (preparation is made within the crown of the tooth) or extracoronal (preparation is made primarily on the outside of the crown of the tooth). An inlay is an intracoronal restoration, whereas an onlay has both intracoronal and extracoronal components in that it has an inlay preparation and also covers the outer surface of one or more cusps. Other extracoronal cast restorations include partial coverage (3/4 and 7/8 crowns) and full coverage crowns (Figure 8-4). Cast metal alloys can also be used to make fixed partial dentures (bridges) and removable partial dentures for replacement of missing teeth.

Gold Dental Casting Alloys   Dental casting alloys have been classified by the American Dental Association as **high noble alloys, noble alloys,** and **base metal alloys.** A noble alloy is one that does not corrode very readily in the oral environment. Gold

(chemical symbol Au) is the most corrosion resistant of the noble metals and has been used in dentistry for centuries. Gold alloy is classified by its gold content as karats (also spelled carats), percentage, or fineness (obtained by multiplying percentage of gold by 10). Pure gold is 24 karat, 100%, or 1000 fine, and half gold is 12 karat, 50%, or 500 fine. Pure gold has limited use in dentistry today but is used in the form of gold foil by a small number of dentists for direct-placement restorations. Pure gold is too soft to use for dental castings, but gold alloys have excellent properties and handling characteristics. Dental gold casting alloys can be classified by their hardness (resistance to penetration), malleability (ability to be shaped as by tapping or pounding), and ductility (ability to be elongated as by stretching or pulling) (Table 8-2). The more ductile the alloy, the more the margins can be burnished (pushing the metal at the margins to close gaps between the restoration and the tooth).

Other Noble Metals for Casting Alloys   Other noble metals include platinum (Pt) and palladium (Pd). Platinum is not used much because of its expense, high melting point, and difficulty mixing

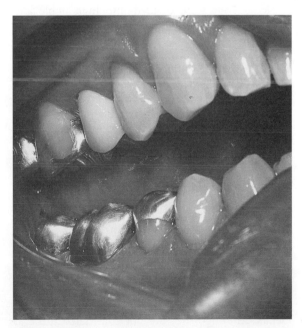

FIGURE 8-4 ■ Partial- and full-coverage cast gold restorations.

TABLE 8-2
Classification of Gold Alloys

Characteristic	Class I	Class II	Class III	Class IV
Hardness	Soft	Medium	Hard	Extra hard
Use	Inlays (not in heavy function)	Inlays, crowns	Inlays, crowns, bridges	Partial denture framework, bridges
Yield strength (amount of stress at which alloy deforms)	Low	Medium	High	High
Wear resistance	Low	Medium	High	High

with gold. Palladium is used widely because it has good corrosion resistance, increases hardness of the alloy, and was less expensive than gold. (Palladium alloys have greatly increased in price due to shortages in the supply of palladium. Currently, it is more expensive than gold.) These noble metals are sometimes referred to as **precious metals** because of their high monetary value. Although silver (Ag) is considered to be a precious metal, it is not considered noble because of its corrosion in the oral cavity.

Noble metals are divided into high noble and noble depending on the percentage of noble elements present. To be in the high noble class they must contain at least 60% noble elements (Au, Pd, and Pt), of which 40% must be gold. Base metals make up the remaining 40%. Noble class alloys contain at least 25% noble elements with no requirement for gold, and the remaining 75% consists of base metals. Because of the lower cost of the metals used in this class, they also have been referred to as *semiprecious* alloys.

Base Metal Dental Casting Alloys The base metal class of dental casting alloys consists of less than 25% noble metals. The primary base metals used in casting alloys are copper (Cu), nickel (Ni), Silver (Ag), zinc (Zn), tin (Sn), and titanium (Ti). Copper and silver are often added to gold alloys to increase their hardness. Zinc is added to reduce oxidation when the alloy is cast. Because of their low cost, base metals have also been called *nonprecious* metals. Although they are not considered to be as good as the noble metals, the base metals are essential for many applications in dentistry. The stiffness

(modulus of elasticity) of base alloys is twice as great as gold-based alloys, so it takes twice the stress to deform them. This property is especially important for use in partial denture frameworks. Drawbacks of base metals include their higher casting temperatures that require different equipment and investing materials than the gold-based alloys and their potential biocompatibility problems. They are much harder than noble metals, making them difficult to cut and to finish. Other base metals used for casting removable prostheses are discussed later in this chapter (see Removable Prosthetic Casting Alloys).

Crystal Formation (Grains) After casting alloys have been melted and cast into the mold, they cool and form crystals (also called grains). Small crystals produce more desirable properties in the metal alloy than large crystals. Some elements such as iridium or ruthenium are added to gold-base alloys to keep the crystals from growing too large. Reheating gold-based alloys (called annealing) can improve some of the properties. However, with base metal alloys reheating will degrade the physical properties.

PORCELAIN BONDING ALLOYS

Porcelain bonding alloys are essentially the same as the other casting alloys with similar physical properties. They are also classified as high noble, noble, and base metal alloys. However, they have minor changes in their composition to make them compatible with dental porcelains. The metals in porcelain bonding alloys are selected and blended so that they have the ability to withstand the high temperatures at which porcelain is fired without distorting or melting. Additionally, small amounts of metals such as indium and tin are added to form the oxides on the metal surface to which the porcelain will bond at high temperature. Alloys that contain silver and copper may cause green staining of the porcelain when fired at high temperatures.

Porcelain-bonded-to-metal crowns have a metal substructure that is covered with layers of porcelain. For porcelain to bond to these metals, after the substructure is cast in metal it is heated at high temperature to form oxides on the surface of the metal. An opaque layer of porcelain is placed (stacked) over the metal to keep the dark color from showing through the porcelain (see Chapter 6, Figure 6-13). The oxidized metal and porcelain are heated at high temperatures (850° to 1350° C depending on the type of porcelain used), and the porcelain chemically fuses to the oxide layer. Then additional layers of porcelain called body and incisal porcelains are built up or stacked to simulate dentin and enamel colors and translucency. They are fired in the oven until they fuse to each other and to the metal. The metal and porcelain must have compatible rates of thermal expansion or the porcelain will crack as it and the metal cool.

REMOVABLE PROSTHETIC CASTING ALLOYS

At one time type IV gold alloys were the main metals used for partial denture frameworks. However, they became quite expensive as the price of gold climbed after deregulation of gold prices in 1969. The metals used today are mostly base metal alloys with or without minor amounts of noble elements (see Figure 13-5 in Chapter 13). These base metals include nickel, titanium, chromium, aluminum, cobalt, vanadium, iron, beryllium, molybdenum, gallium, and carbon. The most common base metal alloys are chrome-cobalt and nickel-chrome. It is the chromium content that gives these metals their corrosion resistance.

Because these metals are very hard and quite difficult to cast, they require special casting machines and are cast by commercial dental laboratories. Other metals may be used for attachments for prostheses such as attachment bars between tooth abutments (see Figure 8-9 later in this chapter), overdenture attachments, and precision and nonprecision attachments for partial dentures. These attachments are made from high noble, noble, or base metals. Attachments are used more frequently with the increasing use of combinations of implants and removable partial or complete denture combinations.

BIOCOMPATIBILITY

Noble metals are more biocompatible with the oral tissues, because they tend to corrode less than base metals. As metals corrode they lose metal corrosion products to the oral cavity. Some of these products are responsible for allergic responses. Of the base metals, nickel has the highest incidence of allergic response. Women have a higher rate of allergy to nickel than do males by a ratio of 10 to 1. A prior exposure to nickel in jewelry is thought to be the likely source of the exposure that sensitizes women to nickel. The overall allergy rate to nickel for the general population is about 9% to 12%. The allergic response is sometimes seen around the free gingival tissues, especially at the margins of base metal crowns. It is less common for removable partial dentures because the metal is often not in direct contact with the tissues and they are not worn constantly as with fixed partial dentures or single crowns. Some responses to nickel cause a skin reaction rather than a response in the mouth even though the oral cavity is the source of the nickel.

Beryllium is a base metal added to nickel-chrome alloys to reduce the fusion temperature for easier casting and to improve physical properties by creating smaller metal crystals when the molten metal cools after casting. Beryllium may also cause allergic responses in susceptible individuals. Laboratory technicians are at risk to nickel and beryllium exposure when casting, grinding, and polishing these metals. Inhalation of beryllium is known to contribute to a lung disease called berylliosis.

Solders

GOLD SOLDERS

Solders are alloys that are used to join metals together or repair cast restorations. Solders used in crown and bridgework are generally gold-based alloys. Gold-based solders are used to join together units of a bridge, add contacts, close holes ground in the occlusal surface by adjusting the bite, or correct small marginal deficiencies on onlays and crowns when they are found to be deficient at the try-in appointment. Gold-based solder is often categorized according to the fineness. The higher the fineness number, the higher the gold content and the lower the melting point of the solder. This is important when soldering two gold castings together or adding a contact to a gold crown, because the solder must melt before the casting. To solder two units of a bridge together, they first must be invested in a special gypsum soldering investment in the proper relationship to each other (see Chapter 12). A flux is applied to the alloy surfaces to be soldered. The flux removes surface oxides so that the solder will flow freely and wet the alloy surfaces as it melts. Flux for gold alloys usually contains borax. The alloys are heated with a torch until they turn red. The solder is added and heated until it melts and flows over the exposed surfaces of the bridge units. Often a contact can be added to a single crown without investing it by holding it over a Bunsen burner.

SILVER SOLDERS

Silver-based solders are used more in orthodontics and pediatric dentistry to solder fixed-space maintainer components (wire loop soldered to an orthodontic band) and to solder wire components to removable orthodontic appliances. Tin is often added to the solder to lower the melting range and improve the flow of the molten metal. Silver solder is selected because it produces a stronger joint than gold solder. Additionally, the heat required to melt gold solder, being greater than that for silver solder, sometimes will degrade the wire adjacent to the solder joint and weaken it.

Wrought Metal Alloys

Wrought metal alloys are different from the casting alloys in that they are formed after the metal is cast. Usually the metal is drawn or extruded through a die or formed in a press to the desired shape, such as a flat plate or a wire or a knife or other instrument shape. So wrought alloys are alloys that have been mechanically changed into

another form. The result is an alloy that is harder and has a greater **yield strength** (point at which a force can create permanent deformation of the metal). Wrought metal has the characteristic of being able to be heat modified, or **annealed,** to create differing resistance to deformity. However, overheating can degrade the properties of the metal.

WIRE

Wire is a wrought metal that may be soft and easily shaped or may resist bending as does a spring. Various degrees of resistance to bending can be created by annealing. Wrought metal is used in removable prosthetic appliances primarily for clasps. It can be either a base metal such as stainless steel or a high noble alloy composed of platinum-gold-palladium (called PGP wire). Stainless steel is composed of iron and carbon with traces of nickel, chromium, and manganese. The addition of the metals other than iron and carbon gives the steel its ability to resist tarnish and rust. Additional examples of wrought wire used in dentistry include arch wires and ligature (tie) wires used in orthodontics and arch bars and ligature wires used in oral surgery for stabilization of a jaw fracture.

ENDODONTIC FILES AND REAMERS

Endodontic files and reamers are other examples of wrought metal used in dentistry. They are made of wrought wire that has been twisted to produce multiple cutting edges (Figure 8-5). Files are made of either stainless steel or nickel-titanium and are used within the root canal to clean and shape it for final filling. Although the nickel-titanium file is far more flexible than the stainless steel file, the stainless steel is sharper and shapes the walls of the canal more easily. Reamers are similar to files except that they have fewer twists in the metal and cut faster.

Metals Used in Orthodontics

WIRES

Orthodontic wires are composed mostly of base metals. They are commonly made of stainless steel,

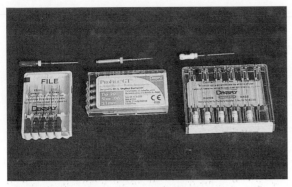

FIGURE 8-5 ■ Variety of endodontic files.

cobalt-chrome-nickel, titanium, or an alloy of titanium and nickel.

As described previously, all arch wires are of the wrought wire variety. Special characteristics are manufactured into these arch wires to create the desired amount of resistance to deformity. The resistance to deformity creates "memory" in the wire so that it tries to reassume its original shape. It is the "memory" that exerts the forces that move the teeth. Stainless steel wire can be bent easily by the dentist. Other wires, such as Nitinol, are nickel-titanium. They are resilient and springy, maintain their shape, and cannot be bent easily at chairside.

The orthodontist will order wires either preformed or in tubes of several straight wires in different lengths and diameters. The diameter of wire is sometimes referred to as **gauge.** The thicker the wire, the smaller its gauge; thus 8-gauge wire is thicker than 16-gauge wire. The diameter of wire is more commonly described in hundredths of an inch (e.g., 0.36 inch). Most orthodontic wires are supplied using the inch diameter classification, although some manufacturers, particularly in Europe, use millimeters as the unit of measure.

BRACKETS AND BANDS

Orthodontic brackets and bands are bonded or cemented on the teeth, and they retain the arch wire that the orthodontist has shaped. The arch wire is shaped into a form that will guide the teeth into their new position. When the wire is tied to the brackets of the teeth the wire tries to assume its ideal form and as a result exerts a force on the teeth that gradually moves them in the desired direction. The arch wire is held to the bracket or band by ligature wire or elastics. Metal orthodontic brackets are cut and shaped from stainless steel alloy and attached to a stainless mesh backing (see Chapter 5, Figure 5-19). They are bonded to the tooth with bonding resin that locks into the mesh backing (see Chapter 5). The edgewise bracket is the most common and has a horizontal slot between four wings. The slot is where the arch wire is placed, and the wings are used to hold the elastics or ligature wire that secures the arch wire. Orthodontic bands are formed from a stainless steel alloy and are preformed or formed at chairside by the dentist. Stainless steel brackets and tubes are welded onto the band or brackets for the purpose of attaching intraoral or extraoral appliances.

LINGUAL RETAINER

A fixed lingual retainer is often placed to help maintain the position of the teeth after orthodontic treatment. It provides long-term stabilization of the anterior teeth. It is often simply a wire adapted to the lingual surfaces of the mandibular anterior teeth and bonded in place with composite resin (Figure 8-6). Occasionally, a similar retainer is used on the palatal surfaces of the maxillary anterior teeth. It may be shortened to include only the maxillary central incisors if its purpose is merely to prevent a midline diastema from reforming after orthodontic closure.

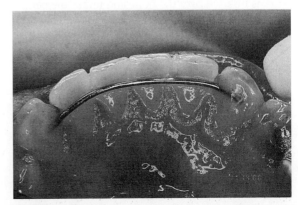

FIGURE 8-6 ■ Orthodontic bonded wire retainer.

Implant Materials

Implant metals have been used in orthopedic medicine for many years and more recently in dentistry. Implants are used as anchors for prosthetic replacement of missing teeth. Their use is expanding as implant materials and techniques continue to improve, and their success rate remains high (90% or more) with careful case selection. Implants can be used to replace one or more single units as individual crowns or as fixed bridges, or they can support a full denture. In the mandible, atrophy (loss through resorption of the bone) of the alveolar ridge is common in patients who have lost teeth at a relatively young age. A complete denture often has very little retention in this circumstance. Implants can help retain and stabilize the denture. Implants are of three main types: subperiosteal, transosteal, and endosteal (Figure 8-7).

SUBPERIOSTEAL IMPLANTS

Subperiosteal implants are placed under the periosteum (a fibrous covering of the bone) and rest on the bone. They are constructed and placed in three stages. First, a surgical incision is made to expose the bony ridge by reflecting the soft tissue and periosteum overlying the bone. An impression is made of the exposed bone. The surgical wound is closed. Second, a metal framework is cast in the laboratory to fit over the bone. It has metal projections on which the prosthesis will be attached that extend through the tissues covering the ridge. Third, a second incision is made to reopen the initial wound and once again expose the bone. The implant framework is inserted over the bone and under the periosteum. The overlying tissues are sutured closed with the metal projections for the prosthesis protruding into the oral cavity. This type of implant is most common in the mandible.

TRANSOSTEAL IMPLANTS

The **transosteal implant** (also called a mandibular staple) is used to support a mandibular denture when the patient has severe resorption and lacks enough support for endosseous or subperiosteal implants. It consists of a horizontal support beam attached to metal rods that are inserted into holes drilled all the way through the mandible from its

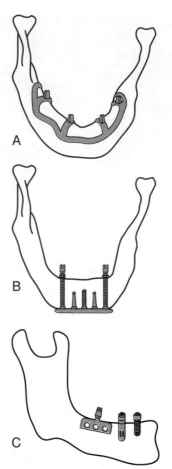

FIGURE 8-7 ■ Implant types. **A,** Subperiosteal. **B,** Transosteal. **C,** Endosteal.

superior border to the inferior border. A metal plate through which the ends of the rods pass is bolted to the underside of the mandible. A transosteal implant requires both intraoral and extraoral incisions for its placement and stabilization. It is seldom used because of its highly invasive nature.

ENDOSSEOUS IMPLANTS

Endosseous (endosteal) implants are surgically placed into the bone. These are the most popular implants currently in use and will be the focus of the implant discussion. Over the years a variety of endosseous implant designs and materials have been used. Today these implants are typically cylinders of various configurations depending on the manufacturer and may include surface irregularities, screw-like threads, or a hollow core with or without holes through its sides. The expectation is that these designs will help the integration of the implant with the bone. Titanium and titanium alloys are the metals most commonly used because of their favorable biocompatibility with the oral tissues. Bone will grow around titanium implants (a process called **osseointegration**) intimately enough to retain them. Pure titanium is not as rigid or strong as titanium alloy, and this property can occasionally lead to failure of the implant if it is placed under heavy loading forces (such as with patients who grind their teeth a lot). Pure titanium quickly forms a thin surface layer of oxides that will integrate with the bone. Some implant metals may have a surface coating of a thin layer of calcium phosphate (in the form of hydroxyapatite) or plasma proteins to enhance osseointegration.

Other materials that have been used for dental implants are ceramics, composites, and polymers. These materials have been used with limited success. One of the negative aspects of the ceramic type is its lack of flexibility, and thus it can transmit greater stress to the implant site.

ENDOSSEOUS IMPLANT PLACEMENT AND RESTORATION

The surgical procedures are done in two stages. The first stage involves exposing the bone at the chosen placement site with a surgical flap. Next a hole is drilled in the bone that is the shape and length of the implant cylinder and a size that is just slightly smaller than the cylinder. When the implant is lightly tapped into place it will have a frictional fit with the bone. Often an acrylic resin surgical guide (called a stent) is made ahead of time with holes drilled through it at the same angulation at which the implant should be positioned. The surgeon places it over the ridge at the time of surgery and inserts a bone-cutting bur through the predetermined holes to cut the hole for the implant at the correct angulation. The stent is particularly helpful when the surgeon has to place several implants that all need to be parallel to each other for purposes of the restoration that will be placed on the implants. It is important that excessive heat not be generated during the drilling of the bone.

The bone can easily be damaged and then will not integrate with the implant cylinder (also called a fixture).

Restoration of the single-tooth implant is usually with a prosthetic crown that is attached to the implant core by means of a small screw often made of gold alloy (Figure 8-8). If the screws are not tightened properly, they may come out. If they are tightened too much, the metal of the screw might be strained to the point of breaking. Special wrenches called torque wrenches are set to deliver the recommended amount of force to tighten the screws. Some implant designs use frictional fit or cement to retain the crown. Implant crowns retained by the latter two methods tend to come off more frequently.

Implants can be used to support a removable prosthesis when there is inadequate alveolar ridge (Figure 8-9). They can also be used to anchor a prosthesis to replace missing facial parts lost to trauma or cancer surgery (see Chapter 13, Figure 13-10).

MAINTENANCE

In addition to its interface with the bone, the implant has an interface with the soft tissues where it protrudes through the gingiva or mucosa. Although there are no connective tissue fibers (i.e., periodontal ligament or junctional epithelium) connecting to the implant surface as there are to the cementum on the root surface of a natural tooth, there is a close adaptation and attachment of the sulcular epithelium to the implant surface. This close adaptation helps develop a biologic seal that prevents microorganisms from invading the tissues. The implant surface can accumulate bacterial plaque and calculus just as teeth do. The tissues surrounding the implant (peri-implant tissues) will become inflamed much like the gingiva around teeth. If not controlled, this inflammation and bacterial invasion can progress into the bone surrounding the implant and contribute to its failure. It is critically important to the success of the implant that the patient employs meticulous oral hygiene techniques and works with the dentist and dental hygienist to implement an effective tissue management program. The dental hygienist plays an integral role in helping the patient maintain the health of the implants and in reinforcing home care techniques. Likewise, the dental assistant can reinforce

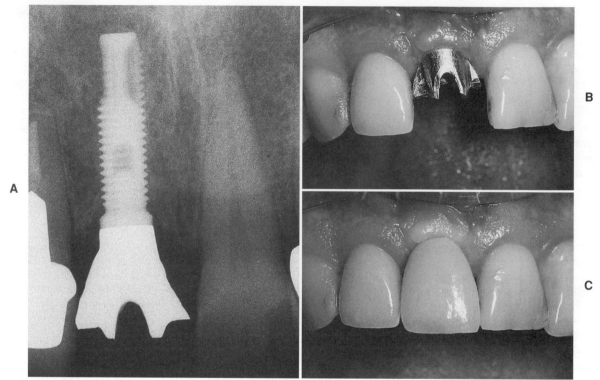

FIGURE 8-8 ■ Single-tooth implant. **A,** Radiograph of implant fixture in bone. **B,** Abutment member to which the crown is attached. **C,** Crown attached to implant.
(Courtesy Dr. Mark Dellinger, University of California School of Dentistry, San Francisco, Calif.)

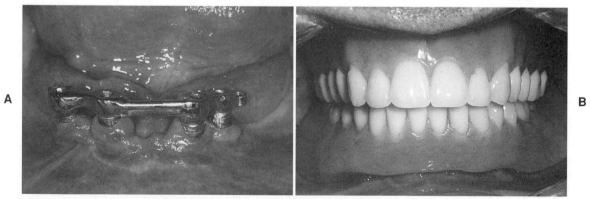

FIGURE 8-9 ■ Implant-supported denture. **A,** Implants supporting a connector bar onto which a lower denture will attach. Implants were used because the ridge had resorbed and was inadequate to retain the denture. **B,** Lower denture supported by the implants. A clip inside the denture slides over the bar (A) to retain the denture.
(Courtesy Dr. Mark Dellinger, University of California School of Dentistry, San Francisco, Calif.)

oral hygiene techniques when the patient comes in for periodic examinations or treatment.

HOME CARE

The number and type of implants and the prostheses used for restoration will vary from patient to patient. Therefore it is important to customize the home care regimen for each patient. Home care aids that are beneficial to patients with implants include a variety of each of the following: disclosing agents, brushes, flosses, wooden plaque removers, and antibacterial agents.

Disclosing Agents   Plaque-disclosing agents can help patients visualize the location of plaque in difficult to reach areas. These agents should be used daily for the first few weeks until the patient becomes more proficient in keeping the implants clean, then periodically to check on effectiveness of hygiene techniques. The patient should be given a disposable mouth mirror to help visualize all areas of the mouth. Adequate lighting is important also.

Brushes   Soft-bristled brushes should be used to avoid scratching the implants. Gentle sulcular brushing is recommended to help maintain peri-implant tissues. Brushes will also need to be positioned at a variety of angles in order to clean around and under the prosthesis. Selection of brushes will depend in part on the number and spacing of the implants. For single-tooth implants, as well as implant-supported fixed bridges, interproximal brushes are helpful for reaching between the implant and the adjacent tooth or pontic. Interproximal brushes that have plastic coating on the wire holding the bristles together are recommended to avoid scratching the implant (Figure 8-10). End-tuft brushes can be helpful when the space between implants is greater than practical for interproximal brushes (Figure 8-11). Most brushes with plastic handles can have the angulation of the brush head altered by heating the handle in hot water and bending it to the desired angle. Patients who have problems with manual dexterity because of arthritis, stroke, or other medical problems can use power brushes. Rotary brushes with bristles forming a point are useful for reaching between implants that are spaced far apart. If a dentifrice is used, one should be selected that is not abrasive.

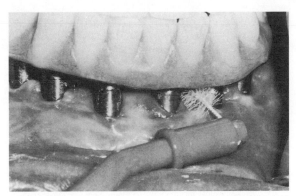

FIGURE 8-10 ■ Interproximal brush used to clean implant. (Reprinted by permission from *Endosteal dental implants*, St Louis, 1991, Mosby, Figure 31-7, p. 404.)

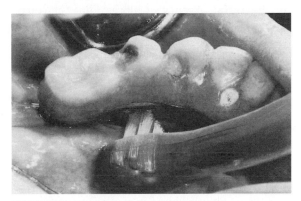

FIGURE 8-11 ■ End-tuft brush used to clean implant. (Reprinted by permission from *Endosteal dental implants*, St Louis, 1991, Mosby, Figure 31-6, p. 404.)

Flosses   A variety of flosses is available. Regular-thickness floss, dental tape, flossing cord, knitting yarn, twill tape (from fabric stores), gauze strips, and fuzzy-type floss with threader (Superfloss) all have applications for plaque removal, depending on the nature of the implants and the overlying prosthesis (Figure 8-12). Floss threaders are helpful to carry floss under prostheses such as complete dentures or fixed bridges, particularly where access is difficult.

Wooden Plaque Removers   Balsa wood triangular sticks and toothpicks can be used with care to aid in plaque removal. These items will not scratch the implants.

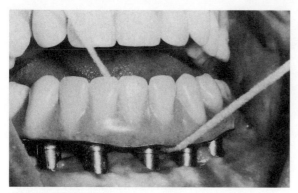

FIGURE 8-12 ■ Superfloss used to clean dental implant. (Reprinted by permission from *Endosteal dental implants,* St Louis, 1991, Mosby, Figure 31-13, page 407.)

Antibacterial Agents   Chlorhexidine gluconate solution is an effective antibacterial agent. It should be used as a rinse for about a week following the second surgical stage when the implant is uncovered. It is also useful to use when inflammation is found in peri-implant tissues after placement of the prosthesis. It is often used as a 30-second twice-daily rinse for 1 to 2 weeks. It can also be applied directly to the problem site on an interproximal brush, end-tuft brush, or cotton swab. Frequent use of chlorhexidine will cause brown staining of the prosthesis and natural teeth. An alternative antibacterial agent that is beneficial in controlling gingivitis but is not as effective as chlorhexidine is a phenolic compound (Listerine) (see Chapter 7). Oral irrigation may be used to deliver the antibacterial solutions, but it should be used at low pressure and not directed into the sulcus. If it is used at too high a pressure, damage to the biologic seal with the epithelium may occur.

HYGIENE VISIT

The patient should return to the dental office at 3- to 4-month intervals for routine implant assessment and maintenance. At the maintenance visit the review of the health history and vital signs and examination of extraoral and intraoral structures are conducted in the same manner as for patients without implants; however, questions specific to implants should be asked, such as implant mobility, soreness, bleeding of peri-implant tissues, and looseness of the prosthesis. The dentist may request peri-

HOME CARE AIDS FOR IMPLANT PATIENTS

Brushes
- Regular soft-bristled toothbrush
- Interproximal brush with plastic-coated wire
- End-tuft brush
- Power brushes: standard or rotary with pointed brush tip

Flosses
- Regular floss or tape
- Yarn or Superfloss
- Cord
- Twill tape
- Gauze strips

Wooden Sticks
- Balsa wood sticks (StimuDents)
- Toothpicks

Antibacterial Agents
- Chlorhexidine solution
- Phenolic compound rinse (Listerine)

odic radiographs to check the bone level surrounding the implants. The hygienist should perform a visual inspection of the peri-implant soft tissues to evaluate for edema (swelling), erythema (redness), bleeding, and other indications of inflammation. Problem areas can be pointed out to the patient, and a review of oral hygiene techniques should be done. If the patient has a particular problem area, alternative cleaning aids and techniques can be recommended. Routine probing is not recommended. When probing of the peri-implant sulcus is done to check the status of an implant, it should be done with a light touch and a plastic probe so as not to disturb the biologic seal and scratch the implant surface.

Recent improvements in single-tooth implants have eliminated exposed metal by covering it with porcelain from the implant crown. In these situations conventional metal curettes and scalers can be used. However, when titanium is exposed, special scaling instruments should be used to avoid damage to the surface of the implant (Figure 8-13). Plastic or graphite curettes and scalers or metal instruments

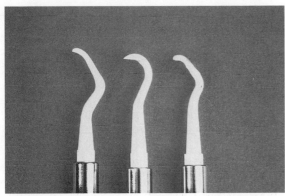

FIGURE 8-13 ■ Plastic scaling instruments for implants. (Courtesy Hu-Friedy Mfg. Company, Inc.)

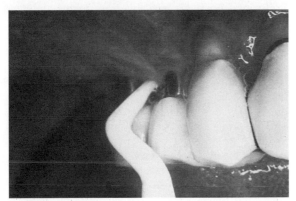

FIGURE 8-14 ■ Use of plastic scaler around posterior implants. (Courtesy Hu-Friedy Mfg. Company, Inc.)

with a Teflon or gold coating are recommended (Figure 8-14). Prophylaxis pastes with coarse or medium grit should not be used on titanium. Even very fine paste can produce some surface scratches on the implant. If polishing is deemed necessary, tin oxide in a rubber cup applied with light pressure may be used. Conventional steel curettes, ultrasonic scalers, and air polishers are not indicated for use against titanium surfaces.

IMPLANT FAILURE

Early failure of an implant is usually due to a failure of the bone to integrate with the implant. Lack of integration can be due to poor surgical technique, with generation of excessive heat when drilling the implant hole in the bone; infection of the implant site; poor quality of bone; or placing loading forces on the implant too soon. Failure of the implant that occurs after the initial integration is usually caused by bacterial infection extending from the peri-implant tissues into the bone or overloading the implant during function, leading to loss of the supporting bone.

Endodontic Posts

Teeth in which the pulpal tissues are infected or die often receive root canal therapy (endodontic treatment). Conventional root canal therapy generally entails making an access preparation through the crown of the tooth to the pulp chamber, removing the diseased pulpal tissue from within the root canal with a series of fine files, and sealing the root canal space with a special sealer (gutta percha) so that bacteria cannot grow in the space.

PURPOSE

Posts are metal or nonmetal dowels or rods placed within the root canal space after a root canal treatment. It once was believed that posts reinforced endodontically treated teeth against fracture, and many posts were placed for this purpose. However, it is now clear that the purpose of a post is to retain the core buildup over which the final restoration (crown) is placed. If there is adequate tooth structure remaining to hold the core buildup without a post, a post should not be used. Although the choice of using posts or other retaining designs is up to the dentist, it is important for all clinicians to be familiar with the various types of posts that might be used. Dental assistants and hygienists are often asked questions by patients about the materials they see in their teeth on the radiographs mounted on the view box. Some patients may confuse the post with an implant and need to be educated as to the differences.

CLASSIFICATION

It is beyond the purpose of this section to discuss retention and post design, but basically posts can be classified as active or passive. **Active posts** engage the root canal surface with threads, and **passive posts** are simply cemented into the canal space without engaging the canal walls. Posts can also be classified by their shape: parallel or tapered. Parallel posts have been shown by in vitro studies (meaning they were not conducted in living creatures but were done in the laboratory) to transmit less stress to the root than tapered posts. Posts can be made of metal or can be nonmetal (Table 8-3). Posts can be custom

---

TABLE 8-3 ▮
Composition of Posts

Custom-Cast Posts

Nickel-chromium alloy (Ni-Cr)
Cobalt-chromium alloy (Co-Cr)
Gold alloy (ADA type IV)
Palladium-silver alloy

Preformed Posts

METAL
Titanium (99% pure)
Stainless steel (Fe-Ni-Cr)
Titanium-aluminum-vanadium alloy (Ti-Al-V)

NONMETAL
Ceramic (Zirconia)
Fiber-reinforced resin

---

made in the laboratory or can be purchased preformed in various sizes and materials.

CUSTOM POSTS

Custom posts are made from a wax or resin pattern made directly on the tooth or made in the laboratory on a replica of the preparation (a die) poured from an impression of the tooth. Custom posts are cast into metal or ceramic using the lost wax technique. Noble or base metal alloys or ceramic-fired materials are used. Cast posts generally are made with the core already attached.

PREFORMED POSTS

Preformed posts are available from many commercial sources and are by far the most commonly used posts (Figure 8-15). The designs of these preformed posts are active or passive, parallel or tapered, and metal or nonmetal. They rely on retention by their length, diameter, and shape and by use of a cementing or bonding medium. (See Chapters 5 and 10 for discussions of bonding and cementing materials.) The preformed posts come in kits with drills specific to the size and style of the post. Preformed metal posts are made of stainless steel, titanium, or titanium alloy. Preformed nonmetal posts are made of fiber-

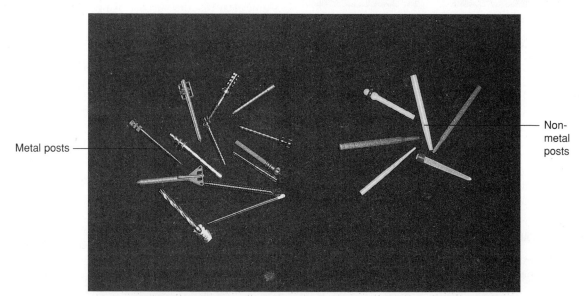

Metal posts —

— Non-metal posts

FIGURE 8-15 ▮ Variety of preformed metal and nonmetal posts.

reinforced resin or ceramic materials. Preformed posts generally do not have a core attached by the manufacturer, so one must be added. The core can be made of amalgam, composite resin, or hybrid glass ionomer.

SUMMARY

Metals play a major role in restorative and corrective dentistry. Amalgam is still an economical and useful restorative material, although composite resins are gaining in popularity and their physical properties are constantly being improved. Gold and alloys of gold are some of the most biologically compatible materials and have many uses, even with the shift toward cosmetic dentistry. Noble and nonnoble metals have a significant role in modern prosthetic dentistry. They are the main support for removable partial dentures, fixed bridges, and prostheses used in combination with implants. Implants are increasing in use, and the titanium implants are enjoying a high degree of success. Titanium is lightweight and has the best characteristics of strength and elasticity of any of the implant materials currently available. However, care must be taken when providing periodontal preventive care around titanium fixtures to prevent scratching their surfaces. Orthodontic treat-ment relies heavily on the use of metal. Brackets are predominantly metal, although some are ceramic. Wrought wire, with its "memory," exerts predictable forces and has made the job of the orthodontic clinician easier, improved comfort for the patient, and reduced the time of treatment. Endodontic treatment has moved into the new millennium with the use of titanium files and the controlled speed of the electric handpiece. Likewise, the restoration of endodontically treated teeth and the use of post and core materials have changed dramatically. There are now both metal and nonmetal posts available for the dentist to select for the process of restoring endodontically treated teeth. The indications for each are important for the clinician to understand.

Patient education is an important aspect of the role of the dental assistant and dental hygienist in dental practice. The ability to describe to the patient the pros and cons of the various materials used in practice and to aid in the treatment process depends on your knowledge of these materials. As new metal-based materials are introduced into dental practice, it is important to stay current on their indications, contraindications, and application techniques. Manufacturers' instructions for their care and use should also be followed. Many manufacturers have Web sites on which they post information relative to their materials.

CHAPTER REVIEW

Select the one correct response for each of the following multiple-choice questions:

1. In the amalgam restoration, which of the following elements has the most effect on corrosion reduction?
   a. Silver (Ag)
   b. Mercury (Hg)
   c. Copper (Cu)
   d. Iron (Fe)

2. In the amalgam restoration the two main components are
   a. Silver and copper
   b. Copper and tin
   c. Silver and mercury
   d. Mercury and zinc

3. Why should all remnants of amalgam be removed from the placement instruments before they are autoclaved?
   a. The steam causes the amalgam to fuse to the stainless steel.
   b. Amalgam corrosion products produced by the steam are toxic.
   c. The heat causes mercury vapor to be released from the amalgam.
   d. The heat melts the silver component and it will clog the drain of the autoclave.

4. **The strength of the amalgam restoration can be affected by**
   a. Overtrituration
   b. Undertrituration
   c. Corrosion
   d. All of the above

5. **A properly mixed amalgam should appear**
   a. Dry and crumbly
   b. Soupy and shiny
   c. As a homogeneous mass with a slight shine
   d. Liquidlike and should pour easily out of the capsule

6. **Scrap amalgam should be**
   a. Autoclaved before sending it to the recycler
   b. Thrown in the incinerator
   c. Stored under water in a sealed container
   d. Put into the general nonmedical waste

7. **With high-copper alloys, which metal reacts with the copper to reduce gamma-2 phase corrosion?**
   a. Tin
   b. Zinc
   c. Silver
   d. Lead

8. **The fact that mercury makes up almost half of the amalgam has caused concerns about**
   a. Its safety for patient use
   b. Risks to the office staff
   c. Environmental effects of improper disposal of amalgam waste
   d. All of the above

9. **Amalgam has been popular for restoration of carious teeth because**
   a. It is economical
   b. It has excellent physical properties
   c. It is easy to manipulate
   d. All of the above

10. **Bonding an amalgam during the placement of a restoration**
    a. Keeps it from corroding
    b. Prevents tarnish
    c. Seals the margins and reduces microleakage
    d. Increases postoperative sensitivity

11. **How does tarnish differ from corrosion?**
    a. Tarnish occurs only on the surface.
    b. Tarnish is more harmful to the restoration than corrosion.
    c. Tarnish contributes to the destructive effects seen in the gamma-2 phase.
    d. Tarnish cannot be removed by polishing, whereas corrosion can.

12. **A gold alloy that is 50% gold has how many karats?**
    a. 24
    b. 18
    c. 14
    d. 12

13. **The ADA recognizes which three major categories of alloys?**
    a. High noble, noble, low noble
    b. High noble, noble, base metal
    c. Precious, semiprecious, and nonprecious
    d. Class I, II, and III

14. **High noble metal classification must contain what percent by weight of gold?**
    a. 40%
    b. 60%
    c. 75%
    d. 90%

15. **Noble metal elements include all of the following EXCEPT:**
    a. Silver
    b. Gold
    c. Palladium
    d. Platinum

16. **Porcelain bonding alloys form oxides on their surface that chemically bond with the porcelain at high temperatures. Which of the following metals may be added to the alloys to help form these oxides?**
    a. Indium or tin
    b. Silver or copper
    c. Cobalt or chromium
    d. Lead or beryllium

17. **Metal that is formed by casting into an ingot or bar and then altered in its form is known as**
    a. Stainless steel
    b. Wrought metal
    c. Milled metal
    d. Transformed metal

18. **High noble alloys usually have which metals added to increase their strength?**
    a. Silver or copper
    b. Nickel or beryllium
    c. Iron or aluminum
    d. Chromium or cobalt

19. **Which type of orthodontic wire is more difficult to adapt as an arch wire because of its springiness and tendency to maintain its original shape?**
    a. Stainless steel
    b. Cobalt-chrome nickel
    c. Gold
    d. Nickel-titanium

20. **Allergy to nickel**
    a. Occurs in less than 3% of the population
    b. Is only seen in the oral cavity
    c. Occurs 10 times more often in women than men
    d. Is associated more often with partial-denture frameworks than with crowns

21. **Solder has all of the following uses EXCEPT:**
    a. Adding a contact to a crown
    b. Joining a pontic to a bridge retainer
    c. Repairing a hole in the occlusal surface of a crown discovered at the periodic oral examination
    d. Joining a wire loop to a band to make a space retainer

22. **The purpose of a flux used during soldering is to**
    a. Lower the melting point of the solder
    b. Make the solder harden quickly
    c. Prevent the solder from flowing to areas where the solder is not needed
    d. Remove oxides from the surfaces of the metals to be soldered so the solder can flow and wet the surfaces better

23. **The most common metal used in implants is**
    a. Gold
    b. Silver
    c. Stainless steel
    d. Titanium

24. **The type of implant that is inserted into a hole drilled into the bone is**
    a. Subperiosteal
    b. Endosseous
    c. Transosteal
    d. Exosteal

25. **Implants can be used to support which of the following prostheses?**
    a. Single crowns
    b. Fixed bridges
    c. Partial or complete dentures
    d. All of the above

26. **Maintenance of the tissues surrounding the implant is crucial to its success. How frequently should patients with implants be seen by the dental hygienist?**
    a. 3-month hygiene visits
    b. 6-month hygiene visits
    c. 9-month hygiene visits
    d. 12-month hygiene visits

27. **The instruments used to clean implants include**
    a. Carbon steel curettes
    b. Air polishers
    c. Ultrasonic tips
    d. Plastic curettes and scalers

28. **Preformed metal posts are available in all of the following materials EXCEPT:**
    a. Gold
    b. Stainless steel
    c. Titanium
    d. Titanium alloy

29. **The purpose of a post is to**
    a. Strengthen the root
    b. Put a permanent seal over the root canal filling material
    c. Strengthen the core material
    d. Retain the core material

30. **Which one of the following statements about cast posts is false?**
    a. They are formed from a wax or acrylic resin pattern.
    b. They can be cast using high noble, noble, or base metal alloys.
    c. They usually have the core attached as part of the casting.
    d. They are used in practice far more than preformed posts.

CASE-BASED DISCUSSION TOPICS

◉ A healthy 23-year-old college student reports to the dental office for a routine examination. It is discovered that she has several class II carious lesions in her molars that require restoration. She does not have a lot of money and wants a durable restoration. She is not concerned if the restorations show when she speaks. *Discuss the advantages and disadvantages of amalgam and composite resin for her situation. Which would you choose for yourself? Why?*

◉ A 43-year-old housewife comes to the dental office and reports that another dentist has told her that all of her old amalgams must be removed because they contain mercury. She asks you about the safety of amalgam fillings. *Discuss the safety issues related to amalgam and the mercury it contains.*

◉ You have just triturated a double-mix capsule of amalgam, and mercury has leaked while the capsule was being shaken and can be seen in small puddles on the outer surface of the triturator. *Discuss the appropriate ways to capture the spilled mercury and dispose of it.*

◉ A 33-year-old school teacher comes to the dental office to have a crown placed on tooth number 18. The dentist has told the patient that she should have a gold crown. After the dentist has left the room, the patient asks you if there are any cheaper metals that could be used. She says that she has no insurance and is short of money at this time. **What can you tell her about the types of metals used for cast crowns and what the pros and cons are for each?**

◉ A 65-year-old retired accountant comes to the dental office with a gold crown for tooth number 19 in his hand. It came off last night while eating sticky candy. The patient complains that since the crown was placed last year he has been packing food between the crown and tooth number 20, which has a disto-occlusal amalgam. The crown has an acceptable fit to the tooth and no dental caries are present. The amalgam is also acceptable. **What can you suggest to solve the food impaction problem? What materials should be used? Describe the correct sequence for the procedure(s).**

◉ As you are preparing for the cementation appointment for a porcelain-bonded-to-metal crown for tooth number 12, you notice several small cracks in the porcelain. **If the crown was not dropped or otherwise mishandled, why did these cracks appear? Discuss compatibility problems as they relate to the physical properties of the porcelain and the porcelain-bonded alloy.**

◉ The dentist has discussed the treatment plan with a patient who is a candidate for implants to support a mandibular complete denture. The dentist has described both subperiosteal and endosseous implants to the patient. After the dentist leaves the operatory, the patient is somewhat confused and asks you to explain the difference. **In layman's terms, describe the difference to the patient.**

◉ A 74-year-old retired grocer comes to the dental office for a maintenance visit. He has several implants supporting two fixed bridges in the posterior part of the maxilla. **As the dental hygienist who will perform the cleaning of his implants, describe the types of instruments you will likely use and the instruments you must avoid. Explain why you have selected these instruments.**

◉ The patient described in the preceding discussion topic is found to have inflammation in the peri-implant tissues around three implants and moderate amounts of calculus and plaque on the approximal surfaces of the implants. He tells you that he had missed his previously scheduled maintenance appointment and that he is just using a regular toothbrush with hard bristles to clean his implants. **What can you do to reinforce regular maintenance visits? What home care aids can you recommend to help him keep his implants clean? Should an antibacterial agent be suggested? If yes, which one?**

REFERENCES
ADA Council on Scientific Affairs: *Products of Excellence ADA Seal Program,* Chicago, 1999, ADA.
Berry TB et al: Amalgam at the new millennium, *J Am Dent Assoc* 129:547, 1998.
Bird D, Robinson D: Restorative and cosmetic dentistry. In *Torres and Ehrlich modern dental assisting,* ed 6, Philadelphia, 1999, WB Saunders.
Christensen GJ: Amalgam vs. composite resin, *J Am Dent Assoc* 129:1757, 1998.
Craig RG, Powers JM, Wataha JC: Dental amalgam; dental casting alloys and solders. In *Dental materials: properties and manipulation,* ed 7, St Louis, 2000, Mosby.

Darby ML, Walsh MM: Dental hygiene care for the individual with osseointegrated dental implants. In *Dental hygiene theory and practice,* Philadelphia, 1995, WB Saunders.

Douglass CW: Dental amalgam: reaching an internal consensus, *Oral Care Rep* 9(1):7, 1999.

Ehrlich A, Torres HO, Bird D: Orthodontics. In *Essentials of dental assisting,* ed 2, Philadelphia, 1996, WB Saunders.

Farah JW, Powers JM, eds: Amalgam alloys, *Dental Advisor* 16(7):1, 1999.

Gladwin MA, Bagby MD: Amalgam; materials for fixed indirect restorations and prostheses; dental implants; specialty materials. In *Clinical aspects of dental materials,* Philadelphia, 2000, Lippincott Williams & Wilkins.

Klein P: Best of both worlds: stainless steel and nickel titanium, *Dentistry Today* 18(7):66, 1999.

Leinfelder K: An evaluation of casting alloys used for restorative procedures, *J Am Dent Assoc* 128:37, 1997.

Marshall GW, Marshall SJ, Baynes SC: Restorative dental materials: scanning electron microscopy and x-ray microanalysis, *Scanning Microsc* 2(4):2007, 1988.

McKinney R: Oral hygiene protocol for implant patients. In *Endosteal dental implants,* St Louis, 1991, Mosby.

Perry DA, Beemsterboer PL, Taggart EJ: Dental implants. In *Clinical periodontics for the dental hygienist,* ed 2, Philadelphia, 2001, WB Saunders.

Phillips RW, Moore KB: Dental amalgam; alloys for dental castings. In *Elements of dental materials for dental hygienists and dental assistants,* ed 5, Philadelphia, 1994, WB Saunders.

US Department of Health and Human Services, Public Health Service: *Dental amalgam: a scientific review and recommended Public Health Service strategy for research, education and regulation,* Washington, DC, Jan 1993, DHHS/PHS.

Xu HHK et al: Three-body wear of a hand-consolidated silver alternative to amalgam, *J Dent Res* 78(9):1560, 1999.

PROCEDURE 8-1 (see p. 331 for competency sheet)

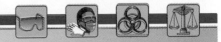

Assist with Placement of Class II Amalgam

EQUIPMENT/SUPPLIES

- Local anesthesia setup
- Operative dentistry setup—assorted burs, excavators, hand-cutting instruments
- Amalgam placement setup—amalgam carrier and well, large and small condensers, ball burnisher; coronal and interproximal carvers; matrix retainer, bands, wedges; articulating paper and holder and dental floss
- Encapsulated amalgam alloy and mercury
- Dental dam setup
- Disposables: gauze, cotton pellets, high-volume evacuation (HVE) tip, air/water syringe tip

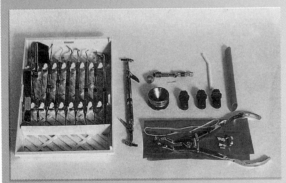

FIGURE 8-16

PROCEDURE STEPS

1 After the administration of local anesthetic, application of the dental dam, and preparation of the cavity, place the preassembled Tofflemire matrix band and retainer on the tooth and insert the wedge firmly in the interproximal space (Figure 8-17).

NOTE: Before placement, the middle of the band should be burnished on a paper pad with a ball burnisher to create the proper contour of the contact area. After placement, the band should be sealed against the tooth at the gingival margin by the wedge, extend approximately 1 mm coronal to the level of the marginal ridge, and be in contact with the approximal surface of the adjacent tooth. The wedge presses the band against the tooth to seal the gingival margin and creates a slight separation of the teeth to make up for the thickness of the matrix band so that a space is not left when the band is removed.

2 Place a base, liner, or cavity varnish, if needed, as directed by the dentist.

NOTE: Copal resin is seldom used as a cavity varnish, because it quickly washes out of the preparation. Some offices have replaced it with dentin sealers or bonding agents that occlude the dentinal tubules. Currently, bases and liners are used less frequently and are applied mostly in deeper cavity preparations, because their need has not been established for use on a routine basis.

3 After the base or liner has set, activate the amalgam capsule (unless it is self-activating), place it into the arms of the triturator, and set for the recommended time and speed (Figure 8-18).

4 When the dentist signals, mix the amalgam, open the capsule, and place the mixed amalgam in the amalgam well (Figure 8-19).

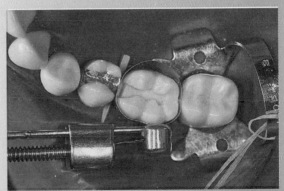

FIGURE 8-17

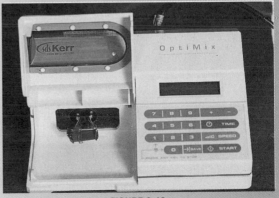

FIGURE 8-18

Continued on following page

PROCEDURE 8-1 (Continued)

5 Fill both ends of the amalgam carrier and place the amalgam in the proximal box from the small end first (Figure 8-20). If access is difficult, the dentist may place the amalgam.

NOTE: Some clinicians who use spherical alloy prefer to place the amalgam in large increments and quickly condense it into the cavity preparation. Spherical amalgam requires much less condensation pressure and displaces easily into the preparation as compared with an admixed amalgam.

6 Continue to fill the preparation with amalgam as requested by the dentist. Ask or anticipate when an additional mix of amalgam is needed to complete the restoration.

NOTE: In some states, dental assistants licensed in expanded functions can place, condense, and carve the amalgam. Usually, the smaller end of the condenser is used first to condense amalgam onto the gingival floor

of the box and against the facial and lingual walls. Both vertical and lateral condensation forces should be used to adapt the amalgam to the preparation.

7 After the preparation has been slightly overfilled, the amalgam is burnished with the ball burnisher over its surface and margins (Figure 8-21). Some clinicians use an anatomic burnisher to begin the initial contour of the occlusal morphology.

NOTE: Burnishing creates a denser surface, adapts the amalgam closely to the margins, and brings excess mercury to the surface that is then carved away.

8 An explorer tip is used to carve excess amalgam away from the band and begin shaping the marginal ridge (Figure 8-22). A discoid carver is used to remove large excesses of amalgam from the occlusal surface.

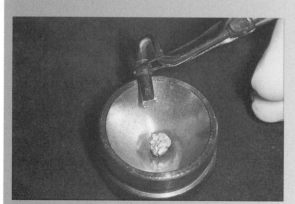

FIGURE 8-19

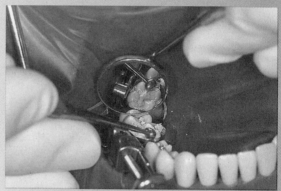

FIGURE 8-21

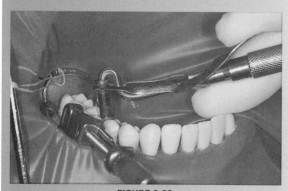

FIGURE 8-20

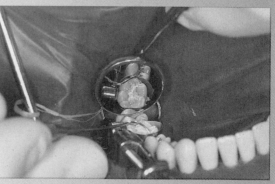

FIGURE 8-22

Continued on following page

PROCEDURE 8-1 (Continued)

NOTE: Removing excess amalgam adjacent to the band helps prevent fracture of the amalgam during removal of the band.

9 Remove the wedge and the matrix retainer. While holding the marginal ridge of the amalgam restoration down with a large condenser, remove the matrix band in an occlusal direction with a gentle rocking motion (Figure 8-23).

NOTE: If the marginal ridge is not held down during removal of the band, the unset amalgam is likely to fracture and require its removal and placement of fresh amalgam.

10 An interproximal carver is used first to carve the gingival margin, then facial and lingual margins to remove any excess. Next, a discoid/cleoid or similar carver is used to carve the occlusal surface (Figure 8-24). The blade of the carver is held partially on the adjacent enamel to act as a guide so that the amalgam margins are not overcarved.

11 Pass dental floss through the contact to clear the embrasure of excess carving debris and to test the adequacy of the contact relationship (Figure 8-25).

NOTE: A weak, open, or poorly contoured contact relationship with the adjacent tooth can lead to food impaction into the gingival tissues and periodontal pocket formation.

12 Remove the dental dam and mark the occlusal contacts with articulating paper (Figure 8-26). High spots as indicated by heavy marks from the articulating paper are carefully carved away. Repeat the process until contact is no longer heavy and the patient indicates that the restoration does not feel high. As a last step, some clinicians smooth the surface of the amalgam with a wet cotton pellet.

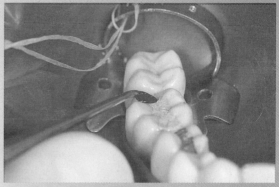

FIGURE 8-24

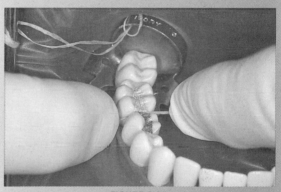

FIGURE 8-25

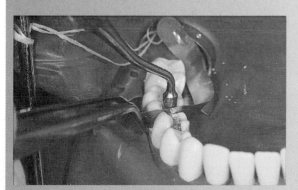

FIGURE 8-23

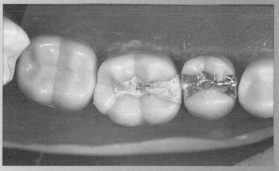

FIGURE 8-26

Continued on following page

PROCEDURE 8-1 (Continued)

NOTE: The patient should be instructed to close very lightly and then open again. If the patient closes too firmly and the amalgam is high, especially at the marginal ridge, it might fracture. When patients are still numb from the local anesthetic, they often cannot judge how hard they are biting. Some clinicians prefer to wait a couple of minutes after completing the carving before checking the occlusal contacts to allow the amalgam to gain some firmness, especially for very large amalgams.

13 Instruct the patient to avoid chewing on the new amalgam restoration for several hours.

NOTE: High-copper amalgams, especially spherical ones, have a high early strength and gain about 80% of their compressive strength in the first 8 hours. The set is usually complete within 24 hours.

9 ABRASION, FINISHING, AND POLISHING

OBJECTIVES

On completion of this chapter the student will be able to:

1. Define *abrasion, finishing, polishing,* and *cleansing.*
2. Discuss the purpose of finishing, polishing, and cleansing of dental restorations and tooth surfaces.
3. Identify the factors that affect the rate and efficiency of abrasion.
4. Compare the relative ranking of abrasives on restorations and tooth structures.
5. Identify methods by which dental abrasives are applied.
6. List the contraindications to the use of abrasives on tooth structure and restorations.
7. Describe the clinical decisions used to determine which abrasive to use when finishing, polishing, or cleansing dental restorations or tooth structures.
8. Describe the abrasives used and procedure for finishing and polishing metals, composite, and porcelain.
9. Describe the abrasives used and procedure for polishing and cleansing metals, composite, porcelain, and gold alloys as part of an oral prophyaxis.
10. Describe the safety and infection control precautions taken by the operator when using abrasives.
11. Relate patient education instructions for prevention and removal of stain from tooth surfaces and restorations.
12. Finish and polish a preexisting amalgam restoration.
13. Polish a preexisting composite restoration.

KEY TERMS

Finishing—A procedure used to reduce excess restorative material to develop appropriate occlusion and contour. This is usually done with rotary cutting instruments. Finishing removes surface blemishes and produces a smooth surface.

Polishing—A procedure that produces a shiny, smooth surface by eliminating fine scratches, minor surface imperfections, and surface stains using mild abrasives frequently found in the form of pastes or compounds. Polishing produces little change in the surface. It may need to be repeated periodically during the life of the restoration if tarnish or stains develop.

Abrasive—A material composed of particles of sufficient hardness and sharpness to cut or scratch a softer material when drawn across its surface.

Grit—The particle size of the abrasive, typically classified as coarse, medium, fine, and superfine.

Cleansing—A procedure that is primarily meant to remove soft deposits from the surface of restorations and tooth structures. Polishing and cleansing are done to remove surface stains and soft deposits from the clinical crowns and exposed root surfaces of teeth after all hard deposits are removed. Aside from abrasives there are also chemical cleansing products that are primarily used for removable appliances.

Margination—A procedure for removal of excessive restorative material from margins of restorations.

Flash—Featherlike excesses of material present on occlusal and proximal surfaces.

Overhang—Excessive material present at the cervical cavosurface margin.

Proper finishing and polishing of tooth structures and restorative materials is clinically relevant because it improves esthetics and surrounding tissue health and increases the longevity of the restorative material.

The goal of finishing and polishing restorations, intraoral appliances, and tooth structure is to remove excess material, smooth roughened surfaces, and produce an esthetically pleasing appearance with minimum trauma to hard and soft tissues. The finishing and polishing of a surface involves removing marginal irregularities, defining anatomic contours and occlusion, removing the surface roughness of the restoration, and producing a mirrorlike surface luster. There are many benefits of smooth tooth surfaces, restorations, or appliances in the intraoral environment. A smooth surface resists accumulation of soft deposits and stains, is less irritating to the gingival or mucosal tissue, and is esthetically pleasing because it reflects light better. A smooth, highly polished restorative surface is more resistant to the effects of corrosion and surface breakdown. A properly finished and polished surface will contribute to the appearance and longevity of the restoration or appliance and the health of the surrounding oral tissues (Figure 9-1). Clinicians performing these functions must have a clear understanding of the factors that cause and control abrasion. Improper use of abrasives can lead to roughening and overreduction of tooth and restorative surfaces. The clinician must be able to recognize that different types of tooth structures and restorative surfaces abrade differently and use the proper protocol for finishing, polishing, or cleansing of that surface. It is also the clinician's responsibility to teach the patient how to properly care for the surface with home care devices and how to prevent the staining habits that diminish their appearance.

Finishing and Polishing

The process of **finishing** and **polishing** is to use a diminishing series of abrasives on a surface to first contour, then smooth, and finally bring a luster to the surface. The effect of abrasion is directly related to the properties of the **abrasive** and the material it is abrading.

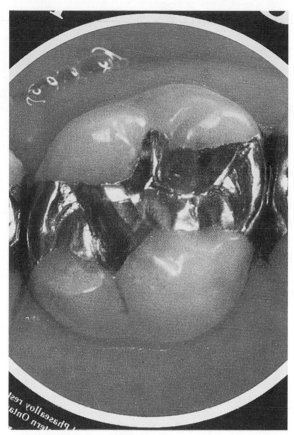

FIGURE 9-1 ■ A finished and polished amalgam restoration.

FACTORS AFFECTING ABRASION

An understanding of the properties of abrasives and the factors that control the rate or efficiency of abrasion will help the clinician make the appropriate clinical decisions. The rate of abrasion is determined by size, irregularity, and hardness of the particles; number of particles contacting the surface; and the pressure and speed with which they are applied. An understanding of these factors will assist the clinician in making the appropriate clinical decisions in the control of abrasion.

Size, Irregularity, and Hardness of the Particles

The size, irregularity, and hardness of the abrasive particle determine the depth of the scratches in the material being abraded and therefore the amount of material being removed. An example is the effect of pumice, which comes in several grades of coarse-ness, on cementum and amalgam. Coarse pumice, a larger and coarser particle, will remove more surface of the softer cementum than the harder amalgam. If flour of pumice were used, a much smaller and more regular particle than coarse pumice, the effect would be to polish the cementum as well as the amalgam. Diamonds are the most abrasive materials used in dentistry. Diamond abrasives can remove large amounts of tooth structure and restorative material, finish restorations, and polish restorations all according to the diamond particle size and irregularity. Their rate of abrasion will also depend on the material being abraded, the pressure applied, and the speed of the rotating device.

If the surface being abraded is harder than the abrasive, there is little or no effect. It is important for the clinician to have an appreciation for the relative hardness of various intraoral materials and abrasives. Hardness is the ability of a material to resist abrasion. The Moh scale ranks materials by their relative abrasion resistance. As seen in Table 9-1 diamond has the highest resistance to abrasion and is therefore considered the hardest; pumice rates a 6 on the Moh scale, which is similar to enamel but harder than amalgam and dentin. Therefore pumice may only polish amalgam whereas it would be abrasive to dentin. It is important to note that porcelain is harder than enamel and dentin. Abrasive wear of tooth structures in contact with porcelain restorations is a problem for many patients. The greater the difference in the abrasive and the surface it is abrading, the faster and more effective the abrasive action is. Compare the Moh hardness ranking for enamel and dentin. You can surmise that exposed dentin is abraded at a much greater rate than enamel during dental polishing procedures. Compare the Moh ranking of composite and gold. If the same polishing agent is used on these as on enamel, the result would be a greater loss of the restorative material.

The size and shape of the particles is an important consideration in manipulating the abrasive. Particles that are large and irregular will cut more efficiently. The sharpness, or efficiency, of the particle is usually lost with use as the edges break down and the particle no longer grabs the surface. Unlike the shape of the particle, the size of the particle does not always break down with use. Abrasive particles are classified from coarse to fine based on their size measured in micrometers (also called microns) One micrometer, or micron, is equal to one thousandth of a millimeter

Table 9-1

Moh Hardness Scale

Diamond	10
Silicon carbide	9-10
Tungsten carbide	9
Aluminum oxide	9
Emery	7-9
Sand—quartz	7
Pumice	6-7
Porcelain	6-7
Tin oxide	6
Amalgam	5-6
Enamel	5
Composite	3-7
Dentin	4
Gold	3

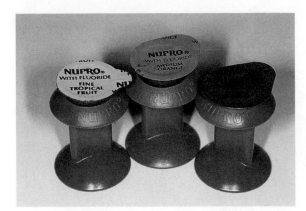

FIGURE 9-2 ■ Different grits of single-dose units of prophy paste in holders.

(10^{-3}) and uses the symbol μm. Abrasives are classified as coarse (100 μm particles and above), medium (20 to 100 μm), and fine (20 μm to submicron particle sizes). Manufacturers use the term **grit** to refer to the size of the abrasive particles. Particles are passed through a standardized sieve that allows specific sizes of particles to pass and then categorizes them from coarse through superfine. Prophylactic polishing pastes are commonly manufactured in various degrees of coarseness, as are abrasive disks and rotary diamonds (Figure 9-2). The clinician must make decisions as to the coarseness of the abrasive and the application method needed for each procedure.

Numbers That Contact the Surface   The more concentrated the particles that contact the surface, the faster the surface will be abraded. If a lubricant is used to dilute the concentration of the particles, the abrasiveness of the material is reduced. Water and saliva are common lubricants used to dilute the effect of abrasion. When using an abrasive, the clinician has control of how much lubricant to add to the material, whether this is before it is put onto the surface or while it is being used intraorally as it picks up saliva. Pumice is manufactured in a powder or paste, giving the clinician the opportunity to further dilute this abrasive. Rotary cutting instruments such as abrasive discs and stones will lose effectiveness as particles break away from their surface or debris

clogs the surface. Many rotary cutting stones and diamonds use the water from the handpiece or three-way syringe to assist in the movement of debris from the cutting edge and act as a surface coolant, thus allowing the surface to maintain its abrasive action much longer.

Speed and Pressure   Increasing the speed and pressure of an abrasive will increase the rate of abrasion. Speed can also produce undesired effects if it results in lack of control. An increase in pressure will cause deeper scratches but also may produce less control of the amount of material being removed. An increase in pressure also decreases the clinician's tactile sensitivity and may produce an undesired overabraded surface. Too much pressure might even reduce the cutting efficiency of the abrasive by decreasing the instrument's torque. Speed and pressure also produce frictional heat, which may produce a detrimental effect on the tooth structure and patient comfort. Care must be taken to control the amount of pressure and speed with which abrasives are applied.

Determining the rate of abrasion is an important consideration when making clinical decisions on what type of material is to be abraded, how much material is to be removed, and the desired outcome.

DELIVERY DESIGN OF ABRASIVES

Dental abrasives are supplied in a number of forms: paste abrasives, loose abrasives, coated abrasives, and bonded abrasives (Figure 9-3).

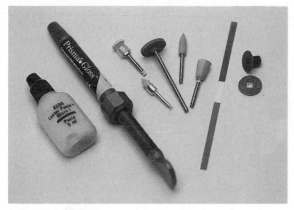

FIGURE 9-3 ■ Different delivery designs of abrasives: paste, bonded, and coated.

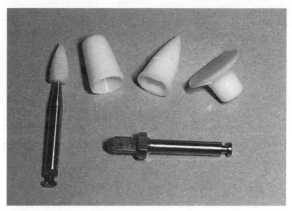

FIGURE 9-4 ■ Shapes of bonded abrasives: reusable point on mandrel and disposable cup, point, and disk with sterilizable mandrel.

Loose Abrasives   Loose abrasives are manufactured in powders and pastes and are classified by their grit or particle size. Grits of coarse, medium, fine, and superfine are available for finishing, polishing, and cleansing surfaces. These may be applied with wheels, brushes, cups, or soft pads. The concentration of particles that contact the surface is clinically controlled. If the clinician uses a coarse, dry paste, rapid removal of surface material will result with possible pulpal damage due to excessive frictional heat. However, if a superfine, highly diluted paste is used, little or no material may be removed. The proper grit and dilution of the loose abrasive must be considered to give the best results in finishing and polishing a given surface.

Bonded Abrasives   Bonded abrasives are rotary instruments that have an abrasive particle uniformly incorporated in a binder to form the shape of the device. Shapes vary in form; points, disks, cups, brushes, and wheels are available. These devices are frequently used for intermediate finishing and initial polishing of restorations (Figure 9-4).

Coated Abrasives   Coated abrasives are supplied on rotary discs and handheld finishing strips. The abrasive particles are secured to one side of a flexible backing with an adhesive. Devices with coating on only one side protect the adjacent tooth from the abrasive and are referred to as *safe-sided*. Flexible backing such as paper or plastic give them the advantage of flexibility but eliminate their ability to be sterilized. Coated abrasives used on rotary devices

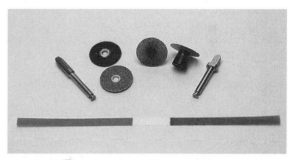

FIGURE 9-5 ■ Different designs of sandpaper disks and mandrels and sandpaper strip.

use sterilizable mandrels for convenience and cost-effectiveness (Figure 9-5).

Abrasives are manufactured for use in the laboratory or at chairside. Some may be used for either purpose. Regardless of how the abrasive material is supplied, the rate of abrasion must be controlled by the clinician.

MATERIALS USED IN ABRASION

Many types of natural and synthetic (human-made) materials are available for use in dentistry. As listed from most to least abrasive, each of these materials leaves the surface of the restoration or tooth structure with varying degrees of roughness.

Diamond   Diamond is the hardest substance known, rating a 10 on the Moh hardness scale. It will efficiently abrade any substance. Rotary diamonds are expensive and are not usually disposable, so they are most often found bonded in varying degrees of coarseness to rotary cutting shanks or disks. They are sterilizable and have the capability of being reused several times before they wear out. Fine-particle diamonds come in a paste for polishing composite and porcelain restorations.

Carbide Finishing Burs   Tungsten carbide finishing burs come in several shapes, with designs ranging from 7 to 30 cutting flutes. The higher the number of flutes the bur has, the finer the final finish. A bur containing only seven flutes will have a very aggressive cutting action. These burs rank up to a 9 on the Moh scale and are primarily used for finishing.

Silicon Carbide   Silicon carbide is a synthetic material that produces an extremely hard and efficient abrasive material, Moh 9-10. Silicon carbide–coated disks and bonded rotary devices are primarily used in finishing procedures.

Aluminum Oxide   Aluminum oxide is a synthetic abrasive often manufactured in a white or tan powder. The powder form is used in sandblasting restorations in preparation for cementation and air abrasion. It is used in bonded and coated rotary devices. Aluminum oxide–impregnated rubber wheels are called Burlew wheels. This popular abrasive comes in several grits and has largely replaced emery.

Sand   Sand is a natural abrasive composed of quartz and silica. This abrasive rates a 7 on the Moh scale and is manufactured as coated disks and hand-held strips used in the finishing process.

Silicon Dioxode   Silicon dioxide (silex) has a Moh ranking of 6-7 and is commonly found in prophylaxis paste.

Pumice   Pumice is volcanic silica manufactured as a loose abrasive. Flour of pumice (Moh hardness scale 6) is extremely fine and a major component of many prophylaxis pastes used to polish tooth structure.

Rouge   Rouge is iron oxide with a Moh hardness value of 5-6. It is frequently found in block form, which is then run onto a rag wheel to polish precious and semiprecious metal alloys in the laboratory.

Tin Oxide   Tin oxide is an extremely fine abrasive used extensively as a polishing agent for enamel and restorations. This abrasive is usually found as a powder that is mixed with water or glycerin.

Calcium Carbonate   Calcium carbonate, also called chalk or whiting, has a low Moh ranking of 3 and is found in prophylaxis paste and dentifrice.

PREPARATIONS USED FOR ABRASION

Prophylaxis Paste (Prophy Paste)   Prophylaxis paste (prophy paste) is a mixture of 50% to 60% abrasive materials such as pumice and tin oxide and lubricants. Preservatives, flavoring agents, coloring agents, and therapeutic agents are also added. The abrasive powder is diluted with a lubricant to reduce the rate of abrasion and amount of frictional heat produced. The lubricant also helps keep the preparation in a paste form by preventing hardening on exposure to air. Perservatives are placed to prolong shelf life, and coloring and flavoring agents are placed to increase patient acceptance. Fluoride is added to many preparations as a therapeutic agent in the prevention of caries.

Prophylaxis pastes are supplied in coarse to superfine commercially prepared pastes for polishing and **cleansing** of tooth structures. The process of polishing requires materials with a Moh hardness of only 1 to 2 rankings higher than the surface to which they are applied. Remember that polishing of tooth surfaces should remove soft deposits and polishable stains without damage to hard tissues. Studies of the amount of tooth structure removed with prophy paste and rubber cup polish have shown that a sufficient amount of fluoride-rich enamel layer and much greater amount of exposed cementum or demineralized enamel is removed to recommend polishing only those surfaces that exhibit stain. This philosophy of "selective polishing" is regarded as the most appropriate approach in the selection of which teeth and surfaces to polish.

> ▶ **CAUTION**
> *There is a significant amount of roughening of composite and gold restorations even by fine prophy pastes.*

When selecting a prophy paste, the least abrasive paste possible should be selected for the existing stains and soft deposits. These abrasives should be applied as wet as possible with a light touch and low speed.

Dentifrice (Toothpaste) Toothpaste, like prophylaxis paste, contains a mixture of abrasive materials to clean tooth structures and restorations to resist discoloration and plaque accumulation. These commercial preparations contain 20% to 40% abrasive agents, coloring agents, and flavoring agents. The lowest possible abrasive rankings are desirable to prevent removal of softer tooth structures and restorations (Figure 9-6). The ADA Seal indicates that the abrasive particles do not exceed the maximum acceptable abrasiveness (Table 9-2).

Denture Cleansers The use of a toothbrush with water and a mild cleansing agent is sufficient to remove most plaque, surface stains, and food debris

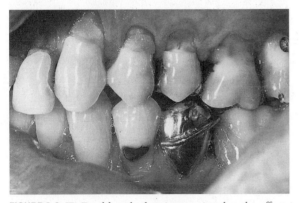

FIGURE 9-6 ■ Toothbrush abrasion; notice that the affects of abrasion are also seen on the amalgam restoration.

Table 9-2
Components of Prophy Paste and Toothpaste

Prophy Paste	Component	Toothpaste
50%-60%	Abrasive	20%-40%
20%-25%	Humectant	20%-40%
10%-20%	Water	20%-40%
—	Detergent	1%-2%
2%-3%	Flavoring/coloring agents	2%-3%
1%-2%	Therapeutic (fluoride)	1%-2%

from removable prosthetic appliances. The immersion of the prosthesis into commercially prepared denture cleansers that loosen stains and deposits that can then be rinsed or brushed away is also appropriate. Commercial denture cleansers should be nontoxic, nonabrasive, and harmless to the components of the prosthesis. Full acrylic prostheses can be soaked in dilute alkaline or acid commercial preparations. Prostheses with metal components should not be placed in dilute acid solutions or hypochlorites (bleach) because of the resultant corrosion of these components.

Finishing and Polishing Procedures

Finishing and polishing procedures follow a similar sequence. Sufficient amounts of material are removed to reproduce the anatomic contours of the restoration/appliance, and finer and finer cuts are then made into the material with diminishing abrasive agents until it takes on a smooth, shiny, mirror-like surface. It is important that the appropriate clinical decision is made as to the choice of abrasive agent, the properties of the surface, and the order in which the abrasive is applied and that attention is given to the thorough removal of each abrasive agent before beginning with a finer one. If abrasive agents are left on structures or on delivery equipment, they continue to abrade even though a finer abrasive is currently being applied.

In addition, care must be taken to consider the anatomic form of the tooth. The finished and polished restoration should have a smooth, continuous line flush with the tooth surface. When restorative margins end at or near the root, instrumentation near or on this cavosurface margin may result in ditching or gouging of the softer cementum surfaces. Contours of teeth must be re-created and should not be flattened or overly rounded. The contact area need not be polished. Polishing this area may remove material, resulting in an open contact that can lead to impaction of food, causing damage to the periodontium, or contribute to caries formation.

MARGINATION AND THE REMOVAL OF FLASH

Before finishing or polishing an amalgam or composite restoration, the clinician should check the integrity of the cavosurface margins for prematuri-

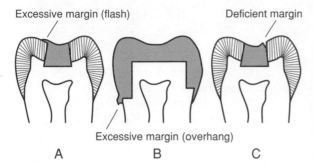

FIGURE 9-7 ■ Drawing of (**A**) excessive occlusal margin (flash), (**B**) excessive proximal margin (overhang), and (**C**) deficient occlusal margin.

Table 9-3

Indications for Margination

- Overhang or flash is not extensive in size.
- Tooth anatomy and contour can be improved.
- Proximal contact is present.
- Restoration is intact; no fractures, open margins, or caries are present.
- The margin is accessible without damage to tissue or adjacent tooth structures.

ties and deficiencies (Figure 9-7). The process of removing restoration prematurities to bring the restoration flush with the cavosurface tooth structure is called **margination**. This process may vary from removal of feathered **flash** to removal of **overhang** (ledges created by overhanging cervical margins). The decision to remove excessive material from a restoration is based on clinical and radiographic findings. Careful evaluation of the restoration is necessary to determine if margination is indicated or if the restoration needs to be replaced (see Table 9-3).

Hand cutting instruments, such as an amalgam knife, scalers and files, or rotary cutting diamonds and carbide burs, are used. When using hand instruments for margination, begin apically to the margin of the restoration using a shaving motion in diagonal overlapping strokes.

AMALGAM

It is generally recommended that amalgam restorations be polished no sooner than 24 hours after

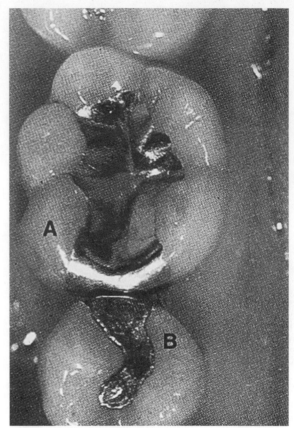

FIGURE 9-8 ■ **A,** Polished amalgam restoration. **B,** Unpolished amalgam restoration.

insertion. The slow final setting of traditional amalgams and potential for chipping the margins of even the new high-copper amalgams prevents immediate polishing. In addition, as many older types of amalgams age, the results of creep and corrosion produce surfaces that may benefit from periodic polishing procedures. This does not seem to be a problem in the newer high-copper amalgams The amount of finishing and polishing required depends on the care taken in carving and burnishing of the amalgam at the time of insertion and the effects of the oral environment on older restorations (Figure 9-8).

Begin by evaluating cavosurface margins for excess material and remove as indicated. Finishing is next, using abrasive devices to remove severe scratches and surface defects. Bonded and coated abrasives greater than 25 μm particle size or special multifluted finishing burs are used. Polishing that is

Table 9-4

Finishing and Polishing Composite Restorations

- *Initial finishing:* bonded and coated rotary abrasives 100 μm or larger or multifluted carbide or diamond finishing burs
- *Intermediate finishing:* bonded and coated rotary abrasives less than 100 μm but greater than 20 μm
- *Final polishing:* bonded and coated abrasives or polishing paste from 20 to 0.3 μm

accomplished with bonded, coated, or loose abrasives ranging from 20 μm to submicron particle sizes gives the amalgam restoration a mirrorlike luster (see Procedure 9-1).

COMPOSITE

Composite restorations are finished and polished as part of the restorative procedure in three steps. Marginal and occlusal excesses are first removed in initial finishing with diamonds or multifluted carbide burs. Intermediate finishing is accomplished with flexible disks, cups, and strips beginning with coarse and sequentially proceeding to superfine. Final polishing is accomplished with a submicron aluminum oxide–based polishing paste applied with soft cups or felt pads (Table 9-4).

GOLD ALLOY

Precious and nonprecious crowns, inlays, and onlays are finished and polished in the dental laboratory before delivery to the dental office for final fitting and cementation. In the process of final fitting, minor adjustments made with abrasive stones and diamonds may be necessary. It is important that the resultant scratches are removed before final cementation. Burlew wheels on a slow-speed handpiece are used, followed by rouge on a rag wheel.

PORCELAIN

Like gold alloys, porcelain restorations are finished and polished in the dental laboratory. Adjustments made during the fitting of these restorations are made with diamonds. Rubber polishing points and wheels designed for porcelain are used for finishing,

and diamond polishing paste is used to polish the restoration to an enamel-like luster.

Polishing During an Oral Prophylaxis (Coronal Polish)

Before the coronal polishing procedure is begun, a careful tactile evaluation of tooth surfaces must be done to correctly identify and remove calculus. If a restoration is incorrectly identified as calculus and aggressively scaled, the restoration may be removed or altered to the point of needing replacement. In addition, all restorative materials must be identified to prevent undesired removal or scratching of the surface by commercially prepared prophy paste. Restorations such as composites glass ionomers, compomers, and gold alloys are much softer than prophy paste and will be adversely affected by their use (see Chapter 3 for identification of restorative materials).

AMALGAM

As previously mentioned, amalgam restorations change over the years from the effects of tarnish and corrosion. Polishing during an oral prophylaxis may greatly benefit these restorations. Use rubber cups or bristle brushes with commercially prepared prophy paste on occlusal and smooth surfaces and dental tape on proximal surfaces, avoiding the contact area.

COMPOSITE

Composite restorations, which become stained after placement, may be polished as part of a regular maintenance appointment. The use of ultrasonic and sonic scalers and air-polishing devices should be avoided on or around these restorations because these instruments may damage the surface of the restoration. The use of traditional prophy pastes may cause excessive wear; typically these restorations should be polished with aluminum oxide polishing paste. It is important that composite restorations are polished only if stain is present and that the appropriate materials are selected and used to avoid scratching or altering the surface of the softer composite materials. Begin with the least abrasive techniques first. If the stain is not easily removed with fine paste, proceed to more aggressive grits or rubber polishing points and finishing disks. Pay close attention to the restoration's contour and marginal integrity, always keeping the rotary instrument moving with a light, sweeping motion. Compete the polishing procedure using light pressure with a very wet, specialized polishing paste on a soft felt pad. Total polishing time should not exceed 30 seconds on any stained surface.

At whatever level of abrasive is chosen, remember to always proceed from most abrasive to least abrasive to finish the restoration. Staining at the margins may also represent microleakage that penetrates under the restoration. These stains cannot be polished away (see Procedure 9-2).

GOLD ALLOYS AND PORCELAIN

Porcelain and gold alloys are extremely resistant to staining. If scratches or irregularities are present, it is usually due to instrumentation that has scratched the outer glaze. Use specially formulated porcelain-polishing paste on porcelain or submicron aluminum oxide on gold. Commercially prepared prophy paste is not recommended.

RESIN CEMENT INTERFACE

Margins on resin-bonded porcelain restorations are more susceptible to staining because of the properties of the resin cements. Stains accumulating at the resin cement interface must be carefully evaluated for actual staining or microleakage. If it is determined that the stain is within the cement and not the result of leakage, it may be removed in the same manner as in composite restoration.

AIR POLISHING AND AIR ABRASION

The use of air to propel very small particles (microparticles) as a replacement for rotary cutting and polishing instruments has gained much popularity. Several in vitro and clinical studies have shown these new delivery systems for abrasives to be both efficient and effective. There is ongoing clinical research to support their use and establish recommendations for specific restorative and other clinical applications. Clinicians should follow manufacturers' recommendations for precautions in safety and contraindications in individual clinical applications.

Air polishing utilizes a combination of sodium bicarbonate, air, and water at a pressure of approximately 40 psi as an effective and efficient means of removing stains and soft deposits from enamel surfaces. Most research results recommend caution near restorations, particularly composite and porcelain surfaces, and on exposed dentin and cementum when using this form of polishing (Figure 9-9).

Air abrasion uses compressed air and a 27 or 50 μm aluminum oxide powder. Cutting can be controlled to remove minimal amounts of tooth and restorative structure. However, this procedure is not recommended for stain removal. This process is used for chairside cleansing of cast appliances before cementation, intraoral repair of porcelain and composite restorations, tooth surface preparations before bonding, and cutting of tooth structure for restorative preparations. Air pressure of 40 to 160 psi and a controlled adjustable-tip orifice allow aluminum oxide particles to strike a tooth or restoration with enough force to effectively cut the surface (Figure 9-10).

The use of appropriate clinician and patient safety equipment and control of aerosols with high-volume evacuation are critical for these procedures.

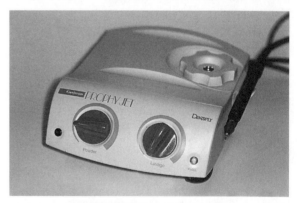

FIGURE 9-9 ■ Air-polishing unit.

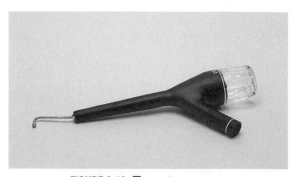

FIGURE 9-10 ■ Air-abrasion tip.

Safety/Infection Control

Aerosols are created whenever a rotary device and moisture are used. These aerosols can provide a means for disease transmission. The use of rotary devices may produce particulate matter and vapors from the substrate being abraded. Silica particles from restorations and mercury vapors pose potential health risks. In addition, splatter from abrasives can produce serious eye damage. The use of precautionary personal protective equipment to include mask and eye protection is essential for the dental team. Protective eyewear is highly recommended for the patient as well. The use of preprocedure antimicrobal rinses has been shown to reduce microbial aerosols, and high-speed evacuation is recommended instead of the saliva ejector.

Maintain dental laboratory asepsis by sterilizing or disinfecting all wheels and rotary cutting devices. Use fresh, dry powders for each procedure, and remove contaminated portions of stick or block abrasives.

Patient Education

Composite restorations and resin-bonded porcelain restorations are particularly susceptible to staining. Effective oral hygiene techniques and awareness of dietary staining and stain-producing habits can prevent a certain amount of surface discoloration.

Thorough removal of plaque from restorative surfaces will prevent staining associated with bacterial accumulation.

Patient education in the effects of staining foods, particularly pigmented beverages such as coffee, tea, and wine, and the result of tobacco stain on composite restorations and tooth surfaces should be part of the original restorative procedure, as well as regular recall appointments. Patients with exposed cementum and dentin are particularly susceptible to staining and the effect of abrasives. In an attempt to improve the color of their teeth, patients may use home remedies or excessively abrasive commercial products. The consequences often are toothbrush abrasion and wear of restorations and tooth surfaces. Patient education should include the use of approved abrasive agents.

SUMMARY

The decision to abrade a surface to contour, finish, polish, or cleanse a structure requires considerable thought. The clinician must have knowledge of the properties of the material being abraded, the abrasive, and the factors that affect abrasion. The process of abrasion can produce undesirable effects if not carefully controlled. The appropriate use of abrasion can also produce a surface that will contribute to the longevity of the restoration and health of the surrounding oral tissues.

CHAPTER REVIEW

Select the one correct response for each of the following multiple-choice questions:

1. **The goal of finishing and polishing of restorations includes**
   a. The removal of excess material
   b. The smoothing of roughened surfaces
   c. The production of better esthetics
   d. All of the above

2. **Cleansing of teeth is primarily meant to**
   a. Remove excess material
   b. Smooth roughened surfaces
   c. Remove soft deposits
   d. Recontour surfaces

3. The depth and space between cuts made by an abrasive is determined by
   a. The properties of the abrasive
   b. The properties of the material being abraded
   c. The contour of the restoration
   d. Both a and b

4. Which of the following represents the correct hardness ranking, from hardest of softest:
   a. Gold, amalgam, composite, enamel
   b. Enamel, amalgam, gold, composite
   c. Composite, enamel, gold, amalgam
   d. Amalgam, enamel, composite, gold

5. The rate of abrasion is determined by all of the following EXCEPT:
   a. The size of the particle
   b. The pressure applied
   c. The speed used
   d. The manufacturer

6. The Moh scale ranks
   a. Materials by their relative abrasion resistance
   b. Hardness of a material
   c. Abrasiveness of a material
   d. Both a and b

7. To control the numbers of abrasive particles that contact the surface,
   a. The operator should increase the speed
   b. The operator should decrease the pressure
   c. The operator should use a lubricant
   d. The operator should not use rotary instruments

8. Loose abrasives
   a. Are safe-sided
   b. Are used on cups and brushes
   c. Come in various shapes
   d. Use sterilizable mandrels

CASE-BASED DISCUSSION TOPICS

◉ Factors that affect abrasion: *Discuss how the operator uses knowledge of the factors that affect abrasion to control the polishing sequence of an amalgam restoration, a composite restoration, and a gold restoration.*

◉ Abrasives: *List two materials used to polish stains from the coronal surfaces of teeth, and discuss the contraindications to using various abrasives on tooth surfaces.*

◉ A 30-year-old computer programmer comes to the dental office complaining of catching dental floss on a new class II distal occlusal (DO) composite restoration on tooth number 29. Examination reveals excess composite at the gingival margin and an overcontoured distofacial surface of this restoration. *Discuss instruments, materials, and techniques for correcting the problem.*

REFERENCES

American Dental Association Council on Scientific Affairs: Products of Excellence ADA Seal Program, *J Am Dent Assoc* 129:1, 1998.

Anusavice K: *Phillips' science of dental materials,* ed 10, Philadelphia, 1996, WB Saunders.

Denture cleansers, Department on Dental Materials, Instruments and Equipment, *J Am Dent Assoc* 106:77, 1983.

Farah JW, Powers JM: Composite finish and polishing, *Dental Advisor* 15:1, 1998.

Goldstein R et al: Patient maintenance of esthetic restorations, *J Am Dent Assoc* 123:61, 1992.

Gutmann M: Air polishing: a comprehensive review of the literature, *J Dent Hygiene* 72:47, 1998.

Introduction to biomaterials properties/biomaterials properties table listing: www.lib.umich.edu/libhome/Dentistry.lib/Dental_tables/toc.html.

Jefferies SR: The art and science of abrasive finishing and polishing in restorative dentistry, *Dent Clin North Am* 42:613, 1998.

Miller B: Dental restorative materials, an update on care, *Dental Hygienist News* 8:9, 1995.

Miller M, editor: *Reality,* vol 13, *Maintaining esthetic restorations,* Houston, Tex. 1999, Reality Publishing.

Nash L: The hygienist's role in aesthetic and cosmetic restorations, *J Practical Hygiene* 3:9, 1994.

Natoli S: Air abrasion in dentistry, *Dental Assistant* Sept-Oct 1997 pp. 11-15.

Tolle-Watts S: Clinical application of the air polisher, *J Practical Hygiene* 1:4, 1992.

Wilkins E: *Clinical practice of the dental hygienist,* ed 8, Philadelphia, 1999, Lippincott Williams & Wilkins.

Yap AU, Lye KW, Sau CW: Surface characteristics of tooth-colored restorations polished utilizing different polishing systems, *Operative Dentistry* 22:260, 1997.

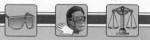

PROCEDURE 9-1 (see p. 332 for competency sheet)

Finishing and Polishing a Preexisting Amalgam Restoration

EQUIPMENT/SUPPLIES (Figure 9-11)

- Mirror and explorer
- Air/water syringe
- Articulating paper
- Isolation materials
- Slow-speed handpiece and attachment
- Finishing burs, stones, disks, and cups
- Dappen dish
- Pumice
- Disposable rubber cup and brush
- Tin oxide

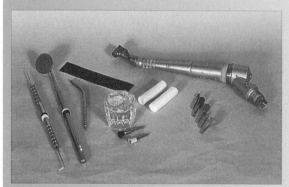

FIGURE 9-11

NOTE: Polish amalgams no sooner than 24 hours after insertion to allow amalgam to develop its maximum strength.

PROCEDURE STEPS

1 Examine cavosurface margins of entire restoration for excess material.

NOTE: Remove excess material to prevent plaque accumulation or gingival irritation.

2 Check occlusion with articulating paper and clinically for premature occlusal contact.

NOTE: Premature occlusal contact can cause sensitivity and excessive wear on the restoration or opposing teeth; the dentist will need to adjust the occlusion.

3 Remove proximal cavosurface prematurities with an amalgam knife or a similar sharp instrument using short, overlapping strokes (Figure 9-12).

4 Isolate the restoration with cotton rolls and saliva ejector.

5 Use pointed stones for occlusal anatomy and disk or cup for smooth surfaces, moving from most to least abrasive (brown first, then green, finally super greenie) (Figures 9-13 and 9-14).

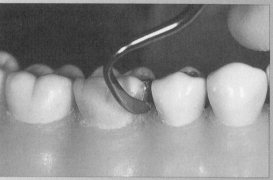

FIGURE 9-12

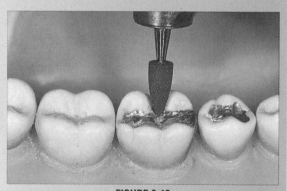

FIGURE 9-13

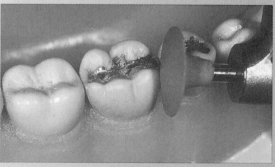

FIGURE 9-14

Continued on following page

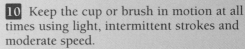

PROCEDURE 9-1 (Continued)

6 Use slow to moderate speed, always moving the stone from tooth to amalgam to prevent ditching the cavosurface margin.

7 Use a light, sweeping motion, keeping the finishing instrument moving to avoid excessive heat and mercury vapor production.

8 Rinse the area thoroughly when changing abrasives to prevent the more abrasive particles from abrading the surface.

9 Use the rubber cup and brush with a slurry of pumice and then tin oxide (Figure 9-15).

10 Keep the cup or brush in motion at all times using light, intermittent strokes and moderate speed.

11 Rinse between pumice and tin oxide.

12 Polish proximal surfaces with a handheld finishing strip or pumice and dental tape.

13 Wrap the strip around the tooth contours to avoid flattening proximal contours (Figure 9-16).

14 Do not polish through the contact (Figure 9-17).

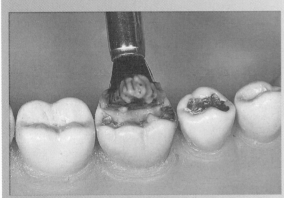

FIGURE 9-15

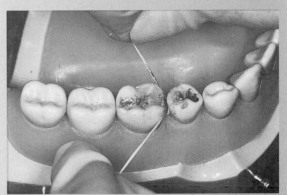

FIGURE 9-16

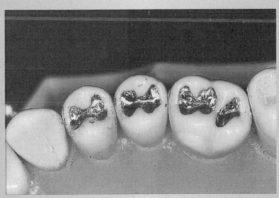

FIGURE 9-17

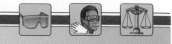

PROCEDURE 9-2 (see p. 333 for competency sheet)

Polishing a Preexisting Composite Restoration

EQUIPMENT/SUPPLIES (Figure 9-18)

- Mirror and explorer
- Air/water syringe
- Isolation materials
- Slow-speed handpiece and attachment
- Abrasive finishing disks
- Sterilizable mandrel
- Abrasive flexible wheels and points
- Polishing paste
- Rubber cup

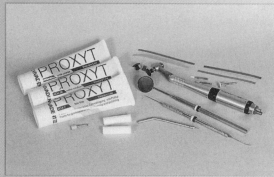

FIGURE 9-18

NOTE: Initial contouring, finishing, and polishing is done immediately after insertion.

PROCEDURE STEPS

1 Examine the restoration for staining.

NOTE: Do not polish if stain is not present.

2 Isolate the area with cotton rolls and saliva ejector.

3 Remove cavosurface flash with a sharp scaler, number 12 scalpel blade, or gold knife.

NOTE: Avoid deeply scratching the restorative material. A shaving motion is used rather than bulk removal because bulk removal may result in voids at the margins if excessive cement is lifted.

4 Use fine to coarse abrasive points and disks on a sterilizable mandrel or flexible wheels and rubber points, rinsing after each.

NOTE: Rinse thoroughly to prevent more abrasive particles from abrading the polished surface (Figures 9-19 and 9-20).

5 Use a light, sweeping motion from enamel to restoration.

NOTE: This prevents ditching of the restorations at the margins (Figure 9-21).

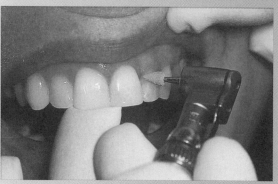

FIGURE 9-19

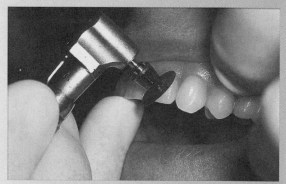

FIGURE 9-20

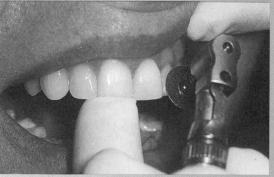

FIGURE 9-21

Continued on following page

PROCEDURE 9-2 (Continued)

6 Keep the rotary device in motion at all times.

NOTE: Smooth surfaces can be polished using cups and disks; occlusal surfaces are better reached with points (Figure 9-22).

7 Finish with sequentially applied abrasive paste on a rubber cup.

NOTE: This must be an abrasive paste designed for polishing composites; begin with coarse and proceed through superfine.

8 Polish proximal surfaces with handheld polishing strips or polishing paste and dental tape.

NOTE: These strips must be very thin to prevent loss of the proximal contact (Figure 9-23).

9 Avoid flattening proximal contours.

NOTE: Keep the rotary polishing device or abrasive strip contoured to the morphology of the tooth.

10 Rinse thoroughly and evaluate for smoothness and luster.

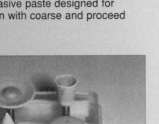

FIGURE 9-22

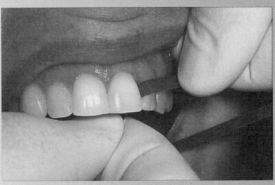

FIGURE 9-23

10 DENTAL CEMENT

OBJECTIVES

On completion of this chapter the student will be able to:

1. Define the key terms.
2. Discuss the uses of cements in dentistry for pulpal protection, luting, restorations, and surgical dressing.
3. Describe the properties of cement and how these properties affect selection of a cement for a dental procedure.
4. Discuss the components of each dental cement.
5. Discuss how these components affect the properties of the cement.
6. Discuss the advantages and disadvantages of each cement.
7. Discuss the manipulation considerations for mixing cements.
8. Describe the procedure for filling a crown with luting cement.
9. Describe the procedure for removal of excess cement after cementation.
10. Apply the mixing technique for each type of cement.

KEY TERMS

Varnish—A thin layer placed on the floor and walls of the preparation to seal the tubules and minimize microleakage.

Liner/low-strength base—A thin layer of material placed to protect the tooth from the components of dental materials and microleakage, stimulate reparative dentin, or act as a pulp capping.

Base/high-strength base—A thick layer of cement used to protect the tooth from chemical and thermal irritation.

Secondary consistency—Thick, puttylike, condensable material that can be rolled into a ball or rope, suitable for use as a base.

Buildup—A thick layer of cement used to replace missing tooth structure in a badly broken-down tooth and act as support for a restorative material such as a crown.

Permanent—Lasting indefinitely.

Temporary Revisions—Materials expected to last from a few days to a few weeks.

Luting—Cementing two components together, such as an indirect restoration cemented on or in a tooth; inlays; crowns; bridges; veneers; orthodontic brackets and bands; posts; and pins.

Primary consistency—Less viscous, flows easily, can be drawn to 1-inch string with a spatula lifted from the center of the mass; suitable for luting.

Intermediate—Materials expected to last from a few weeks to a year.

Sedative—Acting to soothe or relieve pain.

Few materials in dentistry are used as frequently or in as much variation as dental cements. There are many dental cements, and each may have specific or multiple uses (Table 10-1). There is no one universally acceptable cement that fulfills all applications; there are a variety of cements whose properties and manipulation lead them to be an appropriate choice for a given application. In most cases cements have inferior strength and high solubility when compared with other restorative materials and, with the exception of resin and glass ionomer cements, have little or no adhesive properties. However, the use of cements in a wide variety of dental procedures is extensive. With the multitude of cements and their applications, it is easy to become confused as to which cement to select for a given situation. In most cases the dentist will select the cement for the procedure based on mechanical and biologic considerations. It becomes the dental assistant's responsibility to manipulate the cement to the proper consistency within a specific time frame. Many expanded-function auxiliaries may also place the cement and remove it at the end of a procedure. The dental hygienist may place and remove cements, as well as instrument against their surface during periodontal procedures. It is important that the allied oral health practitioner have a thorough understanding of cement uses, properties, limitations, and manipulation to effectively use these materials.

Uses of Dental Cements

PULPAL PROTECTION

The bacterial effects of caries, the biologic response to chemicals contained in restorative materials, and even the cutting of tooth structure may cause pulpal irritation. Pulpal irritation can also occur due to thermal conductivity of metal restorations placed near the pulp and when the dentin remaining over the pulp is too thin to withstand compressive, tensile, and shearing stresses. Cavity varnish, liners, and bases act as protective layers between the dentin and the restorative material (Figure 10-1).

Cavity Varnish   Cavity **varnish** acts as a protective barrier between preparation and restoration.

TABLE 10-1
Uses of Dental Cements

Purpose	Cement
Low-strength base/liner	Calcium hydroxide, glass ionomer, zinc oxide eugenol
High-strength base, buildup	Reinforced zinc oxide eugenol, zinc phosphate, zinc polycarboxylate, glass ionomer
Permanent cementation:	
• Cast crowns	Zinc phosphate, zinc polycarboxylate, glass ionomer, hybrid glass ionomer, resin based
• Porcelain, ceramic, or composite veneers, inlays, onlays, and crowns	Resin based
• Orthodontic bands	Fluoride added to zinc phosphate, glass ionomer
• Orthodontic brackets	Resin based
Provisional cementation	Zinc oxide eugenol, noneugenol
Provisional restorations	Reinforced zinc oxide eugenol, polycarboxylate, zinc phosphate
Surgical dressing	Eugenol and noneugenol surgical dressing

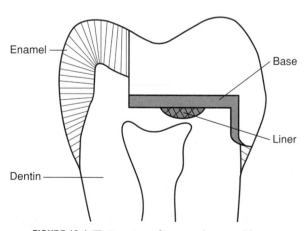

FIGURE 10-1 ■ Drawing of cement liner and base.

Varnish formulations are solutions of natural resins (copal) or synthetic resins dissolved in a solvent such as alcohol or chloroform. The varnish is applied in two or three layers over the surface of the preparation. The solution is placed in a thin film, and evaporation of the solvent is allowed to occur for 5 to 15 seconds before application of the second layer. The remaining resin protects the pulp by sealing the tubules from the penetration of irritating chemicals found in some restorative materials and luting agents. This resin varnish also reduces the amount of microleakage and staining at the restoration-tooth interface. The varnish is supplied in two bottles; the primary bottle is 90% solvent and 10% resin. A separate bottle of solvent is supplied to dilute the material in the primary bottle when it thickens as the solvent evaporates. The lid of the varnish must be kept tightly capped to avoid evaporation of the solvent. Copal varnishes, although popular for many years, are not used much any longer because they wash out within a few months. Today's dentin bonding agents, which also seal enamel and dentinal tubules, have largely replaced the use of varnish.

Liner/Low-Strength Base   Calcium hydroxide is used as a **liner/low-strength base** in cavity preparations where dentin no longer covers the pulp. When very small exposures of the pulp are suspected, this material is used as a direct pulp-capping agent. The two-paste system is composed of calcium hydroxide, zinc oxide, and glycol salicylate. Equal amounts of catalyst and base pastes are incorporated to a creamy consistency.

Calcium hydroxide has an alkaline pH of between 9 and 11. This alkali stimulates secondary dentin when in direct contact with the pulp, providing a barrier between pulp and restoration. It has some thermal insulating properties and provides minimal strength to support the forces of condensation. Questions about the long-term success and retention of these bases and the development of dentin bonding systems have greatly reduced the routine use of this material.

High-Strength Base   A **base/high-strength base** provides thermal insulation and support for restorations. Cements used as bases are mixed to **secondary consistency,** a thick, puttylike consistency that is condensable and can be rolled into a ball or rope. Bases placed in a thickness of 0.5 mm or greater provide protection from the thermal conduction of metallic restorations. When the cavity preparation is so deep that there is 2 mm or less of remaining dentin over the pulp, many clinicians will choose to provide mechanical support for the restoration by first placing a cement base.

Buildup A **buildup,** much like a high-strength base, provides mechanical support for a restorative material when an excessive amount of tooth structure is removed. The remaining tooth structure may first need to be rebuilt to better support the restorative material or to act as a foundation before crown preparation. By placing a cement buildup, the compromised tooth is reinforced.

LUTING-CEMENTATION

Cements used for **permanent** or **temporary luting** (cementing of two components together) of fixed prostheses, orthodontic bands and brackets, and pins and posts must have good wettability and flow to provide a thin film thickness. When the tooth structure and fixed prostheses are in intimate contact a microscopic space exists, the tooth-restoration interface. The primary purpose of luting cement is to fill this space (Figure 10-2). Cements mixed to **primary consistency** must have thin enough viscosity to be able to flow into a film thickness of 0.25 μm or less. If the viscosity of the cement is such that the prosthesis fails to regain intimate contact with the tooth, a thick layer of cement will be exposed at the margin. This may also occur if the margins do not fit precisely before luting. Exposure of cement to oral fluids at the margins results in dissolution of the cement. As cement is lost at the margins, bacterial plaque can accumulate beneath the crown where the patient cannot clean, resulting in recurrent caries. Some cements have the capability of chemically bonding the prosthesis to the tooth. The chemical bond enhances retention by reducing the separation of the tooth-prosthesis interface.

Orthodontic Bands and Brackets Orthodontic bands and brackets are retained on teeth for several months or even years. Brackets are usually bonded directly to the tooth structure (see Chapter 5), whereas bands are luted with a dental cement. The cement must adhere tenaciously to the enamel and the orthodontic appliance to provide leverage for

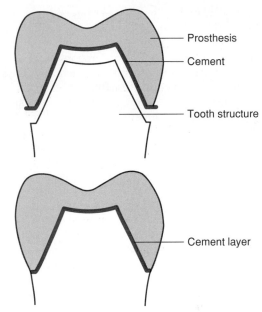

FIGURE 10-2 ■ Drawing of seating a crown and the cement filling the restoration-tooth interface.

tooth movement. Demineralization of the tooth surface caused by solubility of cements, with resultant leakage of bacteria between the bands and the tooth surface, has been problematic for many patients. This concern has been minimized to some extent with fluoride-releasing cements.

RESTORATIONS

Permanent, Temporary, and Intermediate Because of their lower strength and wear resistance and higher solubility, cements are not frequently chosen as permanent restorations. The exception is glass ionomer cement, which, because of its release of fluoride, is used for class V restorations of root caries in adults and for the restoration of primary teeth (see Chapter 6).

As provisional and **intermediate** restorations, dental cements are mixed to secondary consistency. The choice of cement for this type of restoration is largely based on the particular clinical situation. Provisional restorations are used for emergency situations when appointment scheduling does not allow for sufficient time to place a permanent restoration. Provisional restorations are placed when a tooth is symptomatic or deep caries removal is required. By placing a **sedative** provisional restoration, the dentist is able to evaluate the response of the pulp before reappointment for a permanent restoration. Provisional and intermediate restorations are used to restore teeth awaiting treatment such as inlays, between endodontic appointments, or when extensive treatment plans require several weeks or months of coverage before treatment can be completed. See chapter 14 for a discussion of intracoronal cement provisionals.

SURGICAL DRESSING

As a surgical dressing, cements are used to provide protection and support for the surgical site, provide patient comfort, and help in the control of bleeding. Most clinicians prefer a noneugenol dressing, which may be dispensed in both light-cure and chemical-cure formulas. These materials are mixed to a soft, puttylike consistency; they harden when placed over the tissue, forming a rigid covering (Figures 10-3 and 10-4).

Properties of Dental Cements

Properties of dental cements differ from one type of cement to another. No cement is ideal for every clinical situation; for example, a cement may be appropriate for a single crown, but it may not be ideal for a multiple-unit bridge. The clinician must consider both physical and biologic properties when selecting cement for a specific dental procedure. The most important properties are strength, solubility, viscosity, biocompatability, retention, esthetics, and ease of manipulation (Table 10-2).

STRENGTH

Cements are brittle materials with good compressive strength but more limited tensile strength. The strongest cements are resin cements, and the weakest cement is zinc oxide eugenol. Cements used for permanent luting and high-strength bases need good compressive and tensile strength. As can be seen in Table 10-2, resin-based cement is high in mechanical strength and fracture toughness, whereas polycarboxylate cement is low in both. Most cements are a combination of powder and liquid; their ratio determines many of the cement's properties. The

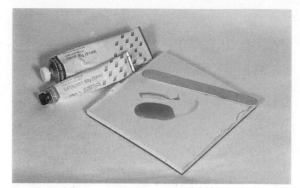

FIGURE 10-3 ■ Materials and supplies for mixing a surgical dressing.

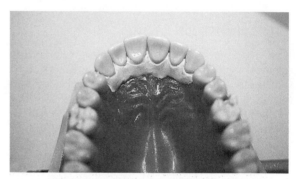

FIGURE 10-4 ■ Surgical dressing in place.

CRITERIA FOR A WELL-PLACED DRESSING

- Smooth with as little bulk as possible
- Covers the surgical site with minimal overextension
- Interlocked interdentally to provide stability

---

strength of a cement is controlled primarily by the amount of powder used in the prepared mix. Generally, an increase in the powder to liquid ratio increases the strength of the cement. However, excessive powder or liquid can weaken the cement.

SOLUBILITY

The tendency of cements to dissolve in the oral fluids, leading to microleakage, recurrent caries, and failure of the restoration, is one of the biggest hurdles for dental cements. Most of the cements

Table 10-2

Properties of Cements

Property	Glass Ionomer Cements	Hybrid Ionomer	Resin	Zinc Phosphate	Zinc Polycarboxylate	Zinc Oxide Eugenol
Mechanical	Moderate	Moderate	High	Low	Low	Low strength
Solubility	Moderate	Low	Very low	High	High	High
Film thickness	Low	Low	Low	Low	Low, medium	Low, medium
Postoperative sensitivity	High	Low	Low	High	Low	Low
Fluoride	High	High	None	None	None	None
Adhesion	Good	Good	High	None	Moderate	None
Esthetics	Good	Good	Good	None	None	None
Manipulation	Moderately easy	Easy	Difficult	Difficult	Moderately easy	Easy

used in dentistry will disintegrate in the oral environment over time. Solubility is important whenever the cement is expected to remain exposed to mouth fluids for prolonged periods of time. Resin-containing cements are as close as possible to being insoluble. The amount of powder incorporated into the final product greatly influences the solubility of the resultant cement.

VISCOSITY/FILM THICKNESS

The consistency of mixed cement is the measure of its ability to flow under pressure. This is particularly important in the case of cement used for luting, because it determines the dentist's ability to seat the indirect restoration properly. For primary consistency, cements should be able to be mixed thin, about the consistency of honey. Low film thickness is critical to seating and retaining indirect restorations. To be an effective luting cement, American Dental Association (ADA) specifications require the cement to be able to flow into a film thickness of 25 μm or less.

Secondary consistency requires the addition of powder to increase strength and bring the cement to a thick, puttylike consistency. Cements mixed to secondary consistency are used as bases and restorations, either temporary or permanent. The addition of powder increases the viscosity and strength and decreases the solubility of the cement.

Several factors influence the consistency of a mixed cement. Temperature has a great effect; a lower temperature will slow the setting reaction, giving the

clinician more working time and allowing incorporation of more powder into the liquid. The amount of powder incorporated into the mix may substantially increase the viscosity of the mixed cement.

BIOCOMPATIBILITY

Many cements are a combination of a powder of zinc oxide or powdered glass and an acid. The pH of the acid both at placement and after complete setting is a concern. Postoperative pulpal sensitivity is related to the pH and manipulation variables of the cement. Other causes are unsealed dentinal tubules, trauma to the pulp during preparation, and bacterial leakage under the provisional restoration. Careful attention to powder/liquid ratios, dispensing technique, and mixing recommendations can minimize this concern. Eugenol, found in the liquid of zinc oxide eugenol cements, has an obtundant, sedative effect on the pulp. Fluoride release from powdered glass formulations reduces secondary caries.

RETENTION

Retention of indirect restorations is accomplished by adhesion, the attachment of one substance to another with an adhesive. The adhesive is a semifluid cement that is able to penetrate into microscopic irregularities in both the internal surfaces of an indirect restoration and the adjoining tooth structure. This produces a restoration that is both resistant to microleakage and highly retentive. One group of cements, glass ionomers, also forms weak chemical bonds to tooth structure that aid in retention and reduce microleakage.

ESTHETICS

Cements are available in a variety of shades and opacities for luting porcelain veneers, ceramic or composite inlays and onlays, and porcelain full crowns. Usually, a shade is chosen to approximate the shade of the restoration so that the appearance of the restoration is not altered by the underlying cement as light passes through the restoration and reflects off the cement. Occasionally, it is necessary to mask the color of the dentin, especially if it is discolored. In this situation an opaque cement of the appropriate shade is selected. Try-in paste is provided by many manufacturers; this water-soluble paste is matched to the base shade of the cement and is used to tack the restoration in place to check the shade of the final product. Try-in paste is recommended to ensure an accurate prediction of the final appearance of the restoration and acceptance of the restoration esthetics by both the dentist and patient.

Manipulation

MIXING

It is important that cements be mixed to their appropriate consistency following manufacturer's recommendations and measuring ratios, with meticulous attention to detail. Cements that are mishandled may lead to difficulties seating or retaining the restoration or pulpal sensitivity. Cements may be hand mixed or come in predosed capsules and syringes. Some cements have been packaged in automixing cartridges similar to those used for impression materials (Figure 10-5). Advantages and disadvantages of each delivery system are listed in Table 10-3.

The working time and setting time are considerations in the choice of cement and the mixing mechanism. The longer working time needed for cementation of longer span bridges versus single crowns, the shorter setting time required for difficult-to-isolate areas, patient considerations, and the dental assistant's mixing skills all play a part in the choice of an appropriate cement. The dental assistant is responsible for delivering the cement in the

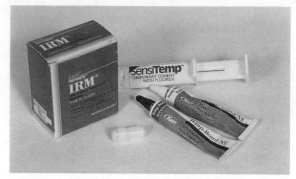

FIGURE 10-5 ■ Hand-mix, dual-syringe dispensed, paste-paste, and predosed systems.

TABLE 10-3

Advantages and Disadvantages of Delivery Systems

Hand Mixing	Automixing	Predosed Capsules
Advantages		
Vary viscosity	Consistent mix	Consistent mix
Vary volume of material mixed	Vary volume of material used	Convenience
		Disposable
No extra equipment	Convenience	
Less expensive	Less cleanup required	
Can mix shades if needed		
Disadvantages		
Inconsistent mix	Unable to vary viscosity	Unable to vary viscosity
Less convenient	Additional equipment needed	Fixed capsule volume
		Cannot blend shades
More cleanup required	Cannot blend shades	Requires extra equipment
	More expensive	

proper consistency within specific time frames. A skilled assistant must be able to routinely mix cements to their proper consistency rapidly.

The setting of cements may be initiated by three means: chemical, light, or combination of chemical

MANIPULATION CONSIDERATIONS

1. Keep powder and liquid separated when dispensing.
2. Fluff powder before dispensing by gently rolling the container in your hand to aerate.
3. Use a level scoop of powder, not heaping.
4. Section the powder into increments according to the manufacturer's directions. When increment size varies, the smallest increments are mixed first.
4. Dispense the liquid by holding the dispenser vertically before squeezing to obtain more uniform drops.
5. Close caps of powder and liquid containers immediately after dispensing to avoid evaporation and contamination.
6. Incorporate powder and liquid thoroughly when mixing. If incremental mixing is used, each increment must be completely incorporated before adding the next.
7. Use moderate pressure on the spatula when mixing.
8. Use both sides of the spatula blade.
9. Mix cement in a figure-eight motion.
10. Gather all the material together to test the viscosity

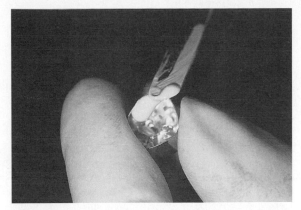

FIGURE 10-6 ■ Loading a crown. Wipe blade of spatula against the margin of the crown.

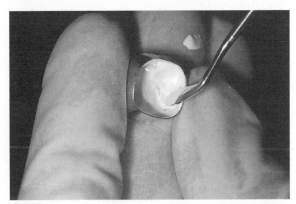

FIGURE 10-7 ■ Loading a crown. Using a flat-bladed instrument, cover all the walls with a thin, even coating of the cement.

and light (dual-cure). The rate of chemical set varies with the different cements. Light-cure cements are popular for porcelain veneers but are contraindicated with thicker ceramic restorations where the light would not penetrate adequately. Dual-cure cements are more appropriate in this case.

LOADING THE RESTORATION

The dental assistant may be responsible for filling the crown with a luting cement before passing it to the dentist. Techniques described in the accompanying box will ensure that the cement is evenly loaded in the crown and that the margins are coated internally (Figures 10-6 and 10-7).

REMOVAL OF EXCESS CEMENT

Allied oral health practitioners may be asked to remove excess cement from crown margins after

LOADING A CROWN FOR CEMENTATION

1. Gather cement from mixing surface with the blade of the spatula or plastic instrument.
2. Wipe the blade against the margin of the crown.
3. Cover all the walls with a thin, even coating of cement.
4. Pass the crown cement-side down on the palm of your hand for the dentist to pick up and seat.

REMOVAL OF EXCESS CEMENT

1. Follow manufacturers' directions for the appropriate consistency at removal. Cement consistencies vary from rock hard to rubbery.
2. Remove cement in bulk when possible.
3. Use an explorer or a scaler to remove cement from smooth surfaces, being careful not to scratch the surface of the restoration or gouge margins.
4. Use a piece of knotted floss to remove cement from interproximal areas.
5. Complete removal of excess cement is essential to maintain gingival health.

seating. It is important to be familiar with the proper consistency of the cement for removal. Some cements should not be removed until completely set, others may be best removed when the cement reaches a rubbery consistency, and others may be best removed while the cement is still tacky.

CLEANUP, DISINFECTION, AND STERILIZATION

The removal of cement before it is set provides for easier cleanup. Clean instruments and equipment that come in contact with cement as soon as reasonably possible with gauze squares saturated with alcohol. If immediate cleanup is not possible, use the ultrasonic cleaner with cement removal solution. Equipment such as amalgamators, cement activators, the outside of cement bottles, dispensing scoops, and syringes must be properly disinfected if barriers have not been used. Sterilization of mixing and delivery instruments is necessary. Glass and plastic mixing slabs are recommended because they can be sterilized in heat sterilizers. Paper pads, although convenient, are a source of contamination, and there is no reliable way to combat this.

CONSIDERATIONS DURING INSTRUMENTATION

Proper instrumentation during prophylactic procedures and appropriate delivery of some therapeutic agents such as fluoride are important considerations for the continuing care of cement margins. Care must be taken to avoid gouging or ditching cement margins during hand instrumentation. Ultrasonic and sonic scalers, as well as air polishing, should be avoided on resin-based cement margins. Fluoride application on resin-based cement margins should be limited to neutral sodium fluoride.

Dental Cements

ZINC OXIDE EUGENOL

Zinc oxide eugenol (ZOE) cements have been widely used for many years. A variety of ZOE cements are available in powder-liquid and paste-paste systems. In the two-paste system, one is labeled a base and the other a catalyst. ZOE cements may be used for temporary cementation, temporary and intermediate restorations, and high- and low-strength bases, as well as root-canal sealers and periodontal dressings.

Composition The principle ingredient of the powder is zinc oxide; resin reinforcers may be added for additional strength for intermediate restorations and high-strength bases. Eugenol, which has the distinct smell of cloves, is a derivative of oil of cloves. Newer formulations have removed the eugenol and are called noneugenol zinc oxide cements.

Properties Eugenol has long been known for its sedative effect on the pulp, largely because of its antibacterial effects. It can also be irritating when in direct contact with oral mucosa or pulp. The mixed ZOE has a neutral pH of 7, which makes it highly biocompatible with tooth structures. The strength depends on the addition of reinforcers. However, ZOE cements are not as strong as other permanent luting agents and are rarely used for this purpose. ZOE cements are ideally suited for temporary cementation; their weaker tensile strength allows them to be easily removed at a second appointment when a permanent restoration is to be placed. Eugenol may interfere with the polymerization process of resins. Cements containing eugenol should not be used under composites or as temporary cements before final cementation with hybrid glass ionomer or resin cements. Noneugenol zinc oxide cements are preferred in these clinical situations. The powder-liquid and paste-paste systems are easily manipulated. The set, strength, and viscosity are controlled by the incorporation of powder or, in the paste-paste system, by changing the ratio of base to catalyst.

ZINC OXIDE EUGENOL

Advantages
1. A wide variety of uses
2. Sedative to the pulp
3. Easily manipulated

Disadvantages
1. Low strength
2. High solubility
3. Unable to be used under composite restorations and indirect restorations cemented with resin or hybrid glass ionomer cements

ZINC PHOSPHATE

Advantages
1. Long clinical history
2. Low film thickness
3. Inexpensive
4. High rigidity

Disadvantages
1. Initial pulpal irritation
2. Mechanical bond only
3. Technique-sensitive mixing
4. Relatively high solubility

ZINC PHOSPHATE

Zinc phosphate is the oldest of the cements. Although it is not as widely used today, it has a long history of success. It is supplied in several brands as a powder-liquid system. These cements are primarily used as permanent luting agents under indirect restorations and for cementation of orthodontic bands. The incorporation of additional powder can provide thermal insulation for use as a high-strength base.

Composition The powder of zinc phosphate cement is principally zinc oxide; fluoride is added by some manufacturers to aid in the prevention of caries under orthodontically banded teeth. The liquid is made from phosphoric acid and water. The chemical reaction, which occurs when the cement powder is incorporated into the liquid, results in an exothermic reaction, the production of heat. Attention to proper mixing technique is required to minimize this reaction. The setting and exothermic reaction of zinc phosphate cement is controlled by time and temperature. Incremental incorporation of the powder into the liquid allows for controlled dissipation of heat. Mixing over a large area of a cooled glass slab also dissipates the heat. The glass slab should be cooled to be effective in dissipating heat but not below the dew point (approximately 65° F) when water condensation would lessen the incorporation of powder and shorten the setting time. Use of a frozen slab can greatly increase the incorporation of powder and increase the working time to help when cementing several orthodontic bands.

Properties Initially the acidity (pH 4.2) of zinc phosphate cement is low and becomes neutral within 24 to 48 hours. The initially low acidity may irritate the pulp in deep preparations. Pulpal protection in deep cavity preparations is recommended with low-strength bases and dentin bonding systems.

The strength, solubility, and film thickness are important properties. The retention of indirect restorations such as crowns, inlays, and onlays can be enhanced by sandblasting the internal surface of the restoration. The cement flows into irregularities in the restoration and on the tooth surface, locking the two together. The low film thickness of properly mixed cements allows for the intimate contact necessary for good retention. Zinc phosphate cement has adequate strength and rigidity for cementation of single-unit and long span bridges, but it is weaker than resin or hybrid ionomer cements. Its solubility is clinically acceptable but higher than other cements. This higher solubility has made it less favorable with clinicians for the cementation of orthodontic bands.

ZINC POLYCARBOXYLATE

Zinc polycarboxylate cements were the first cements developed with an adhesive bond to tooth structures. These cements are primarily used for final cementation of indirect restorations, but they can also be used as high-strength bases with the incorporation of additional powder.

Composition Zinc polycarboxylate cements are supplied as a powder-liquid system. Some manufacturers supply predosed capsules for mixing in an amalgamator. The powder is essentially zinc oxide and the liquid is an aqueous solution of polyacrylic acid. The polyacrylic acid produces minimal irritation to the pulp.

Properties The viscosity of zinc polycarboxylate cement is higher than most other cements. The liquid of this cement should not be dispensed before mixing time because the loss of water from evaporation can adversely increase the viscosity. These cements have lower compressive strength and higher solubility than other cements. The retention of polycarboxylate cements is both chemical and mechanical, making this cement desirable for retention of indirect restorations. The bond is achieved only if the cement still exhibits a glossy appearance when the restoration is seated. The working time can be extended by use of a cooled glass slab.

GLASS IONOMER CEMENTS

Since their introduction in 1969, glass ionomer cements have continued to evolve. Originally developed for esthetic restoration of anterior teeth, glass ionomer cements have become one of the most versatile cements used today. These cements have a chemical bond with tooth structures. Glass ionomer cements are used as permanent luting agents, restorative materials, low- and high-strength bases, and core buildups. In many instances, the same product can be mixed to different viscosities for different uses. This simplifies product selection and inventory control. Glass ionomer cements now include both traditional glass ionomer cements and hybrid ionomer cements (also known as resin-modified glass ionomer cements).

TRADITIONAL GLASS IONOMER CEMENTS

Composition The cement is supplied as a powder-liquid system, with some products coming encapsulated for mixing in an amalgamator and delivered through a gun-type applicator. The powder is a calcium fluoraluminsilicate glass with barium glass added for radiopacity (Figure 10-8). The liquid is a polyacrylic acid copolymer in water. When powder and liquid are mixed, the polyacid attacks the glass to release fluoride ions.

Properties Glass ionomer cements are biologically compatible with the pulp when manipulated properly. Mild to severe postoperative sensitivity has been reported. Overdrying of the preparation and moisture contamination during the first 24 hours of setting have been indicated as possible sources of this sensitivity. Fluoride release during the life of the cement may have an anticariogenic effect. Strength, solubility, and film thickness are comparable with

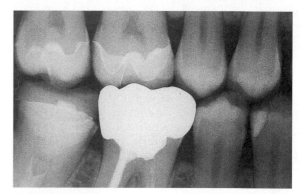

FIGURE 10-8 ■ Cement-filled interface filled with radiopaque cement.

ZINC POLYCARBOXYLATE

Advantages
1. Bonds to tooth structures
2. Nonirritating to the pulp
3. Inexpensive

Disadvantages
1. Higher solubility
2. Lower strength
3. Shorter working time

TRADITIONAL GLASS IONOMER CEMENT

Advantages
1. Chemical adhesion to tooth
2. Fluoride release
3. Easy to mix
4. Moderate strength

Disadvantages
1. History of postoperative sensitivity
2. Moisture sensitive during setting

other permanent cements. An increase in solubility has been demonstrated with early moisture contamination, during the first 24 hours. Teeth restored with glass ionomer restorations, bases, and core buildups must be properly isolated for the 6- to 8-minute setting time. The margins of indirect restorations using these cements should be coated with a coating agent or varnish to protect them from moisture.

HYBRID IONOMER CEMENTS (RESIN-MODIFIED GLASS IONOMER CEMENTS)

The composition of hybrid ionomer cement is similar to glass ionomer cement, but it is modified with the addition of resin. The resin helps improve the bond strength, compressive strength, and tensile strength and decrease the solubility; these cements are virtually insoluble in oral fluids and have excellent film thickness. Fluoride release is the same as that for glass ionomer cements. Expansion of the material as it absorbs moisture after setting is a concern, making the cement less desirable for cementation of all-ceramic indirect restorations because of the risk of fracture.

RESIN-BASED CEMENTS (COMPOSITE RESIN, ADHESIVE RESIN, AND COMPOMER)

Resin cements are basically modified composite used to bond ceramic indirect restorations, conventional crowns, and bridges and for indirect bonding of orthodontic brackets. Temporary resin-based cements have been developed to address the problem that eugenol contamination from ZOE temporary cements causes with bonding agents and composite resin cements. Light-cured, dual-cured, and chemically cured varieties are available; each system has limitations. The dual-cured cements are the most versatile.

Composition   Resin-based cements are similar in composition to composite restorative materials and hybrid glass ionomer cements. Filler particle size is kept very small, similar to microfills or microhybrids (see Chapter 6). Initiators of polymerization are added to change the setting mechanism. Pigments are added to aid in tooth color matching.

Properties   Resin cements are virtually insoluble in oral conditions. They have superior bond strength and are wear resistant at exposed margins. A variety of esthetic shades are available for bonding translucent, all-ceramic restorations.

   Resin cements are used after preparation of the tooth surface and internal surface of the restoration. Prepare the tooth surface for bonding (as described in Chapter 5) with etchant and bonding agent. Prepare the internal surface of the restoration with a solution of acid for ceramics or by sandblasting. It is important to pay attention to manufacturers' directions regarding bonding of the tooth surface and preparation of the restoration surface to achieve a strong bond and eliminate postoperative sensitivity. Removal of excess cement is difficult if the material is allowed to set completely; follow manufacturer directions for removal.

HYBRID IONOMER CEMENTS

Advantages
1. Good strength
2. Fluoride release
3. Insoluble
4. Chemical adhesion to tooth
5. Less postoperative sensitivity
6. Excellent film thickness

Disadvantages
1. Not recommended for all ceramic restorations

TYPES OF RESTORATION AND METHOD OF CURING

Light-cured
Porcelain veneers less than 1.5 mm thick
Orthodontic retainers not containing metal
Periodontal splints not containing metal

Dual-cured (light activated and chemically activated)
Porcelain or indirect resin inlays, onlays, crowns, and bridges

Self-cured (chemically cured)
Metal-based inlays, onlays, crowns, and bridges
Full-metal crowns and bridges
Endodontic posts
Porcelain or indirect resin inlays, onlays, crowns, and bridges

RESIN-BASED CEMENTS

Advantages
1. High strength
2. Insoluble
3. Low wear
4. Excellent bond
5. Esthetic shades available

Disadvantages
1. Requires additional steps in the bonding procedure
2. Requires additional steps in preparation of internal restoration surfaces
3. Removal of excess cement may be difficult

SUMMARY

No single cement satisfies all dental purposes. Cements are chosen for their properties for each different clinical situation. The allied oral health practitioner has responsibility for achieving and maintaining many of these properties. The proper manipulation of the cement before it is delivered to the dentist plays a big part in determining the quality of the physical properties. The use of instruments on a cement margin can directly affect their longevity. Procedures for placement of temporary restorations are important to the success of future permanent ones. The auxiliary must be knowledgeable in uses, properties, handling characteristics, and precautions for all cements used in the office.

CHAPTER REVIEW

Select the one correct response for each of the following multiple-choice questions.

1. **Cements mixed to primary consistency are used for**
   a. Luting and high-strength bases
   b. Luting and low-strength bases
   c. Core buildups
   d. Surgical dressings

2. **It may be necessary to place an insulating base under restorations to**
   a. Encourage secondary dentin formation
   b. Protect the pulp from sudden temperature changes
   c. Reduce acidity
   d. Seal the dentinal tubules

3. **The test for a properly mixed luting cement is**
   a. Putty consistency
   b. Granular consistency
   c. Cement will break and form a drop at the end of the spatula
   d. Cement will hold a thin string, breaking when the spatula is raised an inch

4. **Which cement should *not* be used for temporary cementation of crowns to be permanently cemented with resin cements?**
   a. Zinc polycarboxylate
   b. Zinc phosphate
   c. Zinc oxide eugenol
   d. Any cement is appropriate

5. **Which cement exhibits an exothermic reaction during mixing?**
   a. Glass ionomer
   b. Zinc phosphate
   c. Resin cements
   d. Calcium hydroxide

6. **Which dental cements use the bonding procedure before placement of the dental cement?**
   a. Zinc phosphate and polycarboxylate
   b. Zinc oxide eugenol and glass ionomer
   c. Composite resin and glass ionomer
   d. Calcium hydroxide and zinc oxide eugenol

7. **When luting a crown, it is important to**
   a. Have a film thickness allowing for complete seating
   b. Have a film thickness for proper insulation
   c. Have a film thickness for complete filling of the crown
   d. None of the above

8. **Many cements should not be dispensed until ready to mix because of**
   a. Dehydration from exposure to air
   b. Contamination from moisture in the air
   c. Materials coming in contact with each other
   d. All of the above

9. **Which dental cement bonds to dentin, is kind to the pulp, and resists recurrent decay?**
   a. Zinc oxide eugenol   c. Calcium hydroxide
   b. Polycarboxylate   d. Glass ionomer

10. **Zinc phosphate cement is mixed over a large area of the glass slab to**
    a. Help lengthen the working time
    b. Help neutralize the chemicals
    c. Help dissipate the exothermic reaction
    d. All of the above

11. **Proper instrumentation against cement margins includes all of the following EXCEPT:**
    a. Avoid gouging or ditching cement margins
    b. Use ultrasonic scalers to remove deposits on resin cement margins
    c. Avoid the use of air polishing on resin cement margins
    d. Only neutral sodium fluoride is recommended for use on resin cement margins

12. **Light-cured cements may be used for luting each of the following EXCEPT:**
    a. Nonmetal orthodontic retainers
    b. Nonmetal periodontal splints
    c. Porcelain resin inlays
    d. Porcelain veneers less than 1.5 mm thick

CASE-BASED DISCUSSION TOPICS

◉ A 22-year-old administrative assistant is scheduled for a crown preparation. She has been seen in your office previously for a crown and experienced some difficulty with sensitivity while the provisional crown was in place. **Which cement would be the best choice for luting the temporary crown and why?**

◉ A 40-year-old accountant is scheduled for cementation of an all-ceramic crown on tooth number 5. The provisional crown has been cemented with a noneugenol zinc oxide cement. *Why was this cement chosen for the provisional coverage and which cement would be the best choice for the permanent crown?*

▣ A 9-year-old is scheduled for cementation of orthodontic bands. *Which cement would be the best choice and why?*

▣ You are asked to mix a final luting cement and fill a crown in preparation for seating. Although the crown seated completely on try-in, when the dentist attempts to seat the cement-filled crown the margins remain open and the crown is high. *What might be the explanation for this situation?*

▣ Your office is considering going to a predosed cement system. *What situations can you foresee where this system may be problematic?*

REFERENCES

Anusavice K: *Phillips' science of dental materials,* ed 10, Philadelphia, 1996, WB Saunders.

Christensen G: Success with cements, self-etching primers, *Dental Products Report* p 64, Apr 2001.

Craig RG: *Restorative dental materials,* ed 10, St Louis, 1996, Mosby.

Farah JW, Powers JM: Core materials, *Dental Advisor* 16:6, 1999.

Farah JW, Powers JM: Fluoride-releasing restorative materials, *Dental Advisor* 14:2, 1998.

Farah JW, Powers JM: Permanent and temporary cements, *Dental Advisor* 16:6, 1997.

Fruits T et al: Uses and properties of current glass ionomer cements: a review, *General Dentistry* p 410, Oct 1996.

Helpin M, Rosenberg H: Resin-modified glass ionomers in pediatric dentistry, *Practical Dental Hygiene* p 33, Jan-Feb 1996.

Introduction to biomaterials properties/biomaterials properties table listing: www.lib.umich.edu/libhome/Dentistry_tables/Soldis.html.

Leinfelder KF: Should I change the type of cement I use? *J Am Dent Assoc* 130(10):1492, 1999.

Miller M, editor: *Reality,* vol 13, *Resin cements and resin ionomers,* Houston, Tex., 1999, Reality Publishing.

Wilkins E: *Clinical practice of the dental hygienist,* ed 8, Philadelphia, 1999, Lippincott Williams & Wilkins.

PROCEDURE 10-1 (see p. 334 for competency sheet)

Mixing Zinc Oxide Eugenol Cement: Primary and Secondary Consistency

EQUIPMENT/SUPPLIES (Figure 10-9)

- Cement paste-paste *or* cement powder-liquid and dispensers
- Paper mixing pad or glass slab
- Flexible cement spatula

PROCEDURE STEPS: PRIMARY CONSISTENCY

1 Dispense the recommended amount of base paste and accelerator paste onto a mixing pad.

NOTE: ½ inch of each is usually enough for a single-crown restoration (Figure 10-9).

2 Mix the material using both sides of the flat blade in a figure-eight motion.

3 The mix is in primary consistency when it is smooth and creamy and after gathering together lifts 1 inch off the mixing surface (Figure 10-10).

4 Whenever possible immediately clean the spatula with gauze.

PROCEDURE STEPS: SECONDARY CONSISTENCY (Figure 10-11)

1 Fluff the powder and measure onto one end of the mixing surface.

NOTE: Aerated powder provides for a more accurate measurement.

2 Shake the liquid and dispense at the opposite end of the mixing surface.

NOTE: Hold the dispenser vertical while dispensing to obtain uniform drops.

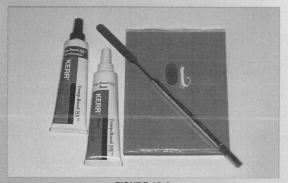

FIGURE 10-9

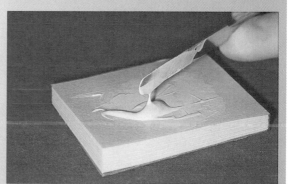

FIGURE 10-10

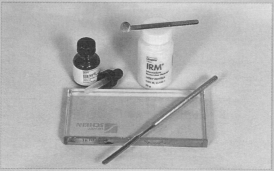

FIGURE 10-11

Continued on following page

3 Incorporate the powder into the liquid in two increments or all at once according to the manufacturer's directions.

NOTE: Incorporate as much powder as possible into the liquid (Figures 10-12 and 10-13).

4 Mix the material using both sides of the flat blade in a figure-eight motion.

5 The cement will be in secondary consistency when it can be rolled into a ball and is no longer tacky (Figure 10-14).

6 Whenever possible immediately clean the spatula with moist gauze.

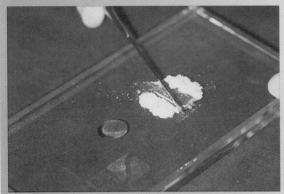

FIGURE 10-12

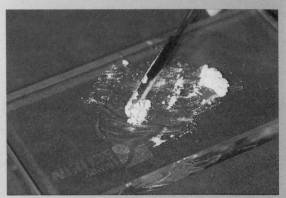

FIGURE 10-13

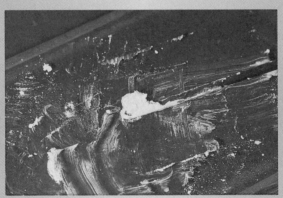

FIGURE 10-14

PROCEDURE 10-2 (see p. 335 for competency sheet)

Mixing Zinc Phosphate Cement: Primary and Secondary Consistency

EQUIPMENT/SUPPLIES (Figure 10-15)

- Cement powder
- Cement liquid and dispenser
- Cool glass slab
- Flexible cement spatula

PROCEDURE STEPS: PRIMARY CONSISTENCY

1 Obtain a cooled glass slab.

NOTE: The frozen slab method may be used for multiple orthodontic bands or long span bridges.

2 Fluff the powder and dispense the recommended amount onto one end of the slab.

3 Divide the powder into four to six increments to include smaller and larger increment sizes.

NOTE: Smaller increments are incorporated first.

4 Shake the liquid and dispense the recommended amount at the opposite end of the slab.

NOTE: Hold the dispenser vertical while dispensing to obtain uniform drops (Figure 10-16).

5 Incorporate the first increment into the liquid.

NOTE: Hold the spatula blade flat against the mixing surface. Use both sides of the spatula in a sweeping figure-eight motion over a large area of the slab (Figure 10-17).

6 Each increment is completely incorporated and mixed for 20 to 30 seconds beginning with the smallest and progressing through the largest.

NOTE: Adding increments of powder and completely incorporating each into the mix will help neutralize the acid, control the setting time, and allow for the completion of the exothermic reaction before use (Figure 10-18).

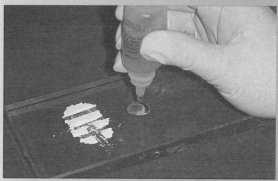

FIGURE 10-16

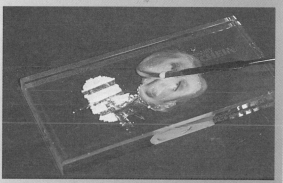

FIGURE 10-17

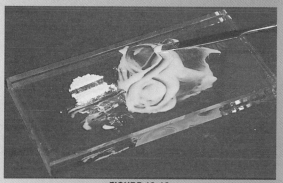

FIGURE 10-18

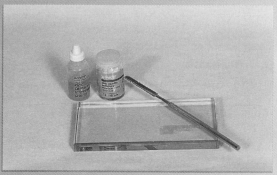

FIGURE 10-15

Continued on following page

PROCEDURE 10-2 (Continued)

7 Place the spatula blade at a 45-degree angle to the slab and gather the mass together to test the consistency.

NOTE: For primary consistency the material should be smooth and creamy. Draw the spatula up from the mix; the cement should follow the spatula, breaking after 1 inch (Figure 10-19).

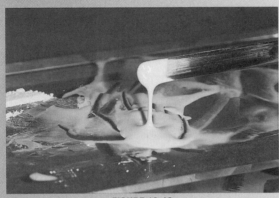

FIGURE 10-19

8 Clean the spatula and slab with moistened gauze and disinfect or sterilize.

NOTE: If the cement is allowed to harden on the slab or spatula, it may be removed in the ultrasonic cleaner or by soaking in a solution of baking powder.

PROCEDURE STEPS: SECONDARY CONSISTENCY

1 Dispense the recommended amount of powder and liquid onto opposite ends of the glass slab.

NOTE: For secondary consistency more powder is required.

2 Divide and mix as previously instructed, incorporating as much powder as possible into the liquid.

NOTE: After reaching primary consistency, larger increments are incorporated in shorter periods of time.

3 The cement has achieved secondary consistency when it can be rolled into a ball and is no longer tacky.

PROCEDURE 10-3 (see p. 336 for competency sheet)

Mixing Zinc Polycarboxylate Cement: Primary and Secondary Consistency

EQUIPMENT/SUPPLIES (Figure 10-20)

- Cement powder and dispenser
- Cement liquid and dispenser
- Paper mixing pad or glass slab
- Flexible cement spatula

PROCEDURE STEPS: PRIMARY CONSISTENCY

1 Fluff the powder and measure onto one end of the mixing surface.

NOTE: Aerated powder provides for a more accurate measurement.

2 Shake the liquid and dispense at the opposite end of the mixing surface.

NOTE: Hold the dispenser vertical while dispensing to obtain uniform drops. If using a syringe dispenser, be careful to note number of lined increments to dispense.

3 Incorporate the powder into the liquid in two increments or all at once according to the manufacturer's directions.

4 Mix the material using both sides of the flat blade in a figure-eight motion.

5 The mix is in primary consistency when it is smooth and creamy and after gathering together lifts 1 inch off the mixing surface.

NOTE: The consistency is somewhat thicker than other cements and appears glossy (Figure 10-21). The cement is too thick if it produces thin, stringy "cobwebs" when lifted off the mixing surface (Figure 10-22).

6 Whenever possible, immediately clean the spatula with moist gauze.

PROCEDURE STEPS: SECONDARY CONSISTENCY

1 Dispense the recommended amount of powder and liquid onto opposite ends of the mixing surface.

NOTE: For secondary consistency more powder is required.

2 Divide and mix as previously instructed, incorporating as much powder as possible into the liquid.

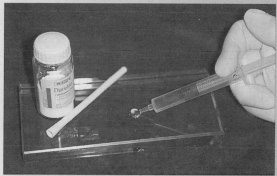

FIGURE 10-20

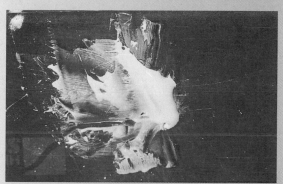

FIGURE 10-21

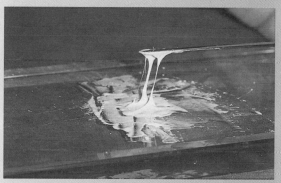

FIGURE 10-22

3 The cement will be in secondary consistency when it can be rolled into a ball and is no longer tacky.

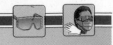

PROCEDURE 10-4 (see p. 337 for competency sheet)

Mixing Glass Ionomer Cement: Predosed Capsule

EQUIPMENT/SUPPLIES (Figure 10-23)

- Predosed capsule of cement
- Cement activator
- Amalgamator
- Cement dispenser

PROCEDURE STEPS

1 Place the predosed capsule in the cement activator and press down on the handle.

NOTE: The activator breaks the seal between the powder and liquid in the capsule, allowing the materials to meet.

Make sure you use sufficient pressure to feel the seal break (Figure 10-24).

2 Place the capsule in the amalgamator and set for the recommended amount of time, usually 10 to 15 seconds.

NOTE: The capsule is similar to an amalgam capsule and must be secured in the arms of the amalgamator before mixing (Figure 10-25).

3 Remove the capsule from the amalgamator and immediately place it into the cement dispenser. Advance the mixed cement to the tip (Figure 10-26).

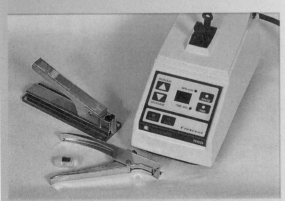

FIGURE 10-23

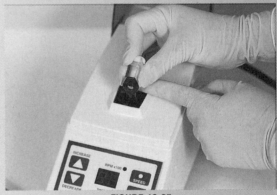

FIGURE 10-25

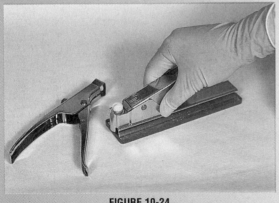

FIGURE 10-24

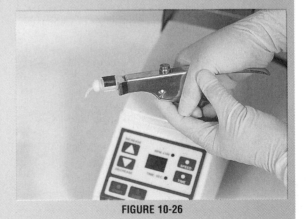

FIGURE 10-26

Contiued on following page

4 Load the crown directly from the dispenser (Figure 10-27).

5 Discard the capsule and disinfect the activator and amalgamator. The dispenser may be sterilized.

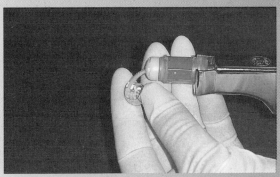

FIGURE 10-27

PROCEDURE 10-5 (see p. 338 for competency sheet)

Mixing Resin-Based Cement: Light-Cured and Dual-Cured

EQUIPMENT/SUPPLIES (Figure 10-28)

- Rubber cup and nonfluoride cleaning paste
- Tooth conditioner
- Primer/bond adhesive
- Disposable brush
- Dispensing dish
- Cement—base and catalyst
- Spatula
- Mixing pad
- Blunt instrument

NOTE: See Chapter 5, Procedure 5-1, for illustrations and further description of steps 1 through 8.

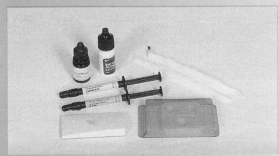

FIGURE 10-28

1 Clean preparation of all provisional material.

NOTE: Materials containing eugenol should not be used in provisional coverage.

2 Clean the dentin with a rubber cup and nonfluoride cleaning paste.

NOTE: Fluoride should not be used before bonding.

3 Rinse thoroughly and lightly air-dry.

4 Clean and dry and prepare the internal surface of the restoration.

NOTE: Organic debris accumulated during try-in must be removed. This can be done by several means (e.g., ultrasonic cleaner, phosphoric acid etchant). Microetching is recommended for preparation of the internal surface of the restoration.

5 Apply tooth conditioner according to the manufacturer's direction.

NOTE: The use of a fine needle tip attached to the syringe of the conditioner will allow control of the conditioner to prevent etching of areas prone to postoperative sensitivity.

6 Rinse and blot dry, leaving a moist, glistening surface.

NOTE: Blot drying provides the correct amount of "wetness" on the tooth surface while avoiding desiccating the tooth surface.

Contiued on following page

PROCEDURE 10-5 (Continued)

7 Isolate area to prevent saliva contamination.

NOTE: If saliva contamination occurs, repeat steps 5 and 6.

8 Apply primer/bond adhesive agent to the tooth and internal surface of the restoration according to the manufacturer's directions.

Light-Cure Technique: Ceramic, Porcelain, and Composite Restorations

• Dispense desired shade of cement base paste into restoration.

• Seat the loaded restoration and remove excess cement at the gingival margin with a blunt instrument. Light-cure the gingival margin, and once restoration is "tacked" in place remove excess cement from proximal surfaces. Continue to light-cure the proximal surfaces of the restoration.

NOTE: The removal of excess cement before curing is necessary.

Dual-Cure Technique: Crown and Bridge Restorations

• Dispense the desired shade of base paste and an equal amount of catalyst paste onto a mixing pad (Figure 10-29).

• Mix the cement for 20 to 30 seconds until you have achieved a homogeneous mix.

• Dispense the cement into the restoration, being careful not to trap air.

• Seat the loaded restoration and remove the gross excess from marginal areas.

NOTE: The removal of excess cement before curing is necessary; a short light-cure to cause the cement to gel allows for easier removal. Pay special attention to interproximal areas using gloss to remove excess cement.

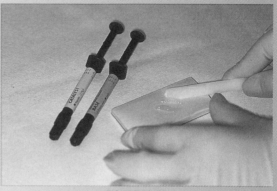

FIGURE 10-29

9 Check the cure and adjust occlusion as necessary.

10 Finish and polish.

Try-in Option

• Dispense the appropriate shade of try-in paste onto a mixing pad. Load the restoration and seat onto the preparation.

NOTE: Try-in paste is matched to the cement base material and is used to obtain the correct shade of cement. Restoration "try-in" is recommended before final cementation to ensure acceptance of restoration esthetics.

• Once restoration fit and esthetics are verified, the try-in paste is removed from the preparation and the restoration is cemented using one of the previously described techniques.

IMPRESSION MATERIALS

OBJECTIVES

On completion of this chapter the student will be able to:

1. Describe the purpose of an impression.
2. List the various categories of impression materials and explain their differences.
3. Describe important characteristics of impression materials.
4. Describe the factors that make agar hydrocolloid a reversible material.
5. List the components of agar hydrocolloid and discuss their functions.
6. Define *sol* and *gel* and describe these states as they occur with the hydrocolloids.
7. Compare the accuracy of agar hydrocolloid with alginate.
8. List the components of alginate impression material and discuss their functions.
9. Explain why alginate is an irreversible hydrocolloid.
10. List the supplies needed to make an alginate impression and explain how they are used.
11. Demonstrate tray selection for alginate impressions for a patient.
12. Demonstrate mixing alginate, loading and seating the tray, and removing the impression.
13. List criteria for an acceptable alginate impression.
14. Demonstrate the proper handling of alginate impressions.
15. Describe the different types of elastomers and explain why they are called elastomers.
16. Discuss similarities and differences among the physical properties of the various elastomers.
17. List the uses of polyether impression material and discuss its advantages and disadvantages.
18. List the uses of polysulfide impression material and discuss its advantages and disadvantages.

19. Explain why polyvinyl siloxane impression material is so popular.
20. Explain the difference between a hydrophobic and a hydrophilic impression material.
21 Explain why some impression materials should be poured immediately and others can wait until later.
22. Discuss the uses of inelastic impression materials and why they are seldom used today.

KEY TERMS

Diagnostic casts—Positive replicas of the teeth produced from impressions that create a negative representation of the teeth. Commonly called *study models* and used for diagnostic purposes and numerous chairside and laboratory procedures.

Bite registration—An impression of the occlusal relationship of opposing teeth in centric occlusion (patient's normal bite).

Colloid—Gluelike material composed of two or more substances in which one substance does not go into solution but is suspended within another substance. It has at least two phases, a liquid phase called a *sol* and a semisolid phase called a *gel*.

Hydrocolloid—A water-based colloid used as an elastic impression material.

Reversible hydrocolloid—An agar impression material that can be heated to change a gel into a fluid sol state that can flow around the teeth, then cooled to gel again to make an impression of the shapes of the oral structures.

Irreversible hydrocolloid—An alginate impression material that is mixed to a sol state and as it sets converts to a gel by a chemical reaction that irreversibly changes its nature.

Agar—A powder derived from seaweed that is a major component of reversible hydrocolloid.

Sol—Liquid state in which colloidal particles are suspended. By cooling or chemical reaction it can change into a gel.

Gel—A semisolid state in which colloidal particles form a framework that traps liquid (e.g., Jell-O).

Hysteresis—The property of a material to have two different temperatures for melting and solidifying, unlike water, which has one temperature for both.

Syneresis—A characteristic of gels to contract and squeeze out some liquid that then accumulates on the surface.

Alginate—A versatile irreversible hydrocolloid impression that is the most-used impression material in the dental office. It lacks the accuracy and fine surface detail needed for impressions for crown and bridge procedures.

Imbibition—The act of absorbing moisture.

Surfactant—A chemical that lowers the surface tension of a substance so that it is more readily wet. For example, oil beads on the surface of water, but soap acts as a surfactant to allow the oil to spread over the surface.

Polysulfide—A rubber impression material that has sulfur-containing (mercaptan) functional groups.

Condensation silicone—A silicone rubber impression material that sets by linking of molecules in long chains but produces a liquid by-product by condensation.

Addition silicone—A silicone rubber impression that also sets by linking of molecules in long chains but produces no by-product. Addition silicones are commonly known as polyvinyl siloxanes and are the most popular materials for crown and bridge procedures because of their accuracy, dimensional stability, and ease of use.

Polyether—A rubber impression material with ether functional groups. It has high accuracy and is popular for crown and bridge procedures.

Impression compound—An impression material composed of resin and wax with fillers added to make it stronger and more stable than wax.

Impression plaster—An impression material composed of a gypsum product similar to plaster of Paris.

Zinc oxide eugenol—A hard and brittle impression material used in complete denture procedures.

In dentistry, an impression material is used primarily to reproduce the form of teeth, including existing restorations and preparations made for restorative treatments, and the form of other oral hard and soft tissues. Impression materials are also used by maxillofacial prosthodontists to make molds of facial defects resulting from cancer and trauma so that they can construct facial prostheses to restore facial form. When used to replicate oral structures the impression materials must be in a moldable or plastic state that can adapt to the teeth and tissues. Usually the impression material in its plastic state is loaded into a tray to carry it to the mouth and support it so that it does not slump and distort. Within a specified period of time the impression material must set to a semisolid, elastic, or rigid state. Elastic impression materials are used more extensively than rigid materials, because elastic materials flex from tissue undercuts when removed from the mouth whereas rigid materials cannot. The completed impression forms a negative reproduction of the teeth and tissues. When plaster or stone is poured into the impression and hardened, the replica that is formed is a positive reproduction of the teeth and tissues (see Chapter 12). The replica is called a cast *or* model. *In the initial diagnosis and treatment planning phase, the dentist may request that the dental assistant or hygienist make impressions of the teeth and surrounding structures so that* **diagnostic casts,** *commonly called* study models, *can be made for further study when the patient is no longer present. When an impression is made of a tooth that has been prepared for a restoration, the replica of the prepared tooth is called a* die *and is used for fabrication of the restoration in the dental laboratory. In some states, dental assistants and hygienists can be licensed in extended functions that*

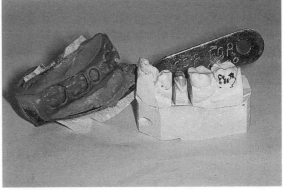

FIGURE 11-1 ■ A double-bite impression and the cast from the impression with a die of the crown preparation that can be removed by the technician to facilitate the creation of a wax pattern.

include making final impressions for crown and bridge procedures. Figure 11-1 shows an impression and the mold and die made from that impression. The use of the die allows the dentist or laboratory technician to perform the procedure by the indirect technique. With the indirect technique the restoration is not made directly on the tooth, as with the direct placement of amalgam, but is constructed in the laboratory (indirectly) and later placed on the tooth.

Many different types of impression materials have been developed over the years, allowing the dentist to select materials according to the demands of the treatment and the oral environment. The participation in the making of impressions is one of the most performed patient contact functions of the dental assistant and is performed increasingly by the dental hygienist. It is important that both have an understanding of the clinical applications, handling characteristics, physical properties, and limitations of these materials.

Impression Trays

Impression trays are used to carry the impression material to the mouth and to support it until it sets, is removed from the mouth, and is poured in dental plaster or stone. They should be rigid to prevent distortion of the impression. They can be made for arches with teeth or for edentulous ridges. Impression trays can be premanufactured trays, called *stock trays,* which are purchased in a variety of sizes for both adults and children (Figure 11-2). Stock trays can be metal or plastic, and each of these can be solid or perforated (has holes in the sides and bottom to help retain impression material that extrudes through the holes). Solid trays often have raised borders on the internal surfaces that help lock in the impression material. These are called *"rim-lock" trays.* Some materials used in solid trays require the application of an adhesive to further retain them and prevent distortion of the impression if they should partially pull out of the tray. Plastic trays are inexpensive and are disposable, whereas metal trays are more expensive and must be cleaned and sterilized between uses. Impression trays can also be custom made. Custom trays are usually constructed in the laboratory with chemically cured, light-cured, or thermoplastic resins on casts of the teeth (see Chapter 13). They are custom fit to the mouth of the individual. They can also be made by lining a stock tray with a putty material that is adapted to the dental arch of the individual, and then an impression is made in this arch-adapted custom tray. Both stock trays and custom trays can be made for full arch impressions or for sectional impressions for part of an arch. The triple tray (also called double-bite or check-bite tray) is a stock sectional tray that is used to make an impression of the teeth being treated and the opposing teeth at the same time and, if used properly, will capture the correct centric occlusion (bite) of the patient. **Bite registration** trays are typically U-shaped plastic frames with a thin fiber mesh stretched between the sides of the frame. The mesh retains the impression material (called bite registration material) and is thin enough so as not to interfere with the closure of the upper and lower teeth in proper bite relationship. Bite registration material is placed on both sides of the mesh, the frame is positioned over the teeth to be recorded, and the patient closes into the normal bite relationship until the material sets.

Elastic Impression Materials

HYDROCOLLOIDS

A **colloid** is a gluelike material composed of two or more substances in which one substance does not go into solution but is suspended within another substance. **Hydrocolloids** are water-based colloids that function as elastic impression materials. The two hydrocolloids used in dentistry are agar hydrocolloid (or **reversible hydrocolloid**) and alginate hydrocolloid (or **irreversible hydrocolloid**). Much like gelatin, when **agar** powder is mixed with water it forms a gluelike suspension that entraps the water (a colloidal suspension called a **sol**). Heating it will disperse the agar in the water faster. When the agar sol is chilled it will **gel**, becoming semisolid or jellylike. When the agar gel is heated it will reverse its state back into a liquid suspension (sol). Therefore it is a reversible hydrocolloid. Alginate powder will also form a sol that gels. However, with alginate a chemical reaction occurs that prevents it from reversing back to a gel when heated. Therefore it is an irreversible hydrocolloid.

Reversible Hydrocolloid (Agar)   Reversible hydrocolloid has been used for over 60 years in dentistry and is the first elastic material to gain popular-

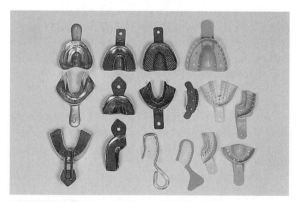

FIGURE 11-2 ■ Variety of metal and plastic impression trays.

ity. It overcame many of the problems with the inelastic materials (discussed later in this chapter) in that it could take accurate impressions of teeth and arches with tissue undercuts and be removed from the mouth without injuring the patient or breaking.

TABLE 11-1

Composition of Agar Hydrocolloid Impression Material

Material	Percentage (Approximate)	Purpose
Agar	12%-15%	Colloidal particles as basis of the gel
Potassium sulfate	1%	Ensures set of gypsum materials
Borax	0.2%	Strengthens gel
Alkyl benzoate	0.1%	Antifungal agent
Water	85%	Dispersing medium for the colloidal suspension

Its main clinical use is for impressions of operative and crown and bridge procedures. It also has uses in the laboratory for the duplication of casts (models). Its use has declined over the years as rubber impression materials have been introduced.

Composition   The agar is derived from an extract of seaweed called agar-agar. The impression material is made from reversible agar gels. The components of the agar gels are 12% to 15% agar, 1% potassium sulfate to ensure proper set of the gypsum material poured in the impression, 0.2% borax as a strengthener for the gel, 0.1% alkyl benzoate as an antifungal during storage, and 85% water. Borax and agar retard the set of gypsum products, so potassium sulfate is added to cancel out their effect (Table 11-1).

Clinical Application   The agar hydrocolloid impression material has been known for many years as simply "hydrocolloid." The use of hydrocolloid requires equipment specific for its use. The impression trays are stock metal trays (called water-cooled trays) with tubing running through them that connects to a water line by rubber hoses to circulate tap

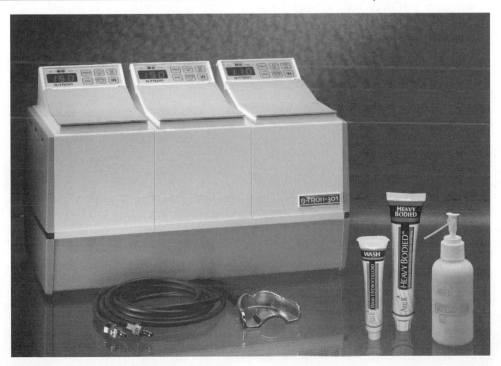

FIGURE 11-3 ■ Hydrocolloid conditioner, water-cooled tray with hoses, impression materials, and wetting agent. (Courtesy Van R Dental.)

water through the tray. The water cools the impression material so that it gels within a reasonable period of time (about 5 minutes). Stock trays also allow for an adequate thickness of material to minimize the dimensional changes seen when hydrocolloid is too thin.

Hydrocolloid is supplied in plastic tubes, as sticks supplied in a glass jar, and as gel in glass cartridges. Two viscosities of hydrocolloid are used to make the impression. The variation in viscosity is achieved by altering the agar content. A stiffer hydrocolloid has more agar. A stiffer hydrocolloid is used to load the tray. A more fluid type is supplied in a glass cartridge that fits the syringe. To prepare the material for making an impression, a special heating unit called a *hydrocolloid conditioner* is used (Figure 11-3). The conditioner has three water bath chambers, each set to a different temperature. When the hydrocolloid gels are heated to 71° to 100° C (160° to 212° F) they become liquid (sol state). The tray and syringe hydrocolloid are liquefied in 8 to 12 minutes in boiling water (100° C) in the first chamber. A second chamber is maintained between 60° and 66° C and acts as a storage chamber where the tray and syringe hydrocolloid can be maintained in a liquid state for several hours, if needed. In a busy dental office the hydrocolloid can be prepared in the morning and kept ready for use all day. A third chamber is kept at 45° to 47° C and is used to temper the tray hydrocolloid for 2 to 4 minutes before the impression is taken. Tempering prevents burns to the oral mucosa or potential pulpal damage to prepared teeth. The syringe hydrocolloid is not tempered, because it is dispensed in such a small stream that it cools quickly as it passes out the needle-shaped dispensing tip and flows around the prepared teeth and into the gingival sulcus. After delivering the syringe material, the tray is quickly connected to the water hoses and seated over the teeth, and then the water is turned on to cool the material. When the hydrocolloid is cooled to 30° to 45° C (86° to 113° F), it returns to a solid (gel). The temperature at which the hydrocolloid liquefies is not the same temperature at which it solidifies (a phenomenon called **hysteresis**) and is unlike other substances, such as water, that have the same melting and freezing points. After the hydrocolloid has adequately gelled, the tray is removed from the mouth quickly with a snap. This allows the material to be removed from undercuts without tearing. Slow removal is more likely to cause the material to tear,

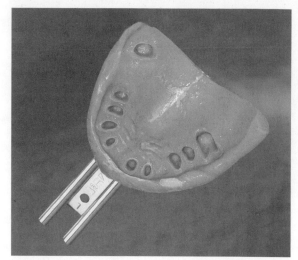

FIGURE 11-4 ■ Impression with agar hydrocolloid in water-cooled tray.
(Courtesy Van R Dental.)

particularly where it is thin. The gel reproduces fine detail of the preparations (Figure 11-4).

An advantage of the hydrocolloid relates to its hydrophilic nature. It can be used in a moist field. The teeth are not dried before the hydrocolloid is placed. In situations where there is a little bleeding or moisture, the hydrocolloid can still obtain an accurate impression, whereas the elastomeric impression materials (discussed later in this chapter) require a dry field. A wetting agent is sprayed on the preparation to aid in establishing intimate contact of the hydrocolloid with the prepared tooth.

Physical Properties The impression must be poured immediately after it is made and disinfected, because it is dimensionally unstable. The gel will lose moisture and shrink if left in the air. If it must be stored for a short period of time, the impression should be placed in a humidor with 100% relative humidity or wrapped in a wet paper towel and sealed in a zippered plastic bag. The risk of distortion of the impression is great if it is not poured within an hour. The impression will imbibe water and swell if left in water or disinfecting liquid for more than a short period of time (10 to 30 minutes). Shrinkage or swelling will result in an inaccurate cast and a poorly fitting restoration. When left standing, many gels undergo a process called **syneresis** whereby they contract and some of the liquid is squeezed out of the gel, forming an exudate on the surface. This loss of water changes the properties of the material. Hydrocolloid impressions can only be poured once to make a cast because they lose water and change dimensionally.

The tear strength for agar hydrocolloid is similar to that of alginate but not as strong as the elastomeric rubber materials discussed later in this chapter. Both agar and alginate hydrocolloid will deform if compressed, but may recover or rebound to the original shape if the compression is not too great. If the compression is too great, the deformation will be permanent.

Although agar hydrocolloid is an inexpensive impression material with excellent accuracy, many practitioners have switched to newer generations of elastomeric impression materials for some of the following reasons: (1) the impressions do not need to be poured immediately; (2) they can be poured more than once; (3) they are highly accurate and dimensionally stable for longer periods; (4) they do not require expensive equipment such as hydrocolloid conditioners; and (5) they do not require the use of water-cooling hoses that sometimes leak.

Irreversible Hydrocolloid   **Alginate,** also called *alginate hydrocolloid* or *irreversible hydrocolloid,* is by far the most widely used impression material. It is inexpensive, is easy to manipulate, requires no special equipment, and is reasonably accurate for many dental procedures. Alginate is used for making impressions for diagnostic casts, partial denture frameworks, repairs of broken partial or complete dentures, fabrication of provisional restorations, fluoride and bleaching trays, sports protectors, pre-

---

COMMON USES OF ALGINATE IMPRESSIONS

- Diagnostic casts (study models)
- Preliminary impressions for complete dentures
- Partial denture frameworks
- Opposing casts for crown and bridge treatments
- Repairs of partial and complete dentures
- Provisional restorations
- Custom trays for fluoride or bleaching
- Sports protectors and night guards

---

liminary impressions for edentulous arches, and a multitude of other uses. However, it is not accurate enough for the final impressions for inlay, onlay, or crown and bridge preparations. It does not capture the fine detail of the preparation needed for a precise fit of the restoration. Also, it is thick and does not flow well into embrasures or occlusal surfaces. Final impressions are taken with more accurate materials such as agar hydrocolloid or one of the elastomers (discussed later in this chapter). Final impressions are used to make detailed replicas of the prepared teeth. It is from these detailed replicas that precisely fitting restorations will be made.

Composition and Setting Reaction   The main active ingredient in alginate is potassium or sodium alginate, which makes up 15% to 20% of the powder (proportions of ingredients vary from manufacturer to manufacturer and with fast-, regular-, and slow-set materials). It is produced from derivatives of seaweed. Other components of the alginate powder include calcium sulfate dihydrate (14% to 20%), potassium sulfate (10%), trisodium phosphate (2%), and diatomaceous earth (55% to 60%). The "dustless" alginate powders have organic glycols added to keep powder from becoming airborne when it is dispensed. Other additives may include flavoring agents, coloring agents, and disinfectants.

When alginate powder is mixed with water, calcium sulfate dihydrate reacts with sodium alginate to form calcium alginate. Calcium alginate is insoluble and causes the sol of mixed powder and water to gel. Because this occurs by a chemical reaction, it cannot be reversed back to the sol state as can agar hydrocolloid. It is a fairly rapid chemical reaction, so trisodium phosphate is added as a retarder to delay the reaction. The amount of retarder that is added will control the time of the set and differentiate between fast- and regular-set alginates. Diatomaceous earth is added as a filler to increase the stiffness and strength and to prevent the surface from being sticky. Potassium sulfate is added to keep the alginate from interfering with the set of the gypsum products used to pour the impression. Some manufacturers have added chemicals to the alginate that change color as the chemical reaction progresses to indicate when it is time to insert the impression and that change again when it is time to remove the impression (Table 11-2).

Working Time   Regular-set alginates have a working time (from start of mix to seating in the mouth) of 2

TABLE 11-2

Composition of Alginate Impression Material

Material	Percentage (Approximate)	Purpose
Sodium or potassium alginate	15%-20%	Colloidal particles as basis of the gel
Calcium sulfate dihydrate	14%-20%	Creates irreversible gel with alginate
Potassium sulfate	10%	Ensures set of gypsum materials
Trisodium phosphate	2%	Retarder to control setting time
Diatomaceous earth	55%-60%	Filler to increase thickness and strength
Other additives: • Organic glycols • Flavoring agents • Coloring agents • Disinfectants	Very small quantities	Reduce dust when handling powder Improve taste of material Provide pleasant colors Antibacterial action

to 3 minutes, and fast-set alginate has a working time of 1.25 to 2 minutes (ADA specification no. 18 sets the minimum at 1.25 minutes). The longer the time used to mix the alginate, the faster it must be loaded into the tray and seated in the mouth.

Setting Time Regular-set alginates set in 2 to 5 minutes, and fast-set alginates set in 1 to 2 minutes. Setting time can be lengthened by using cold water or shortened by using warm water. Adjusting the powder-to-water ratio can affect the set but also adversely affects the physical properties and therefore is not recommended. It is advisable to leave the impression in the mouth for an additional 1 to 2 minutes after it appears set, because the tear strength and the ability to rebound from undercuts without permanent deformation increase during this time.

CLINICAL TIP For patients with sensitive teeth, alginate mixed with cool water can be painful. Use regular-set alginate with warm water. The working and setting times will be shortened, but the patient will be more comfortable.

Permanent Deformation Alginate will be compressed when it is removed from undercuts in the mouth. The greater the compression, the more likely it is that the alginate will be permanently deformed to some degree. A certain thickness of alginate (2 to 4 mm) is needed between the impression tray and the teeth or tissue undercut. Thin alginate will deform more and tear more easily. As

with the reversible hydrocolloid, when removing the alginate impression, it should be removed by a rapid "snap" to prevent the deformation of critical surfaces. If 8 to 10 minutes elapse from the time the impression is removed from the mouth until it is poured, some recovery or rebound will occur from the deformation. That deformation which does not recover is the permanent deformation, and it will be recorded in the poured gypsum cast as a distortion. As long as the distortion is small it may not be clinically significant. Usually, the time needed for disinfecting the impression is at least 10 minutes and most of the rebound will have occurred by then.

Dimensional Stability Like agar hydrocolloid, alginate is very sensitive to moisture loss and will shrink as a result. Once the impression is removed from the mouth it should be rinsed and disinfected (see Procedure 11-4), wrapped in a damp paper towel, and sealed in a zippered plastic bag. Enclosing the impression this way will create an environment with 100% humidity to minimize water loss. Some moisture will be lost from the impression even in 100% humidity from syneresis as with agar hydrocolloid. The paper towel should not be loaded with water or the surface of the impression may become wet. If it imbibes water it will swell and create some distortion. Ideally, the impression is poured after it is disinfected. If the impression must be stored until it can be poured a few hours later, it must be kept in 100% humidity (as with the damp towel and zippered plastic bag).

Tear Strength   The tear strength of alginate is more important than its compressive strength because most commercial alginates far exceed the minimum allowable value for compressive strength. Alginate mixed with too much water will be weaker and more likely to tear on removal from the mouth. Thin sections of alginate are also prone to tearing. Additionally, slow removal of the alginate from the mouth will contribute to tearing. If the impression can be left in the mouth for an additional 1 to 2 minutes beyond the point when it is set, it will increase in tear strength. When properly handled, alginate has adequate tear strength.

Impression Making

Objective   The objective of impression making is to reproduce the oral structures with an acceptable accuracy while practicing good infection control and maintaining patient comfort. In many states the dental assistant and dental hygienist can make alginate impressions for diagnostic casts. In states where this is not permitted, the assistant or hygienist may be called on to prepare the patient for the impressions and to dispense, mix, and load alginate into trays seated by the dentist. Following removal of the impression the assistant or hygienist disinfects and properly handles the impression until it is poured in the appropriate gypsum material. The assistant or hygienist also may be responsible for clearing residual alginate from the mouth and face of the patient.

Tray Selection   Stock trays work well with alginate because they leave plenty of room for an adequate thickness of alginate. Alginate must be tightly adapted to the tray to be accurate. If the alginate pulls loose from the tray, a distortion will occur. If a tray is set on the bench top, unsupported alginate extending from the back of the tray may lift a portion of the impression and dislodge it from the tray. A perforated tray can be used because the alginate oozes through the perforations and locks in place. A solid tray can also be used if an adhesive made for alginate is applied to the inside of the tray before the alginate is loaded. Solid rim-lock trays should also have adhesive applied because alginate will occasionally pull free from the rim-lock on removal of the impression. If disposable plastic trays are used, they should be rigid. Flexible plastic trays have the potential to distort under the weight of the wet gypsum during pouring or when used in areas of undercuts in the mouth.

A properly selected tray will cover all of the teeth and extend into the facial and lingual vestibules without impinging on the tissues. It will extend posteriorly to include the retromolar area for a mandibular tray and the hamular notch area for a maxillary tray. It will be deep enough to provide at least 2 mm of space for alginate beyond the incisal and occlusal surfaces of the teeth. Occasionally, standard stock trays will not cover all of the desired areas for the impression and must be modified with utility wax to create appropriate extensions of the tray and support the alginate. A common area for this to occur is in the third molar area of an individual with large jaws. Wax may also be added to the midpalatal area of the tray to support the alginate when the patient has a very deep palatal vault (see Procedure 11-1, Figure 11-13). Usually, the patient is asked to rinse the mouth to remove loose debris and thick saliva before making the impression. An antimicrobial rinse may be used to reduce the number of oral pathogens.

Dispensing   Manufacturers supply measures for powder and water for their alginates. Use the appropriate ones and adhere to the recommended proportions of powder and water to maintain the desired physical properties of the alginate. Powder measures (also called scoops) will vary among manufacturers, so do not interchange them with other manufacturers' scoops. The same principle also applies to water measures.

> **CLINICAL TIP**   Water and powder measures can vary in size among manufacturers. If your office uses more than one brand of alginate, color-code the measures so they are not intermixed.

During shipping or prolonged periods of sitting, the powder may pack tightly and some of the ingredients may settle out so that they are not evenly distributed throughout the powder. The measure of powder taken will be greater than the manufacturer intended when developing the measuring scoop. When the compacted powder is incorporated into the recommended volume of water, the resulting mix will be too thick and will often set too rapidly. To prevent this from happening, containers of alginate such as cans or plastic containers should be turned end-over-end a few times to decompress (fluff) the powder and mix the ingredients. Some alginates are supplied in premeasured, watertight packages with a quantity suitable for a medium-sized arch (equivalent to two scoops with most manufacturers). This packaging is more expensive, but some practitioners find it to be convenient, to provide a more consistent mix, and to minimize cross-contamination.

> ▶ **CAUTION**
> *Be sure to wear a mask while dispensing and mixing alginate. Alginate dust is potentially hazardous to inhale because it contains silicone dioxide in the diatomaceous earth fillers, as well as other chemicals.*

Mixing   For a moderate to large upper adult arch, 3 scoops of alginate powder is usually required; a small upper arch requires 2 scoops. Most lower adult arches require 2 scoops. One unit of water is required per scoop. Typical water measures are marked to indicate up to three units. Room-temperature tap water is placed in the rubber bowl and the powder is added to it. Cold water retards the set, and warm water accelerates it. The powder is stirred into the water so that the powder is wet. Next, the wet powder is aggressively mixed against the sides of the bowl with a wide-bladed spatula. Some operators prefer to rotate the bowl in one hand while mixing with the other. Some offices use mechanical mixing machines for rapid mixing, ease of use, and a consistent mix. The rubber bowl is attached to the mechanical mixer that spins the bowl. With both mechanical and hand mixing, water-powder mixture is forced against the sides of the bowl to further incorporate the powder into the water and also force out entrapped air. Mixing should be completed within 45 seconds for regular-set alginate and 30 seconds for fast-set alginate. The completed mix should have a creamy consistency. If it appears grainy, it has not been mixed thoroughly.

Loading the Tray   Mixed alginate is picked up on the spatula and forced into the depth of the tray. This action forces out air, thus preventing large voids in the impression. The alginate should be loaded in large increments as quickly as possible. The more

small increments added to the tray, the greater the chance for entrapped air. The tray should be loaded until the alginate is even with the top of the sides of the tray. A wet, gloved finger is used to smooth the surface of the alginate and to create a shallow trough over the ridge area of the alginate that reduces the chance for entrapped air and also helps orient the tray over the teeth when seating it.

Seating the Tray   Once the tray is loaded, the operator should take some alginate from the bowl on the gloved index finger and wipe it on the occlusal surfaces and embrasures of the teeth to force out air from the grooves and embrasure spaces. If regular-set alginate has a 2-minute working time and the alginate was mixed for 45 seconds, the operator has 75 seconds to load the tray, wipe on the alginate, and seat the tray. For fast-set alginate the operator has about 45 seconds for the same process after mixing for 30 seconds.

For the lower impression the operator is usually standing in front of the patient to one side at approximately the 7 o'clock position. The right side of the tray is use to retract the left corner of the mouth and a finger or mouth mirror retracts the right corner. The tray is rotated into the mouth, aligned over the teeth with the tray handle in the midline, and seated in the posterior first. The tray is seated anteriorly, and as it is being seated over the incisors the lower lip is pulled out of the way to allow alginate to flow into the anterior vestibule. The patient is asked to lift the tongue to the roof of the mouth momentarily and then to relax it. This tongue motion allows alginate to flow into the lingual vestibule and defines the lingual frenum attachment. The tray is stabilized by the index and middle fingers of the right hand over the right and left sides of the arch. (All of these procedures should be appropriately repositioned for a left-handed operator.) The procedure is similar for the upper arch with the following modifications. The operator stands just behind the patient at the 11 o'clock position and retracts the right corner of the mouth with the side of the tray while retracting the left corner of the mouth with the index finger of the other hand. The tray is rotated into position, aligned over the teeth, centered with the midline, seated in the posterior first, and gently seated toward the anterior to allow alginate to flow forward and not back into the palate. Trays can also be placed while the patient is in the supine position. A right-handed operator can seat the lower tray from the 8 o'clock position and the upper tray from the 11 or 12 o'clock positions and left-handed operators from comparable positions on the opposite side (4 o'clock for lower and 12 or 1 o'clock for upper). The patient should be seated upright after the tray is placed to minimize the collection of saliva and alginate at the back of the throat. For both upper and lower impressions, the posterior aspect of the tray should be inspected for proper seating and for excess alginate. Excess alginate should be swept away quickly with the mouth mirror or a cotton swab to prevent a gagging or breathing problem for the patient.

Controlling the gag reflex:
- Place topical anesthetic on a cotton swab and put it on the back of the tongue for 1 to 2 minutes or spray back of the mouth with anesthetic spray.
- Place utility wax on the posterior extent of the upper tray to help contain the material.
- Use fast-set alginate. Accelerate the set with warm water, if you can work fast enough to load and seat the tray.
- Properly proportion the water and powder so that the mix is not too runny.
- Do not overfill the tray.
- Seat the tray in the posterior first, then anterior. Look at the palatal area and clear excess material with a quick sweep of the mouth mirror.
- Position the patient's head forward slightly so that saliva will not pool in the back of the throat, and use saliva ejector to keep the mouth clear.
- Use distraction (e.g., have the patient lift one leg during the impression and hold it up, breathe slowly and deeply through the nose).

Removing the Tray   Alginate left in the mixing bowl can be checked for completeness of set. The impression should be left in the mouth for 2 minutes or so after the set, because it gains in tear strength during this time. This may not be possible with patients who gag easily. When ready to remove the tray, use a finger at the side of the tray to apply pressure to break the seal while pulling the tray quickly away from the teeth with a snap. Protect the teeth in the opposing arch with fingers placed on top of the tray.

Handling the Impression   The impression should be rinsed thoroughly under running water to remove adherent saliva. Next, it should be evaluated to determine if the impression is acceptable for its anticipated use. If determined to be acceptable, the impression is sprayed with a suitable disinfecting solution. A laboratory knife is used to remove excess alginate out the back of the tray. Any pooled fluid is drained or shaken off, because the alginate can imbibe moisture and swell. It is wrapped in a damp paper towel and placed into a zippered plastic bag marked with the patient's name until ready to pour. Ideally, the impression should be poured within an hour because it is not dimensionally stable and can lose water by syneresis even in 100% humidity.

Criteria for Clinically Acceptable Alginate Impressions   Alginate impressions should be evaluated immediately after they are removed from the mouth and rinsed. The determination should be made at this point as to whether or not the impression should be repeated so it can be done while the patient is still seated and the operatory is set up for it. An acceptable impression will cover all of the areas of interest (the teeth, ridge form, muscle attachments, palate, etc.). The structures should be recorded with sufficient detail to be clearly identified and should not have a grainy surface, which is usually the result of inadequate mixing. There should be minimal voids caused by entrapped air, especially in areas critical to the use of the impression (e.g., occlusal surfaces if a night guard will be made). The alginate should be fully seated in the tray and should not have pulled free or distorted. The impression should be free of debris. Table 11-3 lists criteria used to assess an alginate impression for clinical acceptability. When problems are found with the impression, refer to Table 11-4 for a troubleshooting guide that suggests possible causes for a variety of problems.

Alginate-Agar Hydrocolloid Combination Technique   Alginate can also be used in combination with agar hydrocolloid for crown and bridge procedures. With this technique a low-viscosity agar hydrocolloid is liquefied and placed in a hydrocolloid impression syringe. The dentist syringes the agar hydrocolloid around the prepared teeth while the dental assistant mixes alginate and loads it into an impression tray. The tray is seated before the

TABLE 11-3

Criteria for an Acceptable Alginate Impression

Both Maxillary and Mandibular Impressions

All teeth and alveolar processes recorded
Peripheral roll and frenums included
No large voids and few small bubbles present
Good reproduction of detai
Free of debris
No distortion
Alginate firmly attached to tray

Maxillary Impression

Palatal vault recorded
Hamular notch area included

Mandibular Impression

Retromolar areas included
Lingual extensions recorded

hydrocolloid sets. If a compatible alginate is used, the alginate and agar hydrocolloid will fuse together. The main advantages of this combination are the accuracy of the agar hydrocolloid, the reduced need for equipment (no water-cooled trays and a simpler and less expensive hydrocolloid conditioner), and the low cost of each of these materials. The main disadvantages are that the impression must be poured up immediately and cannot be repoured for a duplicate cast from the same impression. Dentists and laboratory technicians often like to pour a second cast if the first cast becomes damaged or is found to have voids from entrapped air during the pour. During the construction of a crown or bridge in the laboratory, the replica of the prepared tooth (die) may become damaged or worn. The second pour of the impression permits the technician to work on the second cast. Agar hydrocolloid and alginate do not permit a second pour because they are dimensionally unstable and lose too much moisture during the casting process and become distorted.

ELASTOMERS

Elastomers are highly accurate elastic impression materials that have qualities similar to rubber and, hence, are often called rubber materials. They are used extensively in restorative dentistry for con-

struction of casting, indirect esthetic restorations (see Chapter 6), bridges, implant restorations, partial denture frameworks, and complete dentures. The four most commonly used types of elastomers are polysulfides, polyethers, condensation silicones, and addition silicones. The elastomers have in common a polymerization reaction that involves formation of long-chain polymers and cross-linking of chains. Because they are not water based they are not as sensitive as the hydrocolloids to water loss or **imbibition.** The rubbery nature of elastomers means that they do not adhere well to solid metal or custom acrylic impression trays. An adhesive is placed in the tray to prevent the material from separating from the tray and causing distortion. Each type of elastomer has its own adhesive with which it is compatible; therefore adhesives should not be interchanged among different types of materials. Because of their rubbery nature, elastomers have a certain amount of recovery, or "rebound," from deformation. Rebound reduces distortion in the cast that is poured from the impression. The addition silicones and polyethers have the highest amount of rebound, condensation silicones have moderate rebound, and polysulfides have the poorest amount of rebound. The elastomers generally are not wet well by water (and are called hydrophobic), because water forms a high contact angle with them (see Figure 5-11 in Chapter 5). In other words, water beads on their surface much like raindrops on a newly waxed car. Of the elastomers the polyethers are the most hydrophilic, or wettable. Some of the addition silicones have had substances called **surfactants** added to reduce the surface tension so that they are more hydrophilic and wettable. Wettability can be seen clinically when impression materials are able to capture the detail of a tooth preparation when the surface is moist (but not submerged in water or saliva). It also means that wet gypsum materials will flow better into the fine details of the preparation when the impression is poured. Because most elastomers are not naturally wettable, a surfactant must be sprayed into the impression before it is poured so that the wet gypsum will make good contact with the surface and replicate the fine details.

Polysulfides   Polysulfides are the oldest of the elastomers and are commonly referred to as "rubber base." They are more dimensionally stable and have greater tear strength than alginate or agar hydrocol-

TABLE 11-4

Troubleshooting Alginate Impressions

Problem	Cause	Solution
Premature set	Too much powder in mix Prolonged mixing/loading time Water or room too warm	Fluff powder in container; use correct measures for powder and water Use timer to gauge working time Use cool water to slow the set
Slow set	Water too cold Too much water	Use warmer water Use correct water/powder measures
Grainy, lack of surface detail	Incomplete mix of powder and water	Wet all of powder and mix to creamy consistency
Incomplete coverage of teeth or tissues	Tray too small or short for arch Tray incompletely seated	Select larger tray or extend borders with rope wax Use mouth mirror to check for complete seating of tray
Voids on occlusal surfaces	Trapped air when seating tray	Wipe alginate on occlusal surfaces before seating tray
Large voids at vestibule or midpalate	Trapped air Not enough alginate in tray Improper seating of tray Lip in the way	Place some alginate in vestibule before seating tray Use adequate amount of alginate Seat tray in posterior first, allow alginate to flow forward into vestibule, seat tray in anterior Pull lip out to create room for alginate
Small voids throughout	Air trapped in mix during spatulation	Press alginate against sides of bowl when mixing with wide-blade spatula to force out air
Distortion or double imprint	Impression removed too soon Tray moved while alginate was setting	Check residual alginate in bowl for set; let stand additional 1-2 min Hold tray steady until set; do not have patient hold tray
Torn alginate	Impression removed too slowly Thin mix	Remove impression quickly with a snap Use proper proportions of water and powder
Excess alginate at back of tray	Tray seated in anterior first, then posterior forcing alginate out the back Tray overfilled with alginate	Seat tray in posterior first, forcing alginate anteriorly Load tray level with sides Create shallow trough for teeth Remove excess alginate from back of tray

loids. They are more accurate than alginate but not as accurate as the other elastomers.

Composition and Setting Reaction The polysulfides are supplied as two pastes in tubes marked *base* and *catalyst* that are dispensed in equal lengths and mixed together. The base contains mostly a low-molecular-weight organic polymer that has reactive mercaptan groups and also contains about 20% reinforcing agents in the form of titanium dioxide, zinc

sulfide, or silica. The catalyst is most commonly lead dioxide in an inert oil, but some systems use another form of peroxide. Other substances are added as coloring agents and chemical modifiers to control the polymerization reaction. The catalyst causes the mercaptan groups to form a polymer of polysulfide rubber. The reaction occurs when molecules of the long-chain polysulfide polymer with its functional mercaptan groups react with oxygen from the lead dioxide. The result is a lengthening of the polymer chains and a cross-linking of adjacent chains. Water is produced as a by-product.

Uses and Clinical Handling Polysulfides have been used successfully for crown and bridge impressions and for partial and complete denture impressions. They are usually used in custom impression trays that allow for a thickness of about 2 mm of the material throughout the tray. Custom trays minimize the amount of material used and reduce the dimensional changes that occur in larger volumes of material. A tray adhesive of rubber cement is used to keep the impression material from separating from the tray on removal from the mouth. Polysulfides are supplied in light, regular, and heavy viscosities. Usually, for crown and bridge impressions the light body material is loaded into an impression syringe after mixing, injected around the prepared tooth, and covered with a tray containing the heavy body material. The heavy body material helps force the light body material into the gingival sulcus. The two materials join as they set. The preparation must be thoroughly dried for polysulfides, unlike the hydro colloids, which can be used in a moist field. The polysulfides are hydrophobic (water repelling) and will not flow into areas of moisture. Therefore if there is water, saliva, or blood in the field, the polysulfide materials will not register the surface details needed for accurate dies. Regular body material may also be used in custom trays for crown and bridge and partial and full denture impressions. Light body material is sometimes used over the regular body material as a wash material to correct small deficiencies.

CLINICAL TIP Alginate and agar hydrocolloids can be used in a moist field, because they are hydrophilic. For the most part, elastomers are hydrophobic. Some of them are slightly hydrophilic and are more forgiving of a little moisture, but not to the degree of the hydrocolloids. A well-isolated is essential.

Equal lengths of base (often white) and catalyst (often brown) are mixed to a uniform color without streaks of unmixed material, or the setting reaction will not occur properly (Figure 11-5). A stiff spatula is used to first mix the base and catalyst together with its tip in a circular motion. Then the side of the blade is used to mix the materials using wide sweep-

ing strokes until a homogeneous mix is achieved. The mixing time can easily be accomplished within a minute, but because of the very long working and setting times this step does not need to be rushed as with fast-set alginate.

Properties The setting time of polysulfides ranges from 8 to 14 minutes. Light body material takes longer to set than regular or heavy body. The setting time is very sensitive to moisture and high temperature, as well as the correct ratio of the base and catalyst. On hot, humid days the set may occur more rapidly and the materials may not perform optimally.

Polysulfides have slightly higher permanent deformation than the hydrocolloids but are still in an acceptable range (less than 3%). Their tear strength is approximately eight times that of the hydrocolloids. It is not necessary and frequently not possible to remove the impression with a snap as with hydrocolloids. Although not as sensitive to moisture loss as the hydrocolloids, the polysulfides can lose the water produced as a by-product of the setting reaction, resulting in some degree of distortion. The most accurate dies are obtained when the impression is poured within 30 minutes because of the shrinkage that occurs, about 0.4% the first day. The accuracy of crown and bridge impressions is far more demanding than for complete dentures, so the use of the impression is a factor in deciding how quickly the impression must be poured. Dies made from hydrocolloid impressions are limited to gypsum materials. The polysulfides and the other elastomers can be used to make dies of epoxy or metal (by an electroplating process). The latter two dies are more resistant to abrasion than gypsum dies and are preferred by some laboratories or practitioners. However, the vast majority of dies are made from gypsum materials.

Polysulfide rubbers have a very unpleasant taste and an odor that resembles rotten eggs. They are also messy to work with and hard to clean up. Caution must be taken to not get this material on the operator's or patient's clothing, because it is extremely difficult, if not impossible, to remove. The best solution to use to remove the set material is orange solvent. However, caution should be taken with its use, because it can be irritating to the oral mucosa or even to the skin of sensitive individuals. The polysulfides cost more than the hydrocolloids but are the least expensive of the elastomers. Because of

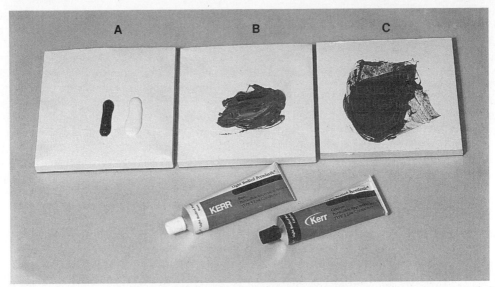

FIGURE 11-5 ■ Polysulfide impression material. **A,** Equal lengths of material dispensed on mixing pad. **B,** Improperly mixed material with streaks. **C,** Properly mixed material with consistent appearance.

their messiness, unpleasant odor, and slow setting time, the polysulfides have largely been replaced by the other elastomers for crown and bridge procedures. Some practitioners still prefer the polysulfides for complete denture impressions.

Silicone Rubber Impression Materials Two types of silicone impression materials have been developed and are named according to the type of polymerization reaction they undergo during setting. The first developed was the condensation silicone. The more recently developed addition silicone is far more popular.

Condensation Silicone Condensation silicone was developed as an alternative to polysulfide. It has more desirable characteristics than polysulfide, such as ease of mixing, pleasant taste, odorless, and shorter working and setting times. It is usually supplied in two tubes, a base and a liquid catalyst. It comes in light, medium, or heavy viscosities, as well as putty. The base is a low molecular-weight silicone called dimethylsiloxane. Silica or copper carbonate is added as a filler to keep the silicone paste from being too runny and to give stiffness to the set impression material. The catalyst contains a suspension of stannous octoate and also contains an alkyl silicate. The material sets in 5 to 7 minutes by a con-densation reaction that produces ethyl alcohol as a by-product. The ethyl alcohol is rapidly lost by evaporation, leading to a relatively high dimensional instability from shrinkage. The dimensional change during the first 24 hours is higher for the condensation silicones than for the polysulfides. The material continues to contract with time and must be poured up within a few minutes to reproduce an accurate cast of the teeth. Their poor wetting characteristics make it difficult to pour casts free of bubbles unless a surfactant is used. Condensation silicones have been used primarily in crown and bridge procedures but have been replaced for the most part by the addition silicones.

Addition Silicone The **addition silicone** impression materials are an improvement over the condensation silicone materials. Their properties provide more dimensional stability and accuracy. They are clean and easy to use, with no foul odor or taste. As a result of these improvements, they have become the most popular materials for crown and bridge procedures. They are also among the most expensive of the impression materials.

Addition Reaction Addition silicone, commonly known as polyvinyl siloxane (PVS), impression material undergoes a polymerization reaction of chain lengthening and cross-linking with reactive vinyl groups that produces a stable silicone rubber. The addition reaction does not produce a low-molecular-weight by-product that can evaporate and cause shrinkage as with the condensation silicones. PVS has the smallest dimensional change (0.05%) on setting of the elastomeric and hydrocolloid impression materials. Some of the addition silicones produce hydrogen gas through a secondary reaction. To counter the release of hydrogen, some manufacturers have incorporated palladium powder that absorbs the hydrogen. When using a PVS material that releases hydrogen, the impression should either be poured immediately before the hydrogen is formed or after 1 to 2 hours when most of the hydrogen has been released. If poured when the hydrogen is being released, the cast that results will have a very porous surface and will be unsuitable for most procedures. PVS impressions can be poured up several times and are dimensionally stable for a least a week without distortion. For this reason many practitioners will send the impression with a prescription to the dental laboratory where the impression may be poured several days later. The PVS materials exhibit less flow (deformation when subjected to a load after setting) than the con-

densation silicones and about 10% of that seen with the polysulfides. This accounts for their accuracy even after repouring.

Dispensing   Like the condensation silicones, the addition silicones are manufactured in light, regular, and heavy viscosities. A monophase viscosity is available from most manufacturers that is slightly more viscous than the regular body material. They are also available in putty form consisting of base and catalyst putty. Powdered silica is added as a filler to give thickness to the base or catalyst pastes or putties. The most popular dispensing system for the light, regular, and heavy materials is in a cartridge with two chambers, one with base and one with catalyst. A mixing tip fits on the end of the cartridge (Figure 11-6). A hand-operated gun-type dispenser or a motor-driven dispenser pushes both the base and catalyst through the mixing tip at the same time. They pass through an intertwined spiral that mixes them together thoroughly by the time they exit the end of the tip. These mixing devices ensure the proper ratio of the two materials without the creation of bubbles or voids. It is important for the operator to make certain that the orifices of the cartridges are cleaned of any residual set material that

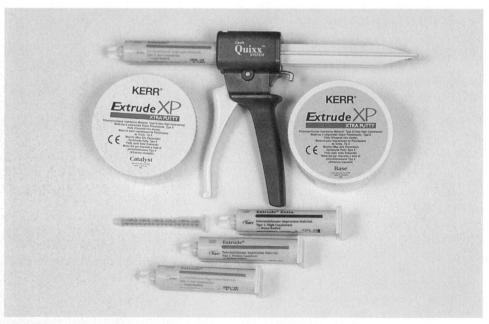

FIGURE 11-6 ■ Polyvinyl siloxane impression material in a variety of viscosities (light, regular, heavy body) in cartridges, putty in plastic jars, mixing gun, and mixing tip.

might block the flow of base or catalyst before applying the mixing tip. Otherwise, the proper amounts of base and catalyst may not be mixed.

Setting Time Because of the popularity of the PVS materials, manufacturers have put much effort into improving their properties to make their product more appealing than their competitors'. Setting times have been adjusted so that the practitioner has an assortment of materials with rapid or regular set. Setting times vary among manufacturers and range from approximately 3 to 7 minutes.

Putty/Wash Technique The PVS putty impression materials are often used as a preliminary impression for the two-step putty/wash procedure. In the first step, the putty is mixed and placed in a stock tray. It is seated over the teeth with a plastic sheet placed between the putty and the teeth to create room for light body material. Some practitioners prefer to cut away some of the putty after it has set to create space for the light body material rather than using the plastic sheet. In the second step, light body material is syringed around the prepared teeth, and some is injected into the space in the putty created by the teeth. The tray with the putty is seated over the teeth. In essence, the putty makes a custom tray from the stock tray. Putty has also been use in a one-step technique where the putty is mixed and loaded into a tray by the assistant while the doctor injects the syringe material around the prepared teeth. The tray is seated while the putty and syringe material are still unset, allowing them to bond together. For subgingival preparations, the stiff putty causes hydraulic pressure that forces the wash material into the gingival sulcus.

Both the one step and two-step putty techniques can result in distortions in the impression if care is not taken. Because putty does not flow well, the one-step technique may result in voids or a pulled appearance of the wash material where wash and putty did not flow and join together completely. With the two-step technique, because the putty is set before the wash is added, any areas where the putty shows through the wash material potentially have distortion. The flexible putty may have been compressed by contact with tooth structure and then rebounded to its original shape when the impression was removed from the mouth. This is particularly critical if it occurs in the area of the prepared tooth. To avoid these problems with putty, some clinicians use a one-step technique in which putty has been replaced with a heavy body material that flows better.

> **CLINICAL TIP** The PVS putty should *not* be mixed with latex gloves on. Sulfur products from the gloves will interfere with the set of the material. Washed hands covered with vinyl gloves should be used.

Putty also has many uses at chairside and in the laboratory. Putty is used in many offices to capture an imprint of a tooth before it is prepared for a crown. After preparation the imprint is used to form a provisional crown using tooth-colored acrylic resin. Some practitioners use the heavy body material instead of putty in the tray and the light body material in the syringe; others select a monophase material to place in the tray and to syringe around the teeth. The monophase material is formulated to have enough body to stay in the tray yet is fluid enough to inject around the teeth. A custom tray provides the most ideal thickness of impression material for accuracy, if not using the two-step putty technique in a stock tray.

Hydrophobic Nature Like condensation silicones, the addition silicones are hydrophobic and must be used in a dry field. A little moisture on the prepared tooth will result in a loss of surface detail in the impression. Some materials are called hydrophilic, but in actuality they are hydrophobic materials to which a wetting agent (surfactant) has been added so that they can tolerate the presence of a small amount of moisture.

Bite Registration Materials Addition silicones are also used as bite registration materials because of their accuracy, dimensional stability, and ease of use. They can be used for this purpose in two ways. Most practitioners prefer to use the automatic mixing cartridge systems and inject the material from the mixing tip directly onto the occlusal surfaces of the mandibular teeth. They then have the patient close into centric occlusion (Figures 11-7 and 11-8). Bite registration materials are viscous materials that stay in place when applied to the occlusal surfaces of teeth. This property makes it easier to register the bite and remove the material from the mouth, because it has not slumped and flowed all over the teeth. Some practitioners use a bite tray that is usually a disposable plastic frame

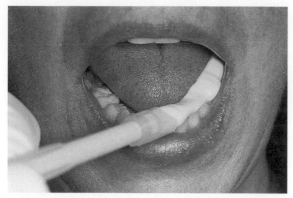

FIGURE 11-7 ■ Applying bite registration material to the teeth.

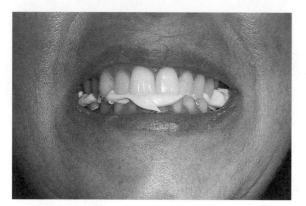

FIGURE 11-8 ■ Patient closed into centric occlusion.

with a gauzelike material stretched between the arms of the frame. Material is dispensed on both sides of the gauze, the frame is seated over the teeth, and the patient closes into centric occlusion (see Procedure 11-3). This system supports the bite registration better than without it. These materials are formulated with a rapid setting time of 1 to 2 minutes. They are relatively stiff materials that exhibit very little flow under loading forces and remain dimensionally stable for at least a week, unlike wax bite registrations, which can warp after removal from the mouth with temperature changes or applied loads.

Silicone Die Technique Some practitioners use a specially formulated addition silicone material in an automatic mixing cartridge system to make dies for indirect composite inlays. A tooth is prepared for a composite inlay, and an alginate impression is made

of the preparation. The silicone die material is injected into the alginate impression and it sets within 2 minutes. That die can be used to prepare the composite inlay at chairside. The completed inlay is cemented in the preparation with resin cement (see Figure 6-15 in Chapter 6). This procedure is relatively quick. It saves the dentist a laboratory bill, the need to tear down and set up an operatory for a second visit, and the need to place and remove a temporary filling, and it saves an additional trip and local anesthetic injection for the patient.

Polyethers Polyethers are rubber impression materials that are very accurate and excellent for use in crown and bridge procedures. They are more hydrophilic than other elastomers unless special surfactants have been added. This gives polyethers good wetting properties for making detailed impressions in the presence of a small amount of moisture and for pouring gypsum products without the formation of bubbles on the surface of the cast.

Consistency and Setting Reaction Polyethers are supplied as light, medium, and heavy body viscosities. Equal lengths of material are dispensed from two unequal-sized tubes of base and catalyst onto a mixing pad. The base is a moderately low-molecular-weight polyether with a cation reactive group. The catalyst contains aromatic sulfonic acid that reacts with ethylene terminal groups to cause cross-linking in a stable rubber material. The catalyst can cause skin and tissue irritation. Therefore thorough mixing of the base and catalyst are necessary to avoid any irritation of the oral tissues. In addition to polyether in tubes, it also comes in pouches of base and catalyst that are placed into a mechanical mixer and delivered directly into the impression tray (Figure 11-9). The mixer handles a much larger volume of material than the cartridges of PVS used in the automatic mixing guns.

Properties The polyethers are the stiffest of all of the rubber impression materials; as a consequence, they can be difficult to remove from the mouth in the presence of undercuts. It is important to have an adequate thickness of material in the tray to allow for more flexibility of the set material. A minimum of 4 mm of space in a custom tray is recommended. Undercuts around bridge pontics, open embrasures around periodontally involved teeth, and fixed implant fixtures should be blocked out with utility wax to prevent the impression material from locking

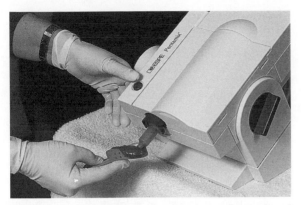

FIGURE 11-9 ■ Polyether impression material mixed and dispensed from mixing machine directly into tray.

under them and preventing removal of the impression tray. Cutting through metal impression trays with burs or diamonds to remove them from the mouth is an unpleasant experience for both the patient and the practitioner.

Polyethers have relatively short working and setting times compared with the other elastomeric materials. The impression tray should be seated in the mouth within about 3 minutes from the start of the mix, because the viscosity increases noticeably during this time. After seating in the mouth, the polyethers set within 3 to 5 minutes. They are also very sensitive to temperature and moisture. Increases in either will shorten the working and setting times even further. Permanent deformation is low com-

pared with the polysulfides but not as low as the silicones. This material is somewhat hydrophilic, so it must not be stored in water or disinfecting solution, because it will swell from the uptake of moisture. Impressions from this material can be poured up repeatedly for up to a week and can be shipped to a dental laboratory and remain dimensionally stable for several days. The fact that their polymerization does not produce volatile by-products contributes to their dimensional stability. Table 11-5 compares features of elastic impression materials.

Inelastic Impression Materials

DENTAL IMPRESSION COMPOUND

Uses Dental impression compound, impression plaster, and impression wax are among the oldest impression materials used in dentistry. **Impression compound** is a rigid thermoplastic material that softens when heated and becomes firm again at mouth temperatures. Impression compound is most commonly used as thick sheets (sometimes called cakes) or sticks (Figure 11-10). It has several uses for impressions. Some dentists use the sheets in stock aluminum trays for making preliminary impressions for complete dentures. Sheets can also be used in complete denture construction to make a custom tray into which a thin, free-flowing impression material (called a wash material) is placed to take a detailed impression of the tissues. Compound used

TABLE 11-5

Features of Elastic Impression Materials

Impression Material	Cost	Surface Detail	Dimensional Stability	Tear Strength	Ease of Use	Pour Within	Ability to Repour
Reversible hydrocolloid	Low	High	Low	Low	Low	Immediately	No
Alginate	Low	Lowest	Low	Low	High	1 hr	No
Polysulfide	Medium	High	Medium	Highest	Medium	30 min to several hours	Yes, second not as accurate
Condensation	Medium	High	Low to medium	Low to medium	Medium	1 hr	Yes
Addition silicone (polyvinyl siloxanes)	High	High	Highest	Medium	High	1 wk	Yes
Polyether	High	High	High	Low to medium	High	1 wk	Yes

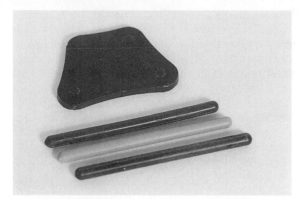

FIGURE 11-10 ■ Types of impression compound sticks.

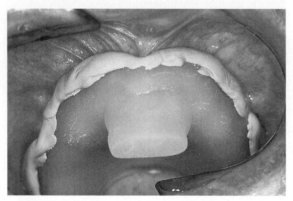

FIGURE 11-11 ■ Stick compound used for border molding of custom impression tray.

(Courtesy Dr. Mark Dellinges, University of California School of Dentistry, San Francisco, Calif.)

for this purpose has been called tray compound. Elastic impression materials in custom acrylic trays have largely replaced the use of tray compound. Compound sticks are often used to mold the peripheral borders of a custom tray and form the palatal seal in impressions for complete dentures (Figure 11-11). After the peripheral borders have been established, an impression is taken in the tray with one of the elastomers.

Composition Compounds typically contain thermoplastic resins and waxes (40%), fillers (50%) of talc or chalk, and plasticizers (10%) to make them less brittle. The talc or chalk used as fillers reduces the flow of the material so it is not too fluid when softened. Organic acids or oils are used to make the compound less brittle. Pigments are added to produce different colors that indicate a certain temperature range at

which compound becomes soft, or simply to differentiate it from that of another manufacturer.

Physical Properties The manufacturer formulates impression compound so that it softens at approximately 60° C (140° F), remains plastic at 45° C (113° F) (with at least 85% flow) when inserted in the mouth, and becomes firm at mouth temperature (37° C [98° F]). Heating in a controlled-temperature water bath is recommended to soften the material evenly throughout. Heating in a direct flame melts the outside rapidly, but the inner core may still be too firm. Too much heat can burn the material and change its properties. If heated in a flame, the compound should be tempered in a water bath of appropriate temperature to keep it from burning the patient. At too cool a temperature, the materials will not be plastic enough to mold to the shape of the tissues, and this will not make an adequate replication of the mouth. The completed impression should be poured with plaster or stone soon after it is taken because stresses induced in the compound as it is heated and manipulated can cause distortion as stresses are released. Additionally, distortion can be minimized by using a rigid tray and by cooling the compound adequately before it is removed from the mouth.

IMPRESSION PLASTER

Impression plaster is seldom used today but was used mainly for complete denture impressions. It is composed of plaster of Paris (calcium hemihydrate) with potassium sulfate or potassium chloride added to accelerate the set (about 3 minutes) and limit the setting expansion to about 0.06% (see Chapter 12). When used as the primary impression material a wet mix (high water/powder ratio) is used. The higher water content makes it more fluid in the mouth and extends the setting time but results in a weaker-set plaster. After it is set in the mouth it is scored with a knife or bur, fractured along the score lines, and removed. The pieces are reassembled in the laboratory with glue or sticky wax, coated with a separating medium (to prevent dental stone from adhering to the plaster), and poured in dental stone to form the cast. Because of the complexity of its technique, impression plaster is rarely used today and has been replaced by elastic materials that are easier to use and that eliminate the potential distortion caused by failure to accurately reassemble the parts of the plaster impression. Impression plaster has also been used as a wash material inside a custom tray made by first adapting softened tray compound in an aluminum tray to the edentulous ridge and then adding a thin mix of plaster to the compound tray. This technique reproduces the details of the oral mucosa well and is dimensionally stable once it has set. Impression plaster is far less costly than the elastomers and is relatively easy to handle. Plaster is used today primarily as a handy utility gypsum in the dental laboratory that has the advantage of a very rapid set. Its shelf life can be extended to approximately 2 years by storing it in airtight containers to prevent absorption of moisture from the air.

ZINC OXIDE EUGENOL IMPRESSION MATERIAL

Zinc oxide eugenol (ZOE) impression material, like impression plaster, is seldom used today. Its use also is limited mostly to impressions of edentulous arches. ZOE impression material is dispensed as a two-tube paste system with two different-colored pastes, one containing zinc oxide (80%), oils (15%), and inert fillers (5%) and the other containing eugenol (15%), oils (65%), resin and fillers, and a chemical accelerator (zinc acetate or magnesium chloride) to speed up an otherwise slow set when the two pastes are mixed. Equal lengths of material are dispensed onto a mixing pad. The manufacturer further controls the ratio of the two pastes by using different-size openings for each tube. The material is mixed to a uniform color and consistency and will have an initial set in 3 to 6 minutes and a final set in about 10 minutes (setting time varies with the manufacturer). A warm or humid day can cause an acceleration of the set. Some clinicians accelerate the set by adding a drop of water to the mix or adding a few zinc acetate crystals. Eugenol and zinc oxide react to form zinc eugenolate and particles of unset zinc oxide. The set material is hard and brittle and will fracture if used in areas of severe tissue undercuts. It is used as a stand-alone final impression material in a custom tray or as a wash material inside of a preliminary compound impression, because it flows readily and picks up fine details in the impression that compound cannot.

In its day ZOE was favored as an impression material for mucostatic impressions. When a patient had loose tissue over an edentulous ridge and the operator did not want to displace these tissues with a stiff or heavy viscosity impression material, ZOE was often chosen. Its thin consistency did not displace the tissue (thus the mucosa was static), as did some of the other impression materials such as compound. It is relatively accurate for its application in complete denture construction and is inexpensive. Nonetheless, ZOE has been replaced largely by elastic materials. The eugenol imparts a somewhat unpleasant taste and can irritate the tissues of some patients. Lubrication of the patient's lips will prevent burning of chapped lips and will keep impression material from sticking to the skin. Once set, ZOE is relatively stable dimensionally (less than 0.1% shrinkage); therefore it does not require immediate pouring as with some of the other materials. Unlike impression plaster impressions, ZOE impressions do not require a separating medium to keep dental stone from sticking to the impression material.

IMPRESSION WAX

Wax is another inelastic material that was used early in dentistry for impressions. Waxes are often stiff at room temperature and become moldable when heated. They lack accuracy for final impressions for restorative treatments and distort easily on removal from tissue undercuts or when affected by temperature fluctuations after removal from the mouth. Some dentists have used them for preliminary impressions of edentulous ridges for complete dentures. Waxes have also been used as bite registration materials. Baseplate wax has been used to form a template for construction of provisional crowns and bridges. Warm baseplate wax is adapted to the teeth, cooled, and removed before crown and bridge treatment. It is flexible enough to pull out of most tooth undercuts. Later it is filled with freshly mixed acrylic resin and reseated over the prepared teeth to form provisional crowns or bridges. Some waxes with low melting temperatures remain moldable at mouth temperatures and are used to correct minor voids in impressions for complete dentures or to build a posterior seal (post dam) for the maxillary denture by adding wax to the impression in the area of the juncture of hard and soft palates (see Chapter 15).

Disinfecting Impressions

Dental impressions always should be considered contaminated. They are usually contaminated with saliva or blood, which may contain viral and bacterial pathogens. Although most infectious agents, such as human immunodeficiency virus (HIV), do not survive for long periods of time outside of the body, many pathogens, such as the hepatitis viruses, can survive for several days. When impressions are not disinfected before they are poured, microorganisms can get into the gypsum and survive for a week or more. Spores can survive much longer.

> **▶ CAUTION**
> *Impressions are potentially infectious. They must be disinfected before being handled in the office laboratory or sent to a commercial laboratory.*

Ideally, disinfection of impressions should begin in the operatory through chairside measures once the impression is removed from the mouth. Dental personnel should wear personal protective equipment until the impressions are properly disinfected. The dental office has the primary responsibility for disinfection. Although the Occupational Safety and Health Administration (OSHA) allows transportation of contaminated items, regulations require proper packaging and labeling of these contaminated items. Dental offices should discuss with the dental laboratory the protocol they will use for disinfecting items sent to the laboratory and how restorations returning from the laboratory should be handled.

The material that is to be disinfected must be compatible with the disinfectant used and the procedure employed. Incompatible disinfection materials and procedures can cause significant distortion of the impression and failure of the restoration to fit correctly.

After removal from the mouth, impressions should be rinsed thoroughly with water to remove saliva, blood, debris, and other loosely attached contaminants. Excess water should be shaken off before using the disinfectant so as not to dilute it. Disinfectants can be applied by immersion of the impression or by spraying its surfaces. Spraying may be preferred for impression materials that tend to distort with immersion, such as the polyethers and alginate. However, spraying has two main disadvantages. First, it creates airborne particles of the disinfecting chemicals that could be inhaled by the staff or patients. Second, it may not adequately reach all surfaces if severe tissue undercuts are present. Immersion can cause distortion of some impression materials, because they are prone to imbibe water and swell. Alginate can be immersed in appropriate

disinfectants for up to 30 minutes. The length of time these sensitive materials are immersed must be monitored carefully, sometimes a difficult task in a busy office. Impressions should be rinsed after the recommended contact time with the disinfectant to remove residual chemicals that can affect the surface of the poured cast. If they are to be transported to the dental laboratory, they should be placed in a closed container or sealed plastic bag.

CLINICAL TIP Spraying of the impression should be done inside a plastic bag or headrest cover to contain the spray and protect the handler from inhaling droplets.

Impression materials are composed of a variety of materials. As such, they often require different materials and handling for disinfection. Manufacturer recommendations for disinfection should be followed. Agar and alginate impressions can safely be disinfected with an iodophor or 1% sodium hypochlorite solution for 10 minutes. Elastomeric impressions can be disinfected with a wide range of solutions. However, each particular material may be adversely affected by some disinfectants. For example, phenols with high alcohol content can dehydrate some of the impression materials. Some of the solutions may also dissolve the tray adhesive that retains the impression material and cause it to come loose from the tray. The silicone, polysulfide, and polyether elastomers can be disinfected with 1:213 iodophors, 1:10 sodium hypochlorite, or complex phenolics. Silicones can also be disinfected with glutaraldehydes. Inelastic impression materials such as ZOE can be disinfected with iodophors or 2% gluteraldehyde solutions. Chlorine solutions should not be used on ZOE impressions but can be used on compound impressions, as can iodophors and hypochlorite. Wax bite registrations, rubber bite registrations, and casts all present different problems for disinfection. Wax may distort when it is immersed. The recommended disinfecting procedure is to rinse-spray-rinse-spray-rinse and then place in the container for transport. Most elastomeric bite registration materials can be safely disinfected by the same solutions as their impression material counterparts. See Table 11-6 for disinfecting times and materials for impressions. Procedure 11-4 describes processing methods for impression materials.

TABLE 11-6
Disinfection of Impressions

Impression Material	Compatible Disinfectants	Immersion Time
Alginate and agar hydrocolloid	1:10 sodium hypochlorite, 1:213 iodophors	10-30 min
Polysulfides	1:10 sodium hypochlorite, 1:213 iodophors, glutaraldehydes, complex phenolics	10-30 min
Silicones (condensation and addition)	1:10 sodium hypochlorite, 1:213 iodophors, glutaraldehydes, complex phenolics	10-30 min
Polyethers	1:10 sodium hypochlorite, 1:213 iodophors, complex phenolics	<10 min or spray
Compound	1:10 hypochlorite, 1:213 iodophors	10-30 min
Zinc oxide eugenol	1:213 iodophors, glutaraldehydes	10-30 min

DISINFECTING CASTS

On rare occasions it may be necessary to disinfect the cast produced from an impression that could not be properly disinfected because of the nature of the contaminants or an impression material that could not be immersed in the proper disinfectant. Casts should be completely set and stored for at least 24 hours before disinfecting to prevent attack by the chemicals on the surface of the cast. Casts seem to be minimally affected by using 1:10 sodium hypochlorite, iodophors, or chlorine dioxide. Casts should be sprayed rather than immersed in disinfecting solutions, because some studies have shown damage to the surface in only a few minutes in water-based solutions. Manufacturers have added antimicrobial agents to some gypsum materials, but studies are not conclusive as to their effectiveness.

STERILIZING IMPRESSION TRAYS

Impression trays must be properly sterilized after their use and after trying the tray in the patient's mouth for fit. Disposable plastic trays are recommended when they can meet the demands of the impression material being used. Flexible materials require a rigid tray to prevent flexing of the tray and distortion of the material. Because of their thickness and rigidity, some putties can better tolerate flexible plastic trays. Inelastic impression materials also may require rigid trays to prevent them from cracking. Plastic trays that are more rigid have been developed and are commercially available. Custom acrylic trays should be discarded when the procedure has been completed or immersed in an acceptable disinfectant if it will be reused at the patient's next appointment. Aluminum, chrome-plated, and stainless steel trays can be sterilized by heated steam or chemical vapors, dry heat, or ethylene oxide after they have been thoroughly cleaned.

SUMMARY

In almost all phases of dentistry, impressions are an integral part of the procedures needed for delivering comprehensive care to patients. In many offices impressions are taken daily, and the various impression materials must be understood by the clinician in order to correctly select, manipulate, and disinfect the materials and to pour casts. Inelastic materials, although not frequently used, still have applications in removable and fixed prosthetics. The most frequently used materials are the elastic materials, including alginate, polyvinyl siloxanes, polyethers, and polysulfides. Reversible hydrocolloid is used much less than the PVS materials but offers similar accuracy for the final impression, but at a much lower cost. Each category of the impression materials has its own handling characteristics that must be considered. Changes in temperature and humidity will influence the materials in different ways, so operators must take these factors into consideration when making impressions. Dimensional changes over time, water loss and gain, deformation, and rebound are among the many physical properties that also must be considered when handling and disinfecting impression materials if the clinician is to meet the objective of producing as accurate a replica of the oral structures as possible.

CHAPTER REVIEW

Select the one correct response for each of the following multiple-choice questions:

1. **A dental impression material**
   a. Forms a positive imprint of the oral structures involved
   b. Allows the creation of a replica of the structures involved
   c. Is always flexible for easy removal from the mouth
   d. Is used only for crown and bridge procedures and for diagnostic casts (study models)

2. **Which of the following impression materials are transformed from a sol to a gel state when set?**
   a. Alginate and agar hydrocolloids
   b. Polysulfides
   c. Zinc oxide eugenol
   d. Condensation silicones

3. **Which one of the following is an example of an inelastic impression material?**
   a. Alginate
   b. Polyether impression material
   c. Dental compound
   d. Polyvinyl siloxane (PVS) impression material

4. **The types of impression materials that are considered hydrophilic are those that**
   a. Have a lot of water in them
   b. Can be immersed in water without absorbing it
   c. Cause water to bead on their surface
   d. Have good surface-wetting characteristics

5. **Hydrophobic impression materials**
   a. Absorb moisture only after their final set
   b. Are the best type of material to use in the mouth because they repel saliva and blood
   c. Need a dry field to get the best results
   d. Provide the best surfaces on gypsum casts, because they resist the uptake of water during the curing of the gypsum

6. **Alginate impression material**
   a. Is accurate enough to be used for crown and bridge procedures
   b. Has very few uses in the modern dental practice
   c. Is dimensionally stable during the first 24 hours
   d. Can be immersed in an appropriate disinfectant for up to 30 minutes without distorting

7. **Agar hydrocolloid**
   a. Works well in a moist field
   b. Is hydrophobic
   c. Has excellent tear strength in deep, narrow spaces
   d. Can be poured up after several days if kept immersed in water

8. **An irreversible hydrocolloid**
   a. Is one that goes from a gel to a sol by heating it
   b. Commonly used in the dental office is agar hydrocolloid
   c. Is hydrophobic
   d. Cannot reverse from a gel to a sol because a chemical reaction prevents it

9. **Polyvinyl impression materials are of the class known as**
   a. Inelastic materials   c. Hydrocolloids
   b. Mucostatics   d. Elastomers

10. **Polysulfide impression materials**
    a. Are easy to mix
    b. Have a rapid setting time
    c. Are the most accurate impression materials
    d. Have excellent tear strength

11. **Which of the following elastomers will imbibe water when immersed in it and swell?**
    a. Polysulfides   c. Addition silicones
    b. Condensation silicones   d. Polyethers

12. **Which one of the following materials produces alcohol as a by-product of its setting reaction and is subject to distortion as it evaporates?**
    a. Agar hydrocolloid   c. Condensation silicone
    b. Polysulfide   d. ZOE

13. **Which of the following statements is true about the addition silicones?**
    a. They are good materials for complete denture impressions but are not accurate for crown and bridge procedures.
    b. They are very dimensionally stable.
    c. They cost about the same as alginate.
    d. They require the use of custom acrylic trays.

14. **The most rigid of the elastic impression materials is**
    a. Alginate   c. Compound
    b. Polysulfide   d. Polyether

15. **The least accurate of the elastic impression materials is**
    a. Agar hydrocolloid   c. Polyvinyl siloxane
    b. Condensation silicone   d. Alginate

16. **Which two of the following elastomers do NOT need to be poured with gypsum material within a few hours after the impression is made?**
    a. Polysulfide and polyvinyl siloxane
    b. Condensation silicone and polyether
    c. Addition silicone and polyether
    d. Condensation silicone and polysulfide

17. **Dental compound impression material can change from a solid to a soft material by heating it. Its greatest use today is for which procedure?**
    a. Border molding custom trays for denture impressions
    b. Making impressions of teeth for single crowns
    c. Making impressions of inlay preparations
    d. Adapted over the teeth before treatment and used after crown preparation to make the acrylic temporary crown

18. Which one of the following, when used for denture impressions, is broken into pieces to remove it from the mouth and reassembled in the laboratory to pour the impression?
    a. Impression plaster
    b. Dental compound
    c. Impression wax
    d. Zinc oxide eugenol

19. Zinc oxide eugenol impression material is
    a. Mixed to the same consistency as the zinc oxide eugenol provisional filling material
    b. Useful for an impression of a crown preparation in the presence of inflamed gingiva because of the healing capacity of the eugenol
    c. Only used as a wash in a compound preliminary full-denture impression
    d. Used alone in a custom acrylic resin impression tray as a wash material

20. Disinfecting of impressions
    a. Is to protect the patient from surface bacteria
    b. Must be done for all impressions
    c. Is done only with impressions for patients with known infectious diseases
    d. Does not need to be done for the new alginates that have bactericidal chemicals incorporated into them

CASE-BASED DISCUSSION TOPICS

◉ A 30-year-old retail store manager comes to the dental office to have impressions made for home bleaching trays. She indicates that she has a moderate gag reflex. *What impression material is well suited for making bleaching trays? What steps can be taken to minimize gagging and to shorten the length of time the impression material remains in the mouth? How should the impression material be handled from the time it is removed from the mouth until it is poured with dental plaster or stone?*

◉ A dentist practicing in California decides to use the services of a dental laboratory located in New York City. He plans to mail his impressions to the laboratory rather than pour them in his office. *What types of impression materials can be used under these circumstances and still produce accurate casts and dies? Which materials definitely cannot be used? What properties of the materials are most important? How should the impressions be handled before they are shipped to the laboratory?*

◉ A 53-year-old mail carrier comes to the dental office with a broken facial cusp on tooth number 31. Adjacent to number 31 the patient has a fixed bridge from number 28 to number 30 that has a pontic replacing tooth number 29. The dentist will prepare the tooth for a porcelain-bonded-to-metal crown and her dental assistant with extended functions will make an impression. Isolation is difficult because the patient salivates profusely and the gingiva is bleeding because the patient is taking blood thinners. The dental assistant will be able to control most of the saliva, and the bleeding will be greatly reduced when the dentist injects a local anesthetic with a vasoconstrictor into the gingival papillae around the tooth. However, the preparation will not be completely dry. *Which one impression material is truly hydrophilic and is accurate enough for crown impressions? Which elastomer, by its nature, is somewhat hydrophilic and could be used? Which materials are not naturally hydrophilic but may have surfactants added to make them more hydrophilic? What precautions should be taken before the impression is taken to ensure that it can be easily removed from the mouth?*

◉ The dentist in your office will replace an existing crown on tooth number 5 for a young female college student because of recurrent caries under the distal margin. He likes to use a two-step polyvinyl siloxane (PVS) putty-wash technique. You will be asked to prepare an acrylic custom provisional crown for the patient. *How should you prepare for this before the dentist removes the crown using the materials at hand? What types of impression trays can the dentist use with this technique? Can a polysulfide tray adhesive be used with the PVS putty? How soon does the PVS impression have to be poured? What disinfectants are safe to use with PVS materials?*

◉ The dentist uses agar hydrocolloid in your office for her crown and bridge impressions. This afternoon she received a call from the dental laboratory indicating that the laboratory's delivery man had been in an automobile accident, and the dies he picked up from your office were broken. *Can the dentist repour the impression and send new dies? Why or why not? Which of the impression materials are good for this purpose? Which elastomer has the greatest accuracy for the longest time?*

◉ A variety of impression materials may be used in the dental office on a daily basis. It is important to protect all dental personnel who might handle the impressions by proper disinfection. Additionally, the accuracy of the impressions might be adversely affected by improper disinfection techniques. *Describe the procedures for disinfecting alginate, agar hydrocolloid, polysulfide, and polyether impression materials.*

REFERENCES

Craig RG, editor: Impression materials. In *Restorative dental materials,* ed 7, St Louis, 1985, Mosby.

Craig RG, Powers JM, Wataha JC: Impression materials. In *Dental materials: properties and manipulation,* ed 7, St Louis, 2000, Mosby.

Ehrlich A, Torres HO, Bird D: Alginate impressions and diagnostic casts: gingival retraction and elastomeric impressions. In *Essentials of dental assisting,* ed 2, Philadelphia, 1996, WB Saunders.

Farah JW, Powers JM, editors: On making good impressions, *Dental Advisor* 1(1):1, 1984.

Farah JW, Powers JM, editors: Crown and bridge impression materials, *Dental Advisor* 6(2):2, 1989.

Farah JW, Powers JM, editors: Impressions and accessories, *Dental Advisor* 9(4):1, 1992.

Farah JW, Powers JM, editors: Bite registration materials, *Dental Advisor* 15(4):2, 1998.

Gladwin MA, Bagby MD: Impression materials. In *Clinical aspects of dental materials,* Philadelphia, 2000, Lippincott Williams & Wilkins.

Gomolka K, editor: Impression disinfection, *Monthly Focus* 7:1, 1998.

Hydrophilic impression materials, *CRA Newsletter* 20(5):3, 1996.

Leinfelder KF, Lemons JE: Impression materials. In *Clinical restorative materials and techniques,* Philadelphia, 1988, Lea & Febiger.

Merchant VA: Infection control in the dental laboratory environment. In Cottone JA, Terazhalmy GT, Molinari GT, editors: *Practical infection control in dentistry,* ed 2, Philadelphia, 1996, Williams & Wilkins.

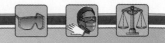

PROCEDURE 11-1 (see p. 339 for competency sheet)

Making an Alginate Impression

EQUIPMENT/SUPPLIES (Figure 11-12)

- Basic setup
- Alginate, powder scoop, and water measuring cylinder
- Rubber bowl, wide-bladed spatula
- Impression trays (perforated) or solid trays including rim-locks require alginate adhesive
- Utility wax ropes
- Saliva ejector, disinfecting solution, zippered plastic bag, paper towels

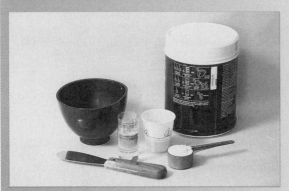

FIGURE 11-12

PROCEDURE STEPS

1 *Patient preparation.* Seat patient. Cover clothes with plastic-backed bib. Explain procedure. Inquire about gag response and ability to breathe through the nose. Remove dental prostheses unless needed in impression. Have patient rinse mouth.

NOTE: If patient has bridges or fixed implant prostheses, block out with wax around pontic spaces likely to lock alginate in place and make removal of impression difficult. Orthodontic bands, brackets, and arch wires may also need blockout wax. If patient has very loose teeth, block out embrasures around these teeth to prevent removing them in impression. Take precautions for gagging (as highlighted in chapter). If not able to breathe through nose, patient may feel threatened if alginate runs out back of tray and blocks airway, so seat tray in posterior first to force material forward. Occasionally, the dentist may want the prosthesis left in during the impression to examine the occlusion later on. Check with the dentist. Rinsing before impression removes debris and ropy saliva. An antibacterial rinse will reduce the number of pathogens.

2 *Tray selection.* Quickly examine patient's mouth, arch size and shape, and palatal depth. Select tray of appropriate size. Try it in for fit. Add utility wax as needed for comfort and extension of tray.

NOTE: If tray border is short or palate deep, add wax to extend tray and support alginate (Figure 11-13).

3 *Mixing alginate.* Tumble container of alginate to fluff powder. Measure 3 level scoops of powder for large upper arch or 2 scoops for smaller arch. Two scoops are adequate for the average lower arch. Place in rubber bowl 1 measure of room-temperature water for each scoop of powder. Add powder to water and stir to wet powder. Vigorously mix and press wet powder against sides of bowl with spatula while rotating bowl with other hand. Final mix should appear smooth and not grainy (Figure 11-14).

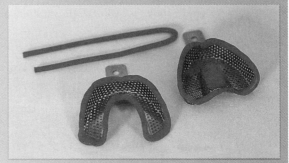

FIGURE 11-13

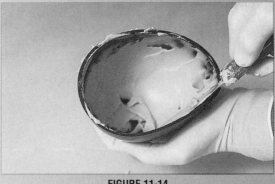

FIGURE 11-14

Continued on following page

PROCEDURE 11-1 (Continued)

NOTE: Prepackaged alginate does not require fluffing because it already is the correct amount. Mix by wiping vigorously against sides of bowl to remove entrapped air and thoroughly mix powder and water. Water cooler than room temperature lengthens working and setting times, whereas warm water shortens them. Complete mix within 45 seconds for regular-set or 30 seconds for fast-set alginate to allow enough time to load tray, paint occlusal surfaces, and seat impression before initial set.

4 *Loading tray.* Load tray in large increments, pressing each into tray until level with sides. Use wet, gloved finger to smooth surface and create a shallow indentation where teeth will go (Figure 11-15). Remove excess alginate.

NOTE: Fewer increments will trap less air. Force out entrapped air by pressing alginate into depth of tray. Indentation for teeth helps orient tray when seating. Extra material added to the anterior part of the tray helps fill the vestibule and get a good peripheral roll.

5 *Seating the tray.* Take alginate from bowl on finger and wipe it over occlusal surfaces and into embrasures. *For upper impression:* From behind and to side of patient (11 o'clock position) retract right cheek with posterior corner of tray and left cheek with index finger. *For lower impression:* From in front and to side of patient (7 or 8 o'clock position) retract left cheek with side of tray and right cheek with left index finger (Figure 11-16). (Left-handed operators make appropriate changes in positions.) Both impressions can be made with the operator seated and the patient reclined or the operator standing with the patient upright.

If the patient is reclined, seat the patient upright after the tray is placed. *For both upper and lower impressions:* Rotate tray into mouth, align tray over teeth with handle in midline. Seat back of tray first and complete seating to the anterior as the lip is gently pulled of the way. Inspect back of tray for excess alginate and remove with quick sweep of mouth mirror. *For lower impression:* Have patient lift tongue once tray is seated and relax it again once alginate has flowed into lingual areas.

NOTE: Seating posterior of tray first allows alginate to flow forward rather than back into the patient's throat. Lifting lip allows alginate to flow into vestibule. Quickly removing excess alginate minimizes gag response. Employ distraction techniques for gaggers. Have them position head forward, breathe through nose deeply and slowly, and use saliva ejector to prevent pooling of saliva.

6 Stabilize tray until alginate is fully set. Allow another 2 minutes before removing tray.

NOTE: Check alginate remaining in the bowl to confirm set. Tray movement during setting will cause distortion in the impression. Allowing 2 minutes after set helps increase tear strength.

7 *Removing tray.* Break seal by pressing down (or up for a lower impression) on side of tray with finger or have patient close lips around tray handle and blow to puff out the cheeks. Hold handle in hand grasped with index finger and thumb and remove tray with a snap.

NOTE: Protect patient's teeth in opposing arch with fingers of other hand. Rapid removal minimizes distortion and tearing of alginate.

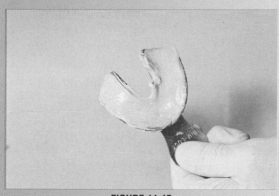

FIGURE 11-15

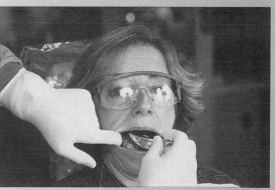

FIGURE 11-16

Continued on following page

PROCEDURE 11-1 (Continued)

8 *Handling impression.* Rinse under running water to remove saliva and debris. Inspect impression using criteria for acceptability (see Table 11-3) (Figures 11-17 and 11-18).

9 *Disinfecting impression.* Spray thoroughly with disinfectant. Drain off pooled liquid.

NOTE: By spraying the impression inside a bag or headrest cover the aerosol is better contained (Figure 11-19). Alginate will imbibe liquid and swell, so pooled liquid should be removed.

10 Cut off unsupported alginate at the back of the tray. Wrap impression in damp paper towel and seal in zippered plastic bag marked with patient's name (Figure 11-20).

NOTE: If tray is laid on the bench top, unsupported alginate at the back of the tray may lift a portion of the impression and dislodge it from the tray. This will cause a distortion in the impression. If alginate is left in air, water will evaporate, causing distortion. Ideally, the impression should be poured within 30 minutes, because it is not dimensionally stable for long periods. It will lose water (by syneresis) even in 100% humidity. Allow 10 minutes before pouring to allow disinfectant to be effective and to allow rebound to occur.

11 Help patient remove alginate from face with damp towel. Have patient rinse mouth. Inspect mouth and remove trapped alginate from embrasures with explorer and floss.

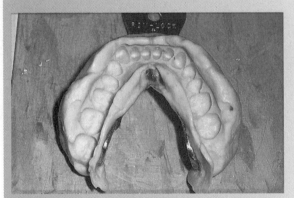

FIGURE 11-17

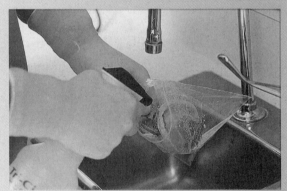

FIGURE 11-19

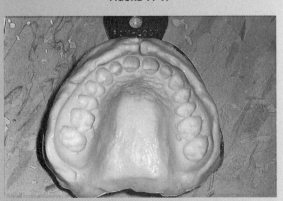

FIGURE 11-18

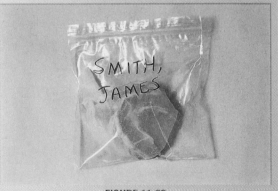

FIGURE 11-20

PROCEDURE 11-2 (see p. 340 for competency sheet)

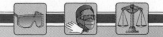

Making a Double-Bite Impression for a Crown

NOTE: In some states the dental assistant or hygienist may be licensed to place retraction cord and make the impression. In states where these functions are not permitted, it is assumed that the dental assistant or hygienist will assist the dentist.

EQUIPMENT/SUPPLIES (Figure 11-21)

- Basic crown and bridge setup
- Double-bite tray (paper insert for metal trays), tray adhesive
- Elastomeric impression material in cartridges: heavy body tray material and light body syringe material
- Dispenser gun and mixing tips
- Impression syringe

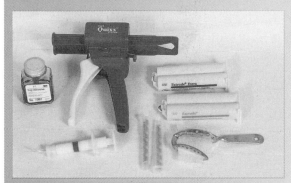

FIGURE 11-21

PROCEDURE STEPS

1 Assemble the cartridge in the gun and extrude a small amount of impression material onto a paper towel to ensure that the orifices are not clogged. Place the mixing tip.

NOTE: Clogged or partially clogged orifices will result in an improper mix of the material with alteration of setting time and physical properties.

2 Inform the patient of the procedure and have patient practice closing into centric occlusion (patient's "normal" bite) with the tray in place (Figure 11-22).

NOTE: Choose opposing teeth that are easily seen, such as the canines on the opposite side of the mouth, and note their position when they occlude. This relationship will be checked when the impression is made to ensure proper closure.

3 Maintain isolation in the quadrant in which the impression will be made.

NOTE: Saliva can saturate the retraction cord and may cause it to displace from the gingival sulcus.

4 Confirm that cord retraction around the crown preparation is adequate (Figure 11-23).

NOTE: The clinician should be able to see the preparation, the cord, and the gingiva displaced from the preparation. In other words, the cord should not be placed so deeply into the gingival sulcus that the gingival crest has collapsed over it and is resting on or near the preparation.

5 Carefully remove the retraction cord after it has been in place for 5 to 8 minutes. Rinse and dry the tooth.

NOTE: If the retraction cord is dry, lightly wet it before removing it. A dry cord may stick to tissues and cause bleeding when removed. To prevent bleeding the cord should be gently lifted from the sulcus rather than ripped out quickly.

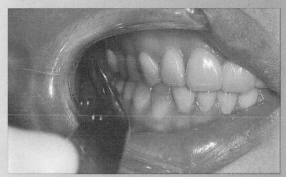

FIGURE 11-22

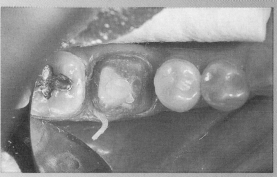

FIGURE 11-23

Continued on following page

PROCEDURE 11-2 (Continued)

6 Inspect the gingiva, sulcus, and preparation before proceeding with the impression. Check to see that the tissue is adequately retracted in all areas around the preparation, that it is not bleeding, and that the margins of the preparation are free of debris.

NOTE: The tissues will stay retracted long enough to control the field. The impression syringe should not be loaded until the field is dry, bleeding is controlled, and retraction is adequate. If a two-cord retraction technique is used in which a smaller cord is left in the sulcus during the impression, check to see that the smaller cord has stayed in place and has not lifted over the margins. If it has lifted, pack it back into place. If blood is oozing from the sulcus, control bleeding by scrubbing the sulcus with a ferric sulfate astringent (such as Astringident) on a small cotton pellet or applicator. Then rinse residual astringent away because compounds containing sulfur can interfere with the set of polyvinyl siloxane impression materials.

7 With the preassembled dispenser gun and mixing tip, load the impression syringe with the light body material. Change cartridges and mixing tips. Load both the preparation and opposing arch sides of the double-bite tray with the heavy body material.

NOTE: Impression putty could be used in place of the heavy body material. The gun-type mixing system ensures a thorough mix with minimal waste of material. For efficiency of time and motion, two guns could be used and preassembled rather than having to unload the light body and load the heavy body with a single gun.

8 Carefully dispense light body material from the syringe to the clean and dry preparation by starting with the tip just apical to the margin. With the material continually flowing, keep the tip in contact with the tooth while slowly tracing the margin and filling the gingival sulcus. Circle the entire tooth to completely cover the margins, and then continue circling while covering the axial walls and finally the occlusal surface (Figure 11-24).

NOTE: Some manufacturers provide a delivery tip that can be attached to the mixing tip to deliver the light body material directly to the preparation from the cartridge. This method can be awkward in the posterior part of the mouth because the end of the long mixing tip is far away from the operator's hand, making fine control of the tip difficult. In this situation the tip frequently bounces out of contact with the preparation during injection of light body material around the tooth, creating air voids in the critical parts of the impression. For retention grooves, the syringe tip should be placed at the bottom of the groove and the groove filled from the bottom to the top.

9 Place the impression tray over the teeth and instruct the patient to close into the rehearsed bite. Check the reference teeth to ensure that the patient has closed into the proper position. Instruct the patient not to shift the bite or open until instructed to do so.

NOTE: A missed bite relation will result in a crown that is grossly high (Figure 11-25).

10 When the two viscosities of impression material have set, remove the impression. Rinse and dry the impression to remove saliva, blood, and debris. Inspect it for completeness of the preparation detail. There should be a slight excess of impression material extending beyond the margins and no folds or voids (Figure 11-26). Minor air bubbles in noncritical areas such as the occlusal surface might be acceptable. Check with the dentist.

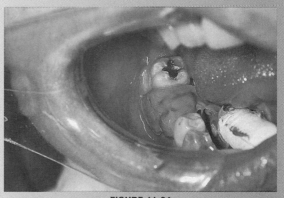

FIGURE 11-24

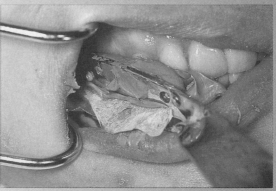

FIGURE 11-25

Continued on following page

PROCEDURE 11-2 (Continued)

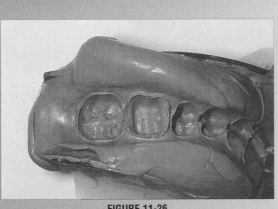

FIGURE 11-26

NOTE: Folds on axial walls are often the result of material that did not join together at the start and end of the circling process around the tooth, because the material had started to set or because the circle was not completed with new material flowing into first-placed material. Air entrapment resulting in small or large voids is often the result of loss of contact of the syringe tip with the tooth during syringing of the material. If a two-cord retraction technique was used and the cord left in place during the impression comes out attached to the impression, do not attempt to remove it. The impression could tear. Cut off any loose ends of cord hanging from the impression with scissors and leave cord that is embedded in the impression material.

11 Spray the impression with a suitable disinfectant, seal it in a zippered plastic bag that has been labeled with the patient's name, and transport it to the laboratory (see Procedure 11-1, Figures 11-19 and 11-20).

PROCEDURE 11-3 (see p. 341 for competency sheet)

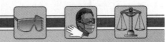

Bite Registration with Elastomeric Material

EQUIPMENT/SUPPLIES

- Basic setup
- Plastic bite tray

- Elastomeric bite registration material in dual cartridge
- Automatic mixing extruder (gun-type) and mixing tips (Figure 11-27)

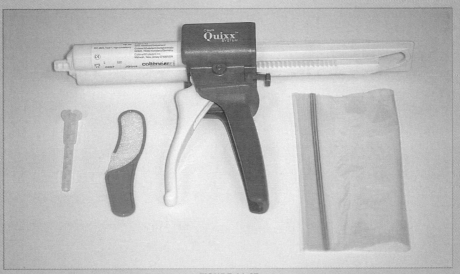

FIGURE 11-27

Continued on following page

PROCEDURE 11-3 (Continued)

PROCEDURE STEPS

1 Assemble the cartridge in the gun and extrude a small amount of bite registration material onto a paper towel to ensure that the orifices are not clogged.

NOTE: Clogged or partially clogged orifices will result in an improper mix of the material with alteration of setting time and physical properties.

2 Place the mixing tip on the cartridge.

3 Inform the patient of the procedure and have the patient practice closing into centric occlusion (the patient's "normal" bite) with the tray in place.

NOTE: Choose opposing teeth that are easily seen, such as the canines, and note their position when they occlude. This relationship will be checked when the bite registration is taken.

4 Dry the teeth to be included in the bite registration.

5 Extrude mixed material onto each side of the bite registration tray until the gauze is evenly covered with material about 2 mm thick (Figure 11-28).

6 Center the tray over the mandibular teeth to be included and have the patient close into the practiced bite (Figure 11-29 and 11-30).

NOTE: Now is the time to check the relationship of the opposing teeth (i.e., canines) to see if they are properly occluded.

7 Instruct the patient to hold the teeth together until the material is set (in 3 minutes or less).

NOTE: If the patient moves the teeth during the setting stage, a distortion will likely occur and will often be seen as imprints wider than the teeth.

8 Remove the bite tray when the material is set. Inspect it to see that all of the teeth needed for the registration are included and that there are no major voids (Figure 11-31).

NOTE: When set, the material should not indent and should feel firm.

9 Check for correct occlusion. Hold the bite registration material to the operatory light and see that light shines through in areas of contacting teeth. The gauze with a thin layer of material should be present in these areas.

NOTE: If the material is thick in areas where there should be contact of opposing teeth, the patient may not have been closed properly. Inspect the patient's occlusion and compare it with the bite registration. If there is an error, repeat the procedure.

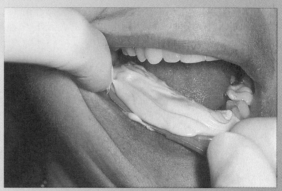

FIGURE 11-29

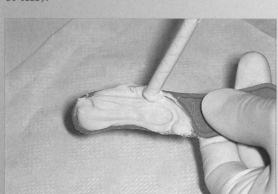

FIGURE 11-28

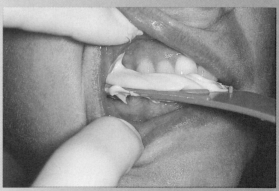

FIGURE 11-30

Continued on following page

PROCEDURE 11-3 (Continued)

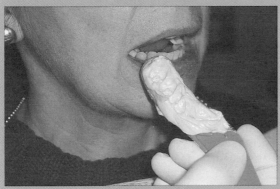

FIGURE 11-31

10 Rinse the material under running water to remove saliva and debris.

11 Spray the bite registration material with a suitable disinfectant while contained within a plastic bag. Seal it in a zippered plastic bag labeled with the patient's name and transport it to the laboratory.

PROCEDURE 11-4 (see p. 342 for competency sheet)

Disinfection of Impression Material or Bite Registration

EQUIPMENT/SUPPLIES

- Impressions/bite registration
- Various disinfecting solutions in appropriate containers
- Zippered plastic bags

PROCEDURE STEPS

1 Rinse impression under running tap water and shake excess off.

NOTE: Rinsing removes much of the saliva, blood, and other biologic debris that can interfere with disinfection.

2 Immerse or spray the impression with an acceptable disinfectant prepared according to the manufacturer's instructions (see Procedure 11-1, Figure 11-19). If spraying, hold impression within a plastic bag to contain the spray.

NOTE: Polyethers can be sensitive to immersion. ZOE should not be disinfected with chlorine-containing solutions because it breaks down the material.

3 Leave solution on sprayed impression or leave immersed impression in solution for the recommended time period.

NOTE: Polyethers should not be immersed for more than 10 minutes because they imbibe water and swell. Spraying is preferred.

4 Rinse with water and gently shake off the excess to remove any residual chemicals.

NOTE: Residual chemicals can adversely affect the surface of the cast when the impression is poured.

5 Package properly for transport (see Procedure 11-1, Figure 11-20). Usually a zippered plastic bag is satisfactory. Label with patient's name.

NOTE: Alginate and agar hydrocolloid should be wrapped in a damp paper towel to keep them from losing moisture and distorting. It is not necessary to wrap the elastomers. They should be dried after the disinfectant is rinsed off.

12 GYPSUM PRODUCTS

CHAPTER OUTLINE

OBJECTIVES

On completion of this chapter the student will be able to:

1. Differentiate between negative and positive reproduction.
2. Differentiate among diagnostic cast, working cast, and dies.
3. Describe the chemical and physical nature of gypsum products.
4. Explain the manufacturing process for gypsum products and how this affects their physical characteristics.
5. Compare the following properties and behaviors of gypsum products: strength, dimensional accuracy, solubility, and reproduction of detail.
6. List the American Dental Association–recognized gypsum products and their most appropriate uses.
7. Explain initial and final set of gypsum and the factors that affect the setting time, setting expansion, and strength.
8. Explain the procedure for mixing and handling gypsum products to create diagnostic casts.
9. Prepare model plaster or stone for pouring.
10. Pour the anatomic portion of maxillary and mandibular diagnostic casts.
11. Pour the base portion of maxillary and mandibular diagnostic casts.
12. Trim maxillary and mandibular diagnostic casts.

KEY TERMS ▪▪▪▪▪

Casts—Hard replicas of hard and soft tissue of the patient's oral cavity made from gypsum products. Also referred to as *models*.

Dies—Replicas of the prepared teeth that are generally removable from the working cast.

Model plaster—The weakest, most porous form of gypsum product used in dentistry.

Dental stone—A stronger, less porous form of gypsum product used in dentistry.

Die stone—The densest form of gypsum product used in dentistry.

Diagnostic casts—Casts generally made from dental plaster or stone and used for patient education, treatment planning, and tracking the progress of treatment, as with orthodontic models.

Working casts—Casts generally made from one of the dental stones that are strong enough to resist the stresses of fabricating an indirect restoration or prosthesis.

Pouring—Pouring the cast refers to the process of vibrating the flowable gypsum product into the impression. This process must produce a cast that is the exact replica of the impression.

Trimming—The process of removing excess hardened gypsum from the cast for ease in working with the cast and appearance in presentation.

Gypsum is a mineral widely found in nature that has been used for making dental casts since 1756. Dental casts and dies are used as replicas of the hard and soft tissues of the patient's oral cavity. First an impression, the negative reproduction of the patient's mouth, is taken using a soft, elastic material. This impression is filled with a flowable gypsum material, which, once hardened, will be the positive reproduction of the hard and soft tissues (Figure 12-1). These hard replicas are used to plan and track the progress of treatment. They are also used in laboratory procedures where they serve as the replicas on which dental procedures unsafe or too difficult to fabricate directly in the mouth are performed. The dental assistant and dental hygienist are frequently called on to produce these replicas. In some states the assistant or hygienist may fabricate intraoral prostheses on these replicas. Both the assistant and hygienist may also find the resultant model useful in presenting information for patient education. The production of gypsum casts requires meticulous attention to detail, a well thought out process in their production, and knowledge of the advantages and limitations of each gypsum material for appropriate selection. Inaccurate, incomplete, or weak casts are of little use and are likely to produce costly mistakes in patient treatment procedures.

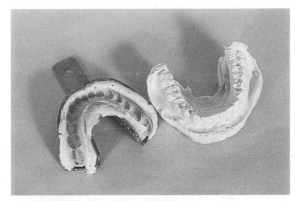

FIGURE 12-1 ▪ Impressions (negative reproductions) are poured in gypsum to form casts (positive reproductions).

Properties and Behaviors of Gypsum Products

CHEMICAL PROPERTIES

Chemically the mineral gypsum is a dihydrate of calcium sulfate ($CaSO_4$—$2H_2O$) and is mined in a solid mass. To form it into a powder, the manufacturer heats this dihydrate, which causes it to lose water. It is then ground to produce a powdered hemihydrate, $CaSO_4—1/2H_2O$. When the hemihydrate is again mixed with water, a product with a viscosity capable of flowing is produced. Once this chemical reaction is complete, the hemihydrate is converted back to a dihydrate and is again a solid mass. The by-product of the chemical reaction is heat, so it is called an *exothermic* reaction. The amount of water required to mix the calcium sulfate hemihydrate is greater than the amount required for the chemical reaction. This excess water produces a mix that can flow into the detail of the impression. The excess water evaporates on setting and a mass of interlocking gypsum crystals is produced. Between the gypsum crystals are small voids of air that were once occupied by the water that has evaporated.

The production of the various forms of gypsum is basically the same. Ground gypsum, calcium sulfate dihydrate, is heated during the manufacturing process until it loses water and becomes calcium sulfate hemihydrate. If the heating process occurs in open vats at a temperature of approximately 115°C, the resulting hemihydrate is porous and irregular in shape. This form is commonly called **model plaster** or *b* hemihydrate. If the heating process is done under pressure and a higher temperature, a more uniformly shaped and less porous form of hemihydrate, *a* hemihydrate, or **dental stone**, is produced. A further increase in pressure and further refining of the powder by grinding results in an even denser stone known as high-strength or die stone (Figure 12-2). This additional refining makes an even more regular particle with better packing ability, thus reducing the amount of water required for mixing and therefore increasing the final density of the

product. When stone is mixed with silica it forms dental investment, a material able to withstand the high heat and stress produced when molten metal is forced into molds to form indirect restorations.

PHYSICAL PROPERTIES

Physically, gypsum products are manufactured as plaster, stone, high-strength stone, and gypsum-bonded investment. The main difference in the physical forms is dependent on the variations of size, shape, and porosity of the powders produced by different manufacturing processes. The larger, more irregular, and porous the particles of powder are, the weaker and less resistant to abrasion the final product becomes. Its properties and behavior determine the specific use of the gypsum product. Properties of strength, abrasion resistance, and solubility and behaviors of setting time and expansion have varying importance depending on the application. Diagnostic casts, for example, are placed under little stress and are usually produced from less expensive materials such as plaster or stone that have lower properties of strength and abrasion resistance. Working casts and dies require materials resistant to greater stresses and thus require higher properties of strength and abrasion resistance and precise accuracy; therefore setting expansion must be carefully controlled.

Strength and Hardness The morphology of the gypsum particles determines the properties and behavior of the gypsum product. Two factors contribute to the strength and abrasion resistance of the final product: shape of the particles and porosity. The strength of gypsum products is related to the amount of water used in producing the study or working cast. Factors that affect the strength of gypsum products also affect their hardness. Increased porosity of the particles makes it necessary to use more water to convert the hemihydrate particles back to dihydrate particles. Because gypsum products require varying amounts of water to wet and incorporate the powder into a workable mixture, it follows that the more water that is used the weaker the cast will be. A product with less water has a higher density of crystals and is therefore a denser and stronger product. The larger, more irregular shape of the particles also prevents them from fitting together densely. For instance, plaster particles are both porous and irregular, requiring more

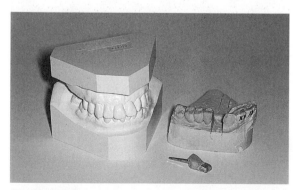

FIGURE 12-2 ■ Diagnostic casts from gypsum, working cast with stone base and high-strength stone anatomic portion, and die from high-strength stone with metal plating.

water to mix. The resulting product has more air space because of less densely packed particles, making plaster considerably weaker than the less porous and more densely packed stone products.

Dimensional Accuracy   Setting expansion occurs with all gypsum products. Plaster has the highest amount of expansion at 0.30% and high-strength stones the lowest at 0.10%. Setting expansion is a result of the growth of crystals as they join. The control of setting expansion is critical for accurate models and dies. It is important that expansion be held to a minimum, particularly when the material is being used to fabricate restorations. If expansion were excessive, the die fabricated from the gypsum material would eventually produce a restoration that was oversized. Although some expansion is acceptable for models fabricated from plaster, expansion of die materials would be a source of costly errors. The strict proportioning of water and powder and the chemical additives placed by the manufacturer are required for dies needing this accuracy. Setting expansion occurs only during the hardening of the gypsum product. No changes occur under normal conditions of use and storage once the product has reached its final set.

Reproduction of Detail   The greater the porosity of the final gypsum product, the less surface detail is produced. Even products that have the least amount of porosity have surface irregularities on a microscopic level. Compatibility of impression material and die material can influence the quality of surface reproduction. Silicone and polyether impression materials generally form the best surface detail with gypsum products. Dies can also be electroplated with metal to produce better surface detail. It is always important to follow the manufacturer's directions in selecting gypsum products that are compatible with impression materials.

Solubility   Set gypsum products are not highly soluble in water. Solubility is directly related to the porosity of the material; therefore plaster is much more soluble than stone. Exposing models to water for prolonged periods should be avoided (Table 12-1).

Classification of Gypsum Products

The desired physical properties and behavior necessary for a particular use determine the criteria for selection of a gypsum product. If strength is desired, the choice of a stone or high-strength stone material is important. If a diagnostic cast is being fabricated, plaster or stone is adequate. American Dental Association (ADA) specification number 25 identifies the following five gypsum products.

IMPRESSION PLASTER (TYPE I)

Impression plaster is rarely used in today's dentistry, having been replaced with the less rigid, elastic impression materials. If selected, it would be used as a final impression wash for edentulous arches.

MODEL PLASTER (TYPE II)

Model plaster is frequently used for diagnostic casts and articulation of stone casts. It has a water-to-powder (W/P) ratio of approximately 0.45 (ml/g), which produces a durable but relatively weak cast when compared with the stone categories. Model

TABLE 12-1
Properties of Gypsum Products

Type	W/P Ratio (ml/g)	Porosity	Compressive Strength	Abrasion Resistance	Setting Expansion
Model plaster	0.45	High	8.8 MPa*	Low	High
Dental stone	0.30	Moderate	20.6 MPa	Moderate	Moderate
High-strength stone	0.23	Low	34.3 MPa	High	Low
High-strength/ high-expansion stone	0.20	Low	48.0 MPa	High	High

*MPa is the abbreviation for megapascal; 1 MPa equals approximately 145 lb/in^2.

> ## USES OF DIAGNOSTIC CASTS
> - Provide a three-dimensional record of the patient's hard and soft tissues
> - Facilitate study of the occlusal relationship of the dental arches
> - Facilitate study of tooth size, position, and shape and arch relations
> - Facilitate study of hard and soft tissues from the lingual view while teeth are in occlusion
> - Provide a record of present conditions for comparison as treatment progresses
> - Provide a visual aid for patient education
> - Provide a legal record of the patient's arches for insurance, legal suits, and forensics

plaster is available in fast and regular sets. This product is traditionally produced in a white color to distinguish it from the dental stones. Because of its simple manufacturing processes, plaster is the least costly of all the gypsum products.

DENTAL STONE (TYPE III)

Dental stone is ideal for making full or partial denture models, orthodontic models, and casts requiring higher strength and abrasive resistance. Because of the particle characteristics, stone requires less water (W/P ratio = 0.30); it therefore packs together tighter and is denser and approximately 2.5 times stronger than plaster. Stone is traditionally colored yellow or white.

DENTAL STONE, HIGH STRENGTH (TYPE IV)

Type IV materials are often referred to as **die stones** because they are especially suited for fabricating wax patterns of cast restorations. A hard, abrasive-resistant surface is necessary to resist the abrasion of sharp instruments used to carve on these stone dies. The product, often colored pink or green, has a W/P ratio of 0.23 and is almost 2 times stronger than type III stones.

HIGH-STRENGTH, HIGH-EXPANSION DENTAL STONE (TYPE V)

This recent addition to the list of ADA gypsum products has been developed in response to the need for even higher-strength and high-expansion dental

stones. Higher expansion may seem to be an undesirable property, but it is needed to compensate for the greater casting shrinkage of newer base metals used for dental castings. The increased strength is obtained from a W/P ratio of 0.20. This material, colored blue or green, is the most costly of all the gypsum products.

Manipulation

SELECTION

As previously mentioned, the selection of a gypsum product should be based on the desired properties of the material. If a **diagnostic cast** were being fabricated, dental plaster would be an appropriate choice because of the lowered needs of physical properties and its cost and ease of manipulation. A **working cast** would require good strength and accuracy and may be formed from dental stone. The dimensional accuracy and strength required for a die would make high-strength stone the best choice. In some instances a combination of one or more gypsum products is appropriate to curtail cost. When working models for cast restorations are being made, a die of high-strength stone is often poured with a base and adjacent teeth of type III stone.

PROPORTIONING (WATER/POWDER RATIO)

The properties of gypsum products are directly related to their W/P ratio. It is important that the mixed material has sufficient flow to reproduce accurate surface detail while remembering that an increase in the recommended W/P ratio will result in a weaker, less accurate model. An increase in water will result in a thin mix that takes longer to set and, because more water is used, is considerably weaker. If too little water is used, the mixture may be difficult to manipulate because it does not produce a flowable mix. Strict adherence to the manufacturer's suggested W/P ratio is recommended.

Water should be measured with a graduated cylinder and powder weighed on a scale. The use of scoops to measure powder is not recommended because of the packing of the powder as it sits in a container. Although it is tempting to rely on experience and eliminate measuring devices, the result may be wasted material and a lack of reliability of the final product. The strength of a stone cast with a high W/P ratio may be no greater than one poured in model plaster. Manufacturers produce preweighed envelopes of powder for critical measurements. This method increases accuracy and saves time but also increases the cost of the material.

MIXING

Most commonly, plaster and stone are mixed in a flexible rubber bowl with a broad metal spatula. Mechanical devices are used when the control of spatulation is critical. The measured amount of water is placed into the mixing bowl and the powder slowly sifted into the water. By sifting powder into water, an even wetting of the powder particles takes place and clumps are avoided. The materials are spatulated by first incorporating the powder and water slightly and then vigorously wiping the mix against the sides of the bowl to force out air and ensure wetting of all the powder particles. Spatulation should continue for 1 minute at 2 revolutions per second until a smooth, homogeneous mix with a glossy surface is produced. An increase in the time and rate of spatulation has a definite effect on setting time and expansion. An increase in the spatulation time and rate will shorten the setting time and increase the rate of setting expansion. Many dental laboratories use mechanical spatulation with a vacuum device to reduce air bubbles and increase consistency and accuracy of mixing. Hand spatulation is the most common means of mixing gypsum materials in private dental offices (see Procedure 12-1).

INITIAL SETTING TIME—WORKING TIME

After mixing for 1 minute, the working time begins. In this time the semifluid mixture is poured into the impression with the help of a mechanical vibrator. As the viscosity of the mixture increases, the material will no longer flow and loses its glossy appearance. This *loss of gloss* indicates that the gypsum has reached its initial set. For regular-set products, the initial set occurs within 8 to 10 minutes from the beginning of the mix. With a mixing time of 1 minute, this gives an ample working time of 6 to 10 minutes to pour the impression.

FINAL SETTING TIME

The final set is reached when the material can safely be handled, but it has minimal hardness and resistance to abrasion. At this time the chemical reaction

is complete and the model is cool to the touch, having completed the exothermic reaction. Most manufacturers recommend 1 hour before the material may be safely separated from the impression.

CLINICAL TIP Before separating the impression from the cast, ensure that no part of the impression tray is connected to the gypsum. Do not pry or rock in one direction too far or the cast will likely break.

Gypsum products continue to harden and are two to three times harder after 24 hours. Failure to separate the model from the impression after 1 hour may have a detrimental effect on the surface characteristics of the model. Always refer to the manufacturer's directions for the impression material to determine contraindications for leaving a gypsum product in contact with the impression material for excessive amounts of time.

CLINICAL TIP If an alginate impression has dried out before the cast has been separated, soak the impression and cast in water for 15 minutes. The alginate will soften, allowing removal of the cast without breaking anatomic structures.

CONTROL OF SETTING TIMES

It is important to keep in mind that it is impossible to accelerate the final set of a mixture without also accelerating the initial set, thereby reducing the working time. If it is necessary to alter the setting time, there are several methods by which this can be accomplished.

Altering the W/P Ratio As previously mentioned, an increase in the amount of water will retard the setting times. However, because an increase of even 1 part of water can reduce the strength by as much as 50%, this is not a recommended control. Decreasing the amount of water will accelerate the setting time, but it also makes the mixture more difficult to manipulate, causing air bubbles and an inaccurate model. Decreasing the amount of water in the W/P ratio is only recommended when the mixture is not being poured in an impression, such as when it is being used as a base to secure models on an articulator.

Spatulation A longer and more rapid spatulation of gypsum results in an accelerated setting time. This

TABLE 12-2
Manipulation Factors

Factor	Working Time	Viscosity	Strength
Increase W/P ratio	Increase	Decrease	Decrease
Decrease W/P ratio	Decrease	Increase	Increase
Increase rate of spatulation	Decrease	Increase	No effect
Increase temperature of H_2O	Decrease	Increase	No effect
Decrease temperature of H_2O	Increase	Decrease	No effect

rapid spatulation will also result in increased setting expansion.

Temperature Within limits, an increase in the temperature of the mixing water will accelerate the setting times. Gypsum is ideally mixed with room-temperature water. Increasing the temperature of the water, not to exceed 100° F, will accelerate the set. Any increase in temperature above 100° F will have a retarding effect, and at 212° F no reaction takes place and the gypsum will not set.

Accelerators and Retarders The most practical way of controlling setting time is by the manufacturer's addition of chemical accelerators or retarders. Manufacturers add accelerators and retarders to change the solubility of the hemihydrate in water. By increasing the solubility of the hemihydrate the added accelerator decreases the setting time, and by decreasing the solubility the added retarder increases the setting time. When accelerators are placed in the gypsum the manufacturer can cut the initial and final set by 50%. These materials are labeled fast set.

The clinician may also add accelerators. Potassium sulfate (K_2SO_4) and set gypsum ($CaSO_4$) particles are examples The water and crystals from ground set gypsum commonly retrieved from the runoff water of model trimmers is called *slurry water.* The dihydrate crystals in the slurry water accelerate the chemical reaction by acting as established sites for crystallization.

Blood, saliva, and alginate are organic substances that can retard the set of gypsum. If these organic components are left in an impression, the surface detail of the resulting model may be easily abraded. All impressions must be rinsed free of any organic matter before the impression is poured. Alginate remains in contact with the gypsum product, so it must be noted that even though the outside surface

of a cast poured from an alginate impression may seem set, the area adjacent to the teeth needs more time to fully harden.

Remember that usually when a change is made in the final setting time a sacrifice is made in the working time, strength, or setting expansion of the final product (Table 12-2).

POURING THE CASTS

Diagnostic and working casts have two parts: the *anatomic portion,* which replicates the hard and soft structures, and the *art portion* or *base,* which aids in handling and articulating the casts. The anatomic portion is poured by vibrating small increments of flowable gypsum into the duplicated oral imprints. The mixture is allowed to flow from tooth to tooth pushing out air as it moves, thus eliminating air voids. The art or base portion can be poured using three methods (Figure 12-3) (see Procedures 12-2 and 12-3).

Double-Pour Method The anatomic portion of one or both arches is poured and left in the upright position. After approximately 10 minutes, a second mix is produced for the art portion(s). This mixture is placed on a glass tile or in a base former. The filled impression is inverted onto the base and the periphery of the two portions is joined. If the cast is being used as a working cast, frequently the anatomic portion is poured in a dental stone and the base portion poured in plaster. This gives the anatomic portion density while allowing for easier trimming of the base portion.

Single-Step Method One mix of gypsum is produced to pour the anatomic and art portions of the cast. After **pouring** the impression, the remaining material is used for the base. This material is placed

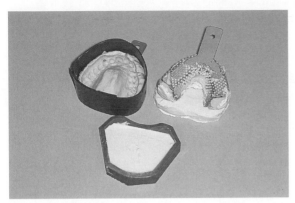

FIGURE 12-3 ■ Pouring the art portion of the cast by boxing, model former, and inversion on patty base.

EVALUATION OF DIAGNOSTIC CASTS

Criteria:

- Anatomic portion is free of all air voids.
- Art portion is free of all air voids greater than 2 mm.
- The union between art and anatomic portions forms a continuous surface.
- The occlusal plane, at the premolar area, is parallel to the bottom of the base.
- The base is of adequate thickness but not so thick as to require excessive trimming.
- There is sufficient material extending past the mucobuccal fold and posterior of casts to replicate all anatomic structures.
- Excess material in tongue area has been smoothed.

---

on a glass tile or in a base former, the impression is inverted onto it, and the periphery of the two portions are joined. This method requires more skill and timing. If the mixture is too wet when you finish pouring the impression, the base may flow excessively when the impression is inverted and the material in the inverted impression may slump away from the impression, causing distortion of the cast or air voids. If the mixture has reached its initial set when inverting, the union between art and anatomic portions will be incomplete.

Boxing Method A strip of wax is used to surround the impression, forming a wall into which the

gypsum is poured. The wax should not distort the impression. It should extend at least 0.5 inch higher than the highest point of the impression and create a base that is parallel to the occlusal plane.

STORAGE

Gypsum products can absorb water from the environment. Humidity and close proximity to water sources will adversely affect the powder. Initially this exposure will accelerate the setting reaction by producing established sites of crystallization. After prolonged exposure, the setting reaction is retarded because of decreased solubility of the crystals by the formation of a dihydrate layer on the hemihydrate particles.

Gypsum should be stored in airtight, moisture-proof containers. To avoid prolonged exposure to moisture, open plaster bins are only recommended if there is rapid turnover of the products.

CLEANUP

Gypsum mixing and handling equipment must be kept meticulously clean. As previously mentioned, set gypsum will accelerate the setting times of a mixture. Bowls, spatulas, mechanical vibrators, and mixing devices should be cleaned of all traces of gypsum as soon as possible after manipulation.

> ▶ **CAUTION**
> *Remember that all excess material should be placed in the trash and not rinsed down drains where it will likely clog pipes. Equipment should then be thoroughly rinsed under running water. Sinks in gypsum-handling areas should be fitted with plaster traps.*

INFECTION CONTROL ISSUES

The need for infection control measures to extend into the dental laboratory has been clearly documented. Routine disinfection of impressions should be done in the dental office. (A discussion of disinfecting agents and procedures for disinfecting impressions is presented in Chapter 11.) If this has not been done, the impression and all equipment, such as plaster spatulas and vibrators, must be handled with proper personal protective equipment or barriers. Casts should be completely set and stored for at least 24 hours before disinfecting to prevent attack by the chemicals on the surface of the cast. Casts should be sprayed rather than immersed in disinfecting solutions, because some studies have shown damage to the surface in only a few minutes in water-based solutions. Solutions such as 1:10 sodium hypochlorite, iodophors, or chlorine dioxide have been shown to have minimal effect on cast surfaces when used in this manner. Gypsum products that contain disinfecting agents placed by the manufacturer are awaiting Food and Drug Administration (FDA) approval.

TRIMMING

Trimming of models with a model trimmer is done to produce an attractive, symmetric model with easy access to all anatomic portions of the model and a base of sufficient bulk for stability. Bases made from dental stones should be soaked in water for 5 to 10 minutes before trimming to saturate the stone, making it easier to trim. Anatomic portions should never be soaked. Saturation of the teeth may lead to a change in surface texture and, in the case of plaster, make the teeth more susceptible to chipping.

The cast should be trimmed so that proportionately the base makes up one third and the anatomic portion two thirds of the total depth. The occlusal plane should be parallel with the base. The periphery of the largest arch is trimmed first, and then the smaller arch is articulated with a wax bite and trimmed to match (see Chapter 15 for fabrication of a wax bite registration). The outer borders should be cut to the depth of the vestibule and include all muscle attachments, retromolar pads, and tuberosities. If there are facially inclined or rotated teeth, the outside borders should be extended symmetrically to include these anatomic structures. The anterior portion of the maxillary arch is cut to a point at the midline, and the anterior portion of the mandibular arch is rounded from cuspid to cuspid (Figures 12-4 and 12-5) (see Procedure 12-4).

EVALUATION OF TRIMMED DIAGNOSTIC CASTS

Criteria:

- Anatomic portion makes up two thirds of the total depth and base portion one third of total depth.
- Bases of the maxillary and mandibular casts should be parallel with the occlusal planes and each other.
- Posterior borders of both casts are at right angles to the base and will stand together when articulated on end.
- Posterior portions include retromolar pads and tuberosities.
- Side borders are perpendicular to the base, symmetric, and trimmed to the depth of the vestibule.
- Anterior borders are perpendicular to the base and are trimmed to the depth of the vestibule.
- Anterior borders of the maxillary cast form a point at the midline and are rounded from cuspid to cuspid for the mandibular cast.
- Mandibular casts have a smoothed tongue space.
- Maxillary and mandibular casts are labeled with the patient's name and date.

▶ **CAUTION**

Exercise care when using the model trimmer. Always wear protective eyewear, establish a flat surface from which to trim, and pay attention to your hand positions. Use even, steady pressure with both hands while trimming. To maintain the abrasive surface of the trimming wheel, maintain an adequate flow of water on the trimming wheel when in use so that it does not clog with gypsum. Clean the wheel and work surface of all gypsum products immediately after finishing.

METAL-PLATED AND EPOXY DIES AND RESIN-REINFORCED DIE STONE

Type IV and V gypsum products are commonly used die materials. These materials are very hard, but they are susceptible to abrasion during carving of wax patterns. Silver or copper plating can create metal-plated dies that are highly resistant to abrasion. The electroplating process forms a shell of metal on the outside of the die.

Epoxy dies use a resin and hardener to produce a die with more abrasion resistance. In addition, some

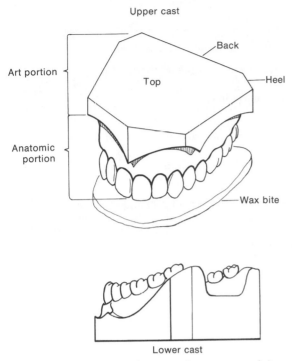

FIGURE 12-4 ■ Drawing of parts and proportion of diagnostic casts. (Reproduced with permission from Bird D, Robinson D, *Torres and Ehrlich modern dental assisting,* ed 6, Philadelphia, 1999, WB Saunders, p 416.)

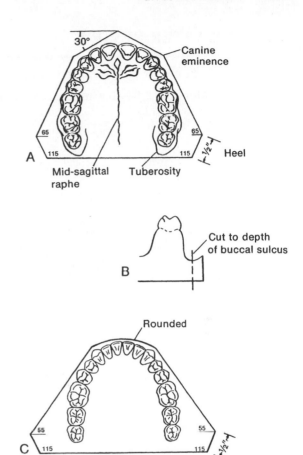

FIGURE 12-5 ■ Drawing of landmarks, angles, and cuts of art portion of diagnostic casts. **A,** Maxillary cast. **B,** Cut to depth of vestibule. **C,** Mandibular cast. (Reproduced with permission from Torres HO, Ehrlich A: *Modern dental assisting,* ed 6, Philadelphia, 1999, WB Saunders, p 212.)

gypsum die stones have resin particles added to make them more abrasion resistant.

INVESTMENT MATERIALS

Investment materials are used to form metal castings through the lost wax technique (see Chapter 15). These materials, which combine gypsum and silica, are able to produce models sufficiently strong to allow molten metal to be poured into them. Investment materials have increased expansion on setting; this expansion is necessary to compensate for the shrinkage of metal castings.

SUMMARY

Gypsum products are used to produce diagnostic and working models of the patient's hard and soft tissues. The properties of strength and hardness, setting expansion, and solubility are directly related to the amounts of water used in their construction. The density of the final product is related to these water amounts and the size and shape of the particle that is manufactured. Manipulation factors such as W/P ratio, rate of spatulation, and mixing water temperature have a great effect as well. The clinician must have a clear understanding of how these variables can be appropriately manipulated. Pouring of models requires meticulous attention to detail to produce a replica that accurately reflects the hard and soft tissues of the patient's oral cavity.

CHAPTER REVIEW

Select the one correct response for each of the following multiple-choice questions:

1. All of the following are considered positive reproductions of the dental structures EXCEPT:
   a. An impression
   b. A diagnostic cast
   c. A working cast
   d. A die

2. The manufacturing process for gypsum products includes all of the following EXCEPT:
   a. The use of heat
   b. The use of pressure
   c. The addition of water
   d. Grinding of particles

3. To decrease the working time of a gypsum product without a change to any physical properties, it is best to
   a. Decrease the water-to-powder ratio
   b. Increase the rate of spatulation
   c. Increase the water temperature
   d. Decrease the water temperature

4. All of the following are differences between plaster and stone EXCEPT:
   a. Different setting time
   b. Different color
   c. Different mixing technique
   d. Different particle size

5. The most appropriate type of gypsum product to use for orthodontic casts is
   a. Type I
   b. Type II
   c. Type III
   d. Type IV

6. Initial setting can be detected clinically by
   a. Loss of gloss
   b. The end of the exothermic reaction
   c. A change in color
   d. Testing to see if the material is hard enough to separate from the impression

7. The area of the diagnostic cast that records the hard and soft tissues is called the
   a. Art portion
   b. Base
   c. Anatomical portion
   d. Impression

8. All of the following statements are true of gypsum products EXCEPT
   a. Excess water makes it easier to mix and manipulate gypsum products.
   b. Excess water is lost in evaporation upon final set.
   c. Excess water is water in excess of what is necessary to complete the chemical reaction.
   d. Excess water will improve the strength of gypsum poured models.

9. It is important to consider all of the following statements when pouring an impression EXCEPT
   a. Alginate impressions should only remain unseparated from the model for 1 hour.
   b. When using the single-step method, the material poured in the impression must reach the initial set before pouring the base.

c. Gypsum material should not be allowed to extend over the edge of the impression tray.

d. Excess gypsum should be wiped from equipment and placed into the trash.

10. **Diagnostic casts are used for all of the following EXCEPT:**
    a. Patient education
    b. Legal documents
    c. Tracking treatment progress
    d. Fabricating orthodontic appliances

CASE-BASED DISCUSSION TOPICS

◉ For each of the following situations, which gypsum material would be the best choice? *(1) The assistant has taken an impression for an orthodontic case study. (2) The dentist has taken an impression for a space maintainer. (3) The hygienist has taken an impression for a custom bleaching tray. (4) The expanded-function assistant has taken an impression for a full gold crown.*

◉ How would each of the following situations be best handled? *(1) You need to make a custom tray for an appointment in progress and have just taken the alginate impression. How would you accelerate the setting time of the gypsum product you select? (2) You have fast-set plaster in your office and wish to mix enough material to pour two arches. How would you increase the working time? (3) Several air voids are present on the surfaces of the teeth. What factors may have caused this? (4) When working on a cast, the teeth chip and crumble easily. What factors may have caused this?*

REFERENCES

Anusavice K: *Phillips' science of dental materials*, ed 10, Philadelphia, 1996, WB Saunders.

Bird D, Robinson D: *Torres and Ehrlich modern dental assisting*, ed 6, Philadelphia, 1999, WB Saunders.

Brukl CE et al: Influence of gauging water composition on dental stone expansion and setting time, *J Prosthet Dent* 51:218, 1984.

Council on Dental Materials, Instruments and Equipment: American Dental Association specification no. 25, *J Am Dent Assoc* 102:351, 1981.

Council on Scientific Affairs and Council on Dental Practice: American Dental Association, infection control recommendations for the dental office and dental laboratory, *J Am Dent Assoc* 127:672, 1996.

Craig RG: *Restorative dental materials*, ed 10, St Louis, 1996, Mosby.

King BB, Norling BK, Seals R: Gypsum compatibility of antimicrobial alginates after spray disinfection, *Journal of Prosthodontics* 3:219, 1994.

von Fraunhofer JA, Spiers RR: Accelerated setting of dental stone, *J Prosthet Dent* 49:859, 1983.

Wilkins E: *Clinical practice of the dental hygienist*, ed 8, Philadelphia, 1999, Lippincott Williams & Wilkins.

PROCEDURE 12-1   (see p. 343 for competency sheet)

Mixing Gypsum Products

EQUIPMENT/SUPPLIES (Figure 12-6)

- Gypsum product
- Scale
- Water (room temperature)
- Water-measuring device
- Flexible mixing bowl
- Broad-blade metal spatula
- Mechanical vibrator

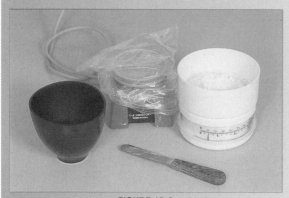

FIGURE 12-6

PROCEDURE STEPS

1 Measure recommended amount of room-temperature water into a clean, flexible rubber mixing bowl.

NOTE: Increase or decrease the water temperature to control the working time.

2 Weigh recommended amount of gypsum powder onto scale, use another bowl or weight onto a paper towel. Make sure to account for the weight of the bowl if you are using this method to transfer powder.

3 Sift the powder gradually into the water allowing the particles to become wet, about 30 seconds.

NOTE: This minimizes the amount of air trapped in the mix.

4 Vigorously mix about 60 seconds by wiping the spatula against the sides of the bowl to incorporate all the powder and remove excess air until a smooth, homogeneous mixture is obtained (Figure 12-7).

NOTE: The viscosity of the mix should be sufficient to allow the material to flow only under mechanical vibration.

5 Turn the vibrator on low and place the bowl on the work surface.

6 Press the sides of the bowl inward with the palms of your hands, at the same time pressing the bowl downward on the work surface of the vibrator to remove all air incorporated during the mixing procedure.

NOTE: This helps remove air trapped during mixing.

7 Complete preparation of the gypsum material in no more than 2 minutes.

NOTE: This includes mixing and initial vibrating and allows for sufficient working time in pouring.

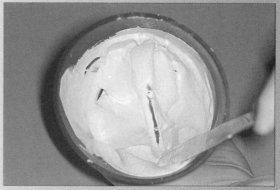

FIGURE 12-7

PROCEDURE 12-2   (see p. 344 for competency sheet)

Pouring the Anatomic Portion of Diagnostic Casts

EQUIPMENT/SUPPLIES (Figure 12-8)

- Mechanical vibrator
- Gypsum mixture
- Broad-blade metal spatula
- Disinfected impression

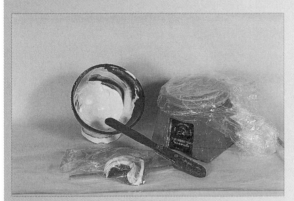

FIGURE 12-8

PROCEDURE STEPS

1 Rinse the impression of all traces of disinfecting solution and tap over the sink until no more water can be shaken out.

2 Holding the handle of the impression tray, place the tray onto the work surface of the mechanical vibrator.

NOTE: To facilitate cleanup, cover the working surface of the mechanical vibrator with a disposable cover such as a plastic bag. Hold the tray on an angle to the working table of the vibrator to aid in the flow of the material.

3 Pick up a small increment of gypsum mixture, no greater than a large pea, on the end of the spatula.

NOTE: This allows for control of the amount of material flowing into the tooth indentations.

4 Place the increment of mixture at one posterior corner of the impression (Figure 12-9).

5 Allow the mixture to flow into the tooth indentations from one side to the next of each indentation, controlling the flow of the mixture to force air out of each indentation.

NOTE: Air bubbles are formed when the mixture moves too fast over the tooth indentations, trapping air in the impression, or if the mixture will not flow sufficiently to fill the indentations. Use small enough increments to control the flow and tilt the impression as needed to aid the speed of the flow.

6 Continue adding increments of mixture, watching the material flow toward the anterior portion of the impression (Figure 12-10).

7 Tilt the impression forward and continue adding increments across the anterior portion of the impression, making sure to control the flow so that air is not trapped.

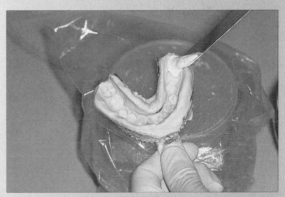

FIGURE 12-9

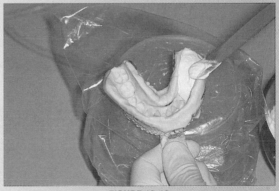

FIGURE 12-10

Continued on following page

PROCEDURE 12-2 (Continued)

8 Tilt the impression toward the opposite posterior portion and continue the addition of increments until the flow reaches the other end of the impression (Figure 12-11).

9 When all of the tooth indentations are filled with the gypsum mixture, begin adding larger increments until the impression is filled (Figure 12-12).

NOTE: Lift the impression from the vibrator to prevent the material from flowing over the impression tray.

10 Vibrate the entire tray for 2 to 3 seconds to settle all increments. Do not smooth the surface of the material.

NOTE: A roughened surface will allow for better attachment with the base.

11 Clean up; wipe all excess gypsum from the bowl and place in the trash. Rinse the bowl and spatula under running water in a sink fitted with a plaster trap. Remove the plastic bag from the mechanical vibrator and clean the vibrator with a wet paper towel.

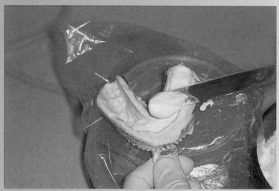

FIGURE 12-11

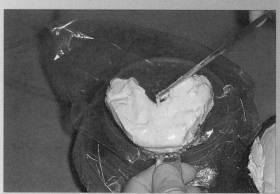

FIGURE 12-12

PROCEDURE 12-3 (see p. 345 for competency sheet)

Pouring the Base Portion of Diagnostic Casts

EQUIPMENT/SUPPLIES (Figure 12-13)
- Glass tile or base former
- Broad-blade spatula
- Gypsum mixture
- Poured impression

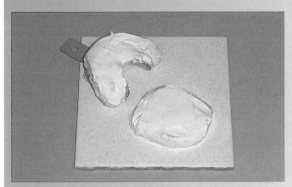

FIGURE 12-13

PROCEDURE STEPS (DOUBLE-POUR METHOD)

1 Allow the poured impression to set for at least 10 minutes.

NOTE: This prevents the gypsum material from "slumping" away from the impression when it is inverted, causing distortion in the cast.

2 Prepare a mixture of gypsum using less water for the W/P ratio.

NOTE: This will produce a thicker mix necessary to accommodate the weight of the poured impression when it is inverted.

NOTE: You may use plaster to pour the art portion of a model even if the anatomic portion is poured with a different product. By using plaster, you will save the cost of the more expensive stone products and, if model trimming is necessary, save time because plaster trims much easier than stone.

3 Place the mixture onto the glass tile or into a base former. You should have a mass at least 0.5 inch thick and slightly larger than the dimension of the filled impression and tray.

NOTE: If using a base former, make sure you choose one large enough for the impression and select the correct arch shape for your impression (pointed for maxillary and rounded for mandibular).

4 Invert the poured impression onto the base, making sure the occlusal plane remains parallel with the base.

NOTE: If using a base former you will also need to make sure you keep the midline centered.

5 Gently move the impression back and forth to bring the anatomic and art portions together.

6 Bring the base material up with a spatula to fill the heels and sides of the impression and along the tray periphery, being careful not to lock the tray in with excess material (Figures 12-14 and 12-15).

NOTE: Make sure there are no large air pockets trapped between art and base portions.

7 Smooth the tongue area of the mandibular impression level with the tray periphery.

8 Allow the gypsum to set completely before separating the model for the impression, 45 to 60 minutes.

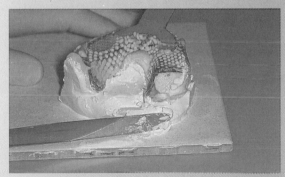

FIGURE 12-14

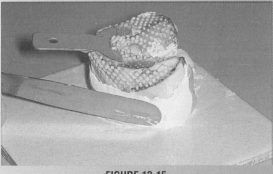

FIGURE 12-15

Trimming Diagnostic Casts

EQUIPMENT/SUPPLIES (Figure 12-16)

- Maxillary and mandibular diagnostic casts
- Wax bite registration
- Measuring devices; millimeter ruler and compass
- Pencil
- Laboratory knife
- Plaster nippers
- Model trimmer

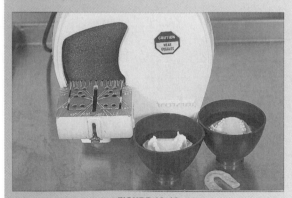

FIGURE 12-16

PROCEDURE STEPS

1 Soak art portion of casts for 5 minutes in water.

NOTE: Do not allow teeth to soak in water because it may cause chipping of plaster or surface roughness of plaster or stone.

2 Cut excess gypsum distal to retromolar pads and tuberosities with plaster nippers (Figure 12-17).

NOTE: Excess gypsum in this area may prevent models from being articulated.

3 Remove small bubbles of gypsum on occlusal surfaces with laboratory knife.

NOTE: This allows for complete articulation with wax bite.

4 Check working table of model trimmer to be sure it is secure and at a 90° angle to the trimming wheel.

5 Adjust water flow over trimming wheel to allow for sufficient water to clean wheel.

Base Cut

6 Place maxillary cast teeth-side down on laboratory bench and rock forward so that anterior teeth touch laboratory bench. Measure from teeth to base of cast; the anatomic portion of the cast should be two thirds of the total height, with the art portion making up one third of the total height. Mark models with compass to this line (Figure 12-18).

NOTE: The occlusal surfaces are parallel to the laboratory bench with anterior teeth touching the surface.

7 Trim bases to the marked line.

NOTE: You may first need to make a flat back cut to secure casts on the working table of the trimmer.

8 Repeat with the mandibular cast.

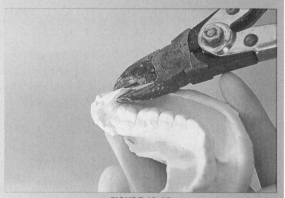

FIGURE 12-17

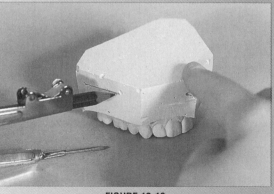

FIGURE 12-18

Continued on following page

PROCEDURE 12-4 (Continued)

Side and Back Cuts

9 Measure back by making a straight line 3 mm behind retromolar pads of mandibular cast or tuberosities of maxillary cast.

10 Trim back to this line (Figure 12-19).

NOTE: Trim the longest cast first; then articulate casts with wax bite and match opposite cast's back cut (Figure 12-20).

11 Measure sides 3 mm from buccal bone at widest portion of arch (usually molar area) and 3 mm at canine eminence. Mark cast with straight edge to connect these points.

12 Trim side cuts symmetric to these lines (Figure 12-21).

NOTE: Do not trim past the depth of the vestibule.

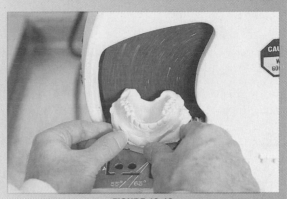

FIGURE 12-19

Anterior Cut: Maxillary Cast

13 Measure 3 mm labial to midline between central incisors. Measure from depth of vestibule or most facially inclined tooth. Mark casts with straight edge to connect this point and the point 3 mm from the canine eminence.

14 Trim anterior cuts symmetric to form a midline point.

NOTE: Maxillary cast forms a point between the central incisors.

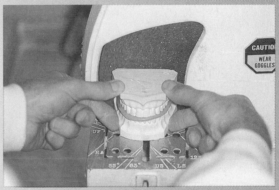

FIGURE 12-20

Anterior Cut: Mandibular Cast

15 Measure as previously instructed 3 mm from several places in anterior region of mandibular arch, and connect these points with the point of the canine eminence to form a curved line. Trim anterior cut of mandible to this curved line.

Heel Cuts

16 Trim heel cuts at a 90° angle to a line formed connecting the canine eminence point to the side/back cut of the opposite side.

NOTE: This line is approximately 0.5 inch and symmetric on each side.

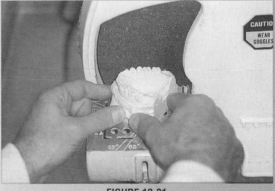

FIGURE 12-21

Continued on following page

PROCEDURE 12-4 (Continued)

OPTIONAL STEPS

Finishing/Polishing

17 Inspect models for small air voids. Small voids may be filled in with a paint brush and a fresh mix of gypsum.

NOTE: Unless requested by the dentist, do not fill in air voids in areas critical to the case.

18 Using model polish and a soft buffing cloth, polish the cast to a shine (Figure 12-22).

Labeling/Storage

19 Using an indelible ink marker, label the base or back cut of the cast with the patient's name and date.

20 Place the cast in a model box labeled with the patient's name, date of the impression, and case number.

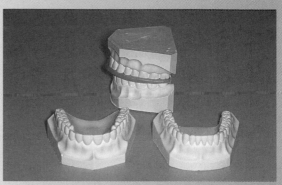

FIGURE 12-22

13 POLYMERS FOR PROSTHETIC DENTISTRY

CHAPTER OUTLINE

Review of Polymer Formation
Cross-linked polymers
Polymerization reactions

Acrylic Resins (Plastics)
Properties
Acrylic resin for denture bases
Polymerization reaction

Denture Liners
Soft lining materials
Hard lining materials
Infection control procedures
Over-the-counter liners

Plastic (Acrylic) Teeth

Characterization of Dentures

Plastics for Maxillofacial Prostheses

Denture Repair
Chemical-cured acrylic repair material
Light-cured repair material

Custom Impression Trays and Record Bases
Chemical-cured tray and record base
   material
Light-cured tray and record base
   material

Care of Acrylic Resin Dentures
Home care
In-office care
Storage of dentures

Summary

Chapter Review

Case-Based Discussion Topics

References

Procedures
Fabrication of custom acrylic
   impression tray
Fabrication of record bases with light-
   cured acrylic resin

OBJECTIVES

On completion of this chapter the student will be able to:

1. Describe the formation of long-chain polymers from monomers.
2. Explain the effect cross-linking has on the physical properties of polymers.
3. Describe the stages of addition polymerization.
4. Explain the function of a free radical.
5. List the important properties of acrylic resins.
6. Describe the procedure for heat processing a denture.
7. Explain the importance of control of heat and pressure when processing a denture.
8. Explain the differences between hard and soft lining materials.
9. List the indications for long- and short-term soft liners.
10. Describe the advantages and disadvantages of chairside and laboratory hard liners.
11. List the indications for the use of acrylic teeth versus porcelain teeth.
12. Describe the process for repairing acrylic dentures.
13. Describe the use of the ultrasonic cleaner for cleaning complete and partial dentures in the office.
14. Describe the home care regimen for complete and partial dentures that patients should follow.

15. List the precautions patients should take when cleaning their dentures.
16. Fabricate custom acrylic impression trays.
17. Fabricate record bases for complete denture procedures using light-cured material.

KEY TERMS

Prosthesis—A device used for the replacement of missing tissues. It can serve both cosmetic and functional roles.

Polymer—A long-chain, high-molecular-weight molecule produced by the linking of many low-molecular-weight monomer molecules.

Monomer—Low-molecular-weight molecules that are joined to form polymers. As used in dentistry, monomers are usually liquids.

Polymerization—The act of forming polymers.

Cross-linked polymers—The joining of adjacent long-chain polymers by bonding of short chains along their sides.

Addition polymerization—Common form of polymerization of dental materials. Monomer molecules are added one to another sequentially as the reactive group on one molecule initiates bonding with an adjacent monomer molecule and frees another reactive group to repeat the process.

Free radical—A reactive group on one end of a monomer that initiates the joining of adjacent monomer molecules to form a polymer.

Poly (methyl methacrylate)—A polymer composed of numerous methyl methacrylate monomers linked together into a long chain.

Plasticizer—Liquid added to acrylic resin to soften it and make it more pliable.

Porosity—Numerous microscopic holes or voids within a material. Often caused during polymerization of resins when monomer vaporizes and is lost.

Long-term soft liner—A soft liner that is used in patients who have problems with hard acrylic denture bases. It is expected to last for 1 to 3 years.

Short-term soft liner—A soft provisional liner used to improve tissue health. Also called a *tissue conditioner.* Typically, it lasts from a few days to a few weeks.

---

*Acrylic resins are polymers that play an important role in removable prosthetics. The resins are used in the construction of complete and partial dentures, as well as maxillofacial **prostheses** (used to replace missing oral or facial structures). They can be used to simulate the oral mucosa and the teeth. They are also used to reline these prostheses to improve their fit and to repair them when they break. Even though a commercial dental laboratory fabricates most of the removable prostheses, the allied oral health practitioner needs to be familiar with the materials and their uses, care, and repair. She or he must understand the materials used in prosthetic dentistry to better care for the patient and to assist the dentist. Patients who wear removable prostheses will often ask the dental assistant or hygienist questions that* relate to the fit or home care of their prosthesis. This chapter covers the uses of acrylics for construction of complete and partial dentures and for relining, tissue conditioning, and repairing these prostheses. It also covers the use of acrylic denture teeth, porcelain denture teeth, and acrylic repair techniques. The instructions to be given to the patient for the care of these prostheses are presented.*

Review of Polymer Formation

Polymers are large, long-chain molecules formed by chemically joining together smaller molecules, called **monomers.** When two or more different types of monomers join together, the polymer formed from them is called a *copolymer.* Copolymers are produced to enhance the physical properties of the material. The act of forming polymers is called **polymerization.**

CROSS-LINKED POLYMERS

The polymer chains often have short chains of atoms attached to their sides. When the side chains of adjacent polymers bond together, the polymers are termed **cross-linked polymers** (see Chapter 6, Figure 6-4). When side chains of adjacent polymers are joined by weak bonds, the polymers are easily manipulated, bent, or stretched. When adjacent polymers are joined by highly charged side chains, the bond is stronger, and the cross-linked polymers are stronger and stiffer.

POLYMERIZATION REACTIONS

There are two types of polymerization: addition and condensation. The reactions are the same as for the impression polymers, addition silicones, and condensation silicones (see Chapter 11).

Addition Polymerization Addition polymerization is the most common form of polymerization for dental materials. It occurs in three stages: initiation (or induction), propagation, and termination. Monomers have a core unit of two carbon atoms joined by a double bond. One carbon atom has two hydrogen atoms attached, and the other carbon atom has attached to it one hydrogen atom and one reactive group called a **free radical.** The free radical is made reactive by the chemical reaction of an organic peroxide, such as benzoyl peroxide, with an activator or accelerator, such as a tertiary amine, or by heating. The free radical initiates the reaction by opening the bond between the two carbon atoms of the monomer. The broken carbon bond causes the monomer molecule to bond to another monomer. Each linkage leaves a free radical available for further reaction. This process of linking monomer units is termed *propagation,* and it continues until the monomer units are used up or until a substance reacts with the free radical to tie it up. When the free radical is tied up or destroyed, the process is terminated. The materials that react by chemical means are called chemical-curing, self-curing, or autopolymerizing. Materials that use heat to initiate the reaction are called heat-curing polymers. Whether

initiated by chemical means or heat, the polymerization process itself releases heat. The heat must be controlled during the process. If the temperature becomes too great, the monomer will vaporize and produce porosity in the material. Porosity weakens the material, causes it to discolor as stains are absorbed into the pores, and can lead to retention and growth of oral microorganisms.

Condensation Polymerization   Materials formed by a condensation reaction do not have many uses in dentistry. The condensation silicone impression materials are the most commonly known, and even they are not used much today. Typically, more than one type of monomer is used. The reaction itself produces by-products such as water, hydrogen gas, or alcohol that may compromise the physical properties or handling characteristics.

Acrylic Resins (Plastics)

Synthetic polymers used in prosthetic dentistry are called *acrylic resins,* because they are derived from acrylic acid. Acrylic resin forms when a liquid monomer is mixed with a powder of small polymer beads, and the mixture undergoes polymerization (Figure 13-1). The polymerized resin is **poly (methyl methacrylate)** (PMMA). It is composed of numerous methyl methacrylate (MMA) monomer units linked together to form a long-chain polymer. The resins are used for denture bases, denture teeth, reline and repair of prostheses, provisional acrylic partial dentures (flippers or stayplates), tissue conditioners, and custom impression trays. They also have uses for orthodontic retainers and removable tooth movement devices (Figure 13-2), bruxism mouth guards, fluoride and bleaching trays, facings on esthetic crowns, and provisional restorations (see Chapter 14). Specialized acrylic resins are used in esthetic tissue replacement for severe gingival recession and for facial reconstruction due to trauma, surgery, or birth defects. Acrylic resins are especially

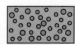

Polymer powder beads in denture resin material

FIGURE 13-1 ■ Acrylic resin beads and monomer in the polymerized stage.

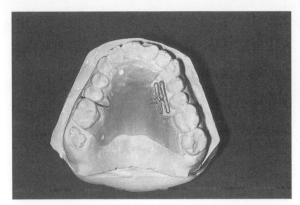

FIGURE 13-2 ■ Removable acrylic orthodontic tooth-movement device.

useful because they can be shaped to any contour and custom colored to match the shade of the teeth, gingiva, or skin. Acrylic resins used in dentistry are often modified by the addition of plasticizers, rubbers, and fillers to change their physical properties. **Plasticizers** are liquids added to soften the acrylic plastics. Oily liquids called aromatic esters are often used as plasticizers. Rubbers may be added to increase the impact fracture resistance of the acrylic resin, and fillers are added to strengthen the resin.

PROPERTIES

Polymerization Shrinkage Polymers undergo shrinkage as a result of the polymerization process. Heat-cured acrylic resins shrink about 6% by volume and about 0.2% to 0.5% linearly (from one point on the denture to another).

Dimensional Change Sources of dimensional change in addition to polymerization shrinkage include water sorption and thermal expansion. A denture base will increase slightly in its overall size when it absorbs water. This expansion may help offset some of the shrinkage that occurs during polymerization. The coefficient of thermal expansion is more than twice that of composite resins (see Chapter 6).

Strength The strength of the acrylic resins is fairly low, with a compressive strength of approximately 11,000 psi (76 MPa) and a tensile strength of 8000 psi (55 MPa). By comparison, amalgam has a com-

pressive strength of about 60,000 psi (415 MPa). Acrylics are not very hard materials (Knoop hardness number 16 to 18) and as a consequence are not very wear resistant. Although they have a fairly good resistance to fatigue failure (can be flexed repeatedly before they break), they will break if dropped on the floor or in an empty sink during cleaning. To combat the brittleness and breakage problem, some manufacturers add butadiene-styrene rubber to the MMA to create a high-impact acrylic resin.

Thermal Conductivity Denture bases do not conduct temperature well. Patients wearing dentures will notice a marked difference when they eat foods such as ice cream or drink hot beverages. Because the denture partially insulates against the temperature of the food or beverage, patients may burn themselves when they attempt to swallow foods that are too hot.

Chemical-Cured versus Heat-Cured Acrylics The type of processing has some effect on the properties. Polymerization is never 100% complete, and varying amounts of free monomer may be present in the polymerized material. In general, the chemical-cured acrylic resins are weaker, softer, more porous, and less color stable than heat-cured acrylic resins. After polymerization there is more residual monomer in the chemical-cured acrylic (up to 5%), and it initially adversely affects many of the physical properties until the monomer leaches out in minute amounts over several days or weeks. The tissues of some patients react to the residual monomer and become inflamed. Some dimensional change can occur during the first 24 hours in chemical-cured acrylic. For this reason, custom acrylic trays should not be used immediately, but should sit for 12 to 24 hours to allow most of the dimensional change to occur so the impression will not be distorted. Heat-cured acrylics are harder, stronger, and less porous and have less than 1% residual monomer that leaches out of the surface relatively quickly. Properties of heat-cured acrylic resins are summarized in Table 13-1.

Porosity. Porosity in polymerized acrylic resin is characterized by the presence of many small or microscopic voids or pores. Porosity in the acrylic weakens it and makes it prone to collect debris and microorganisms. Denture odor and stains develop more readily. Porosity is a result of loss of monomer or inadequate pressure during processing. The

TABLE 13-1 ■
Properties of Heat-Cured Acrylic Resins (PMMA)

Polymerization shrinkage (by volume)	6%
Polymerization shrinkage (linear)	0.2%-0.5%
Coefficient of thermal expansion	More than twice that of composite
Compressive strength	76 MPa (11,000 psi)
Tensile strength	55 MPa (8000 psi)
Hardness (Knoop)	15-18 kg/mm^2
Biocompatibility	Good
Thermal conductivity	Poor
Wear resistance	Fair
Fatigue resistance (to flexing)	Good
Impact resistance (to breakage when dropped)	Poor

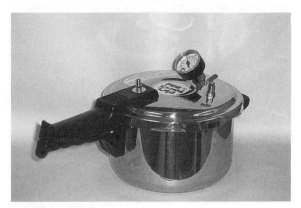

FIGURE 13-3 ■ Pressure pot used to provide a denser chemical-cured acrylic.

monomer is highly volatile and can evaporate rapidly at room temperature during the handling of the mixed powder and liquid. Monomer can vaporize during heat-curing of the resin if the temperature rises too much. Curing under pressure helps keep the monomer from evaporating during polymerization and creates a denser acrylic. When the chemical-cured acrylic is cured in room-temperature water and 15 to 20 pounds of air pressure in a pressure pot (Figure 13-3), the resulting acrylic is stronger and has less porosity and shrinkage. A pressure pot is a laboratory device that resembles a pressure cooker. It is a thick-sided metal pot that seals well and can be pressurized by the addition of air through a one-way valve in its lid.

> ▷ **CAUTION**
> *When using a pressure pot it is not necessary to pressurize it with air to more than 20 psi (pounds per square inch). Although the pressure pot is constructed of heavy materials and can usually withstand high pressure and has a pressure release valve, excessive pressure, more than 30 psi, increases the risk of a mishap should the release valve malfunction.*

ACRYLIC RESIN FOR DENTURE BASES

The primary function of the acrylic resin denture base is to retain the artificial teeth in the prosthesis. It also serves to distribute forces of mastication over a wide area so as to reduce pressure on the ridges that might contribute to resorption of the underlying bone. Additionally, the denture base replaces missing tissues or rebuilds the contours of tissues lost when the underlying bone resorbs. In complete dentures, the base establishes a seal along the periphery of the denture that aids in retention.

POLYMERIZATION REACTION

Acrylic resins polymerize by an addition reaction. Acrylic resins are supplied as a powder and liquid. The powder is composed mostly of small beads of PMMA and benzoyl peroxide (the initiator). Inorganic pigments are added to give the acrylic resin colors resembling oral mucosa, and titanium dioxide is added to keep the acrylic from being too transparent. Small, colored fibers may be added to simulate small blood vessels. Several shades of acrylic are available so that the clinician can attempt to match the variations of racial pigmentation that can occur in the gingiva and mucosa of patients (Figure 13-4). The liquid contains MMA, hydroquinone as an inhibitor or preservative to prevent polymerization of the MMA during storage, and glycol dimethacrylate as a cross-linking agent. Cross-linking of the acrylic polymer chains helps prevent surface cracks, and it improves the resistance to

STEPS IN COMPLETE DENTURE FABRICATION

1. Make preliminary alginate impression of edentulous ridges (by dental assistant).
2. Pour impressions in stone for preliminary casts (by dental assistant).
3. Fabricate custom impression trays from preliminary casts (by dental assistant or laboratory technician).
4. Border mold trays with compound and make final impressions with elastomer (by dentist or extended-function dental assistant).
5. Box impressions with utility wax and pour in die stone for master cast (by dental assistant).
6. Fabricate record bases (wax rims) (by dental assistant or laboratory technician).
7. With record bases, record jaw relations and lip line. Make facebow transfer—not used by all dentists (by dentist).
8. Select shade and mold of teeth (by dentist with help from assistant and patient).
9. Mount casts on articulator and set teeth in wax of record bases (by dentist or laboratory technician).
10. Try teeth in wax in patient's mouth to check appearance and occlusion (by dentist).
11. Return wax try-in to laboratory for final processing in acrylic resin.

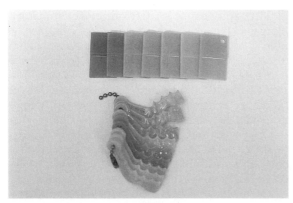

FIGURE 13-4 ■ Acrylic shade guides (also refer to Color Plate 10 at the front of the book).

structural fatigue that can lead to fracture. The liquid is supplied in dark brown bottles to prevent ultraviolet light from initiating polymerization during storage. When the powder and liquid are mixed, the chemical- and heat-cured materials go through a similar reaction, except that chemical-cured materials have a tertiary amine in the liquid as an activator whereas heat-cured materials do not (Table 13-2).

> ▶ **CAUTION**
> *Liquid monomer should be considered a hazardous material. It vaporizes easily when the lid is off of the container. Use in a well-ventilated area, ideally under a vapor hood. Avoid prolonged direct breathing of the vapor. Because all of its potential hazards have not been defined, it is advisable for pregnant workers and patients to avoid breathing the fumes.*

The first stage seen when the powder (polymer) and liquid (monomer) are mixed is called the *sandy stage* because the mixture looks grainy, similar to sand and water, and has a runny consistency. The second stage occurs when the powder particles

TABLE 13-2 ■

Ingredients of Acrylic Resin and Their Function

Component	Function
Liquid	
Methyl methacrylate	Monomer
Hydroquinone	Inhibitor to prevent polymerization of monomer during storage
Glycol dimethacrylate	Cross-linking agent
Tertiary amine	Activator for chemical-cured resin
Powder	
Poly (methyl methacrylate)	Polymer beads
Benzoyl peroxide	Initiator
Titanium dioxide	Reduces translucency
Pigments	Simulate tissue colors
Colored fibers	Simulate small blood vessels

absorb the liquid into their surface. It is called the *stringy stage* because the mixture is stringy when handled and is thicker in consistency. In the next stage, called the *dough stage*, more of the powder goes into solution and the mixture changes from stringy to doughy and is more easily manipulated. In the final stage, called the *rubber stage*, the mixture has a rubbery consistency that can no longer be manipulated for forming the denture base.

Chemical-Cured Resins Polymerization of chemical-cured acrylic resins is set into action when the tertiary amine in the liquid activates the benzoyl peroxide in the powder to produce free radicals. The hydroquinone initially inhibits the reaction from progressing by destroying the free radicals. This inhibition increases the working time so that the materials can be manipulated for a reasonable period of time, usually while the material progresses from the stringy stage to the dough stage. As the hydroquinone is depleted, the reaction proceeds more rapidly and goes from the dough stage to the rubber stage. The reaction is exothermic and goes from warm to quite hot. When the reaction is complete, the material is hard and stiff.

Pour Technique Some of the chemical-cured materials can be mixed to a thin, fluid consistency and poured into a mold and cured under pressure.

Heat-Cured Resins The most common method for processing denture bases uses heat and pressure during polymerization of the acrylic resin. Heat-cured acrylic resins go through similar initial stages of polymerization as the chemical-cured resins. After the dentist has tried in the denture teeth set in wax and the patient approves the appearance, the denture is returned to the laboratory and the technician places the cast of the edentulous arch, along with the denture setup (teeth mounted in wax on a record base), in a specially designed processing flask. The flask separates in the middle into two sections. The denture setup mounted on the cast is invested in a plaster investing material in the flask in such a manner that the flask can be opened in the middle to allow removal of the wax and record base after heating in a water bath. The teeth are held in place by the plaster. All remnants of the wax are removed. A liquid, called a separating medium, is placed and air-dried on the plaster and the cast to prevent the acrylic resin from sticking or absorbing moisture from the gypsum materials. Mixed acrylic resin in the dough stage is placed in the space created by removal of the wax and record base. (It has a longer dough stage than chemical-cured acrylic, because it does not have the tertiary amine activator.) This space is where the denture base will be formed. A sheet of polyethylene material is placed over the resin and the flask is reassembled and closed under pressure. The flask is reopened to remove excess material that exudes out of the sides of the flask. This process is repeated until no excess material appears. The flask is put into a device called a press that maintains pressure on it, and it is placed into a temperature-controlled water bath for at least 8 hours. Heat activates the benzoyl peroxide, causing the formation of free radicals and allowing polymerization to occur. Applying pressure and controlling the heat minimizes porosity by preventing the monomer from vaporizing. More of the monomer is consumed during the polymerization, so less free monomer is present in the cured denture base with heat-processed dentures. Like the chemical-cured resins, the material is hard and stiff when the polymerization is complete. It also shrinks when it is polymerized. The shrinkage is seen most readily in the palatal area and can cause the acrylic to lift from the cast as much as 0.25 mm. If a room-temperature processing technique is used, shrinkage is less, but the properties of the denture are poorer initially because of the presence of much more free monomer. The properties improve as the free monomer leaches out.

A similar process is performed for applying a denture base to a removable partial denture, except that the partial denture will have a metal framework invested in the mold, as well as the teeth set in wax. Because the acrylic resin does not adhere well to the metal, a retentive mesh or lattice is made as part of the partial denture framework to lock the acrylic in place (Figure 13-5).

Injection Molding Some vinyl acrylic resins can be processed by injecting the material into a mold when it is in a doughy form. With some materials shrinkage and porosity are reduced by injection molding. Some laboratories use this technique, because it is faster than the traditional heat processing.

Light-Cured Resins In addition to heat- and chemical-curing, dental resins can also be light-cured. The light-polymerized resins have photo

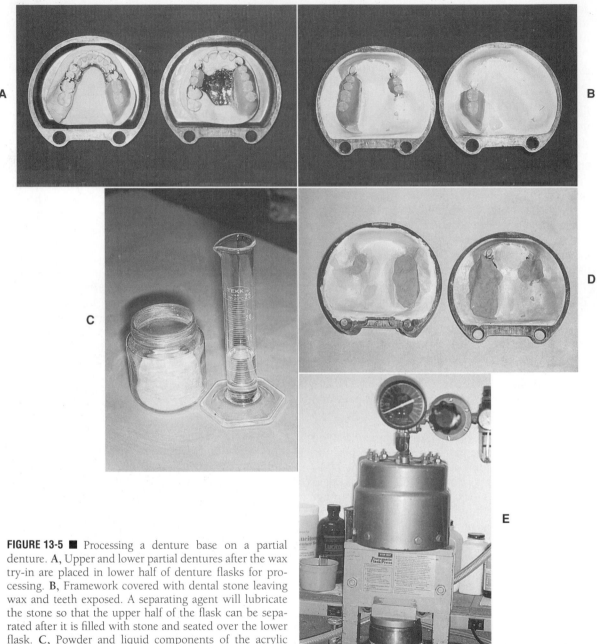

FIGURE 13-5 ■ Processing a denture base on a partial denture. **A,** Upper and lower partial dentures after the wax try-in are placed in lower half of denture flasks for processing. **B,** Framework covered with dental stone leaving wax and teeth exposed. A separating agent will lubricate the stone so that the upper half of the flask can be separated after it is filled with stone and seated over the lower flask. **C,** Powder and liquid components of the acrylic resin proportioned for mixing. **D,** Resin in the dough stage has been placed into the space created after the wax has been softened and removed. The resin will chemically join with acrylic denture teeth. **E,** Assembled denture flask placed in a pneumatic press that pressure packs the acrylic into the space left by the wax. Excess acrylic can be seen extruding from the flask. It will be cut away.

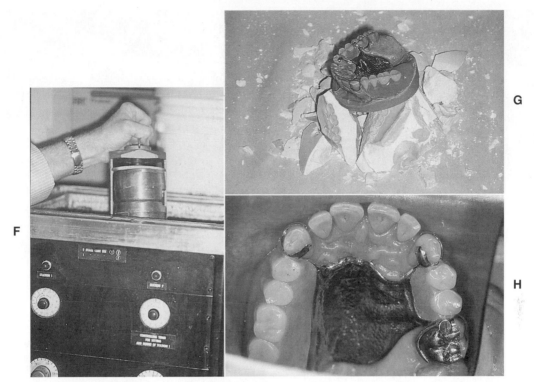

FIGURE 13-5 ■ *Continued*. **F,** Flasks containing upper and lower partial dentures are placed into a temperature-controlled water bath to heat-cure the acrylic. **G,** Upper partial denture with acrylic denture base after removal from the stone encasement that was in the flask. Finishing and polishing of the acrylic is needed. **H,** Completed upper partial denture in the patient's mouth. (Courtesy of Dr. Mark Dellinges, School of Dentistry, University of California, San Francisco.)

initiators such as camphoroquinone and amine activators. These react to form free radicals when exposed to blue light and initiate the polymerization reaction (see Chapter 6). One material contains dimethacrylate resin and silica fillers. The light-cured materials are fast and easy to use but require the purchase of an expensive light-curing unit. The material is available in limited acrylic colors. It is used mainly for record bases, custom trays, and denture repairs.

Denture Liners

SOFT LINING MATERIALS

Complete and partial dentures sometimes have a soft lining material placed on the tissue-bearing surface of the denture base. Soft liners may be used as short-term treatments for a few days up to a few weeks to allow tissues to heal following surgery or when denture sores have formed. Soft liners may also be used for long-term treatment for patients who have chronic soreness with hard denture bases because of sharp bony spicules or thin mucosa over the ridges. Patients feel more comfortable with a lining that has a cushioning effect. Soft liners are also used for patients with tissue undercuts that cannot be surgically corrected. A hard denture base rubs the mucosa in the area of the undercut, whereas a soft liner cushions the tissues and will flex in and out of the undercut when the denture is placed and removed. On average, they last about 1 to 3 years.

Long-Term Soft Liners Long-term soft liners are made from silicone rubber or acrylics such as ethyl or methyl methacrylate that have been made pliable by the addition of plasticizers such as

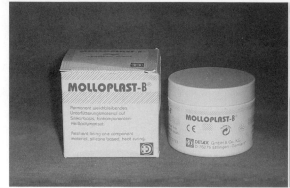

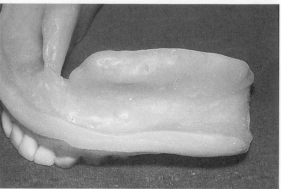

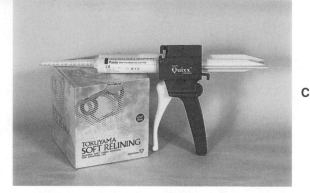

FIGURE 13-6 ■ Long-term soft liners. **A,** Heat-cured, silicon-based soft liner. **B,** Soft liner processed in lower denture. **C,** Chairside, chemical-cured, silicon-based soft liner in cartridges dispensed with a mixing gun and tip.

(Courtesy Dr. Mark Dellinges, School of Dentistry, University of California, San Francisco.)

aromatic esters and alcohol (Figure 13-6). Long-term liners may be processed at room temperature or with the application of heat. Although some long-term silicone and acrylic liners can be placed at chairside, most are placed at the commercial laboratory. Heat-cured silicone liners are processed in the laboratory, because they release acetic acid that can cause tissue burns. Long-term liners composed of acrylic will harden over time as the plasticizers (esters and alcohol) leach out and will need replacement. The silicone liners are more stable over the long term, because they do not have softeners to leach out. However, they can be difficult to adjust. Special burs and stones are needed to make these adjustments. Another problem with long-term soft liners is that they often do not form a good bond to old acrylic. Therefore they may separate from the denture base at the edges and leak between the liner and the denture base. Silicone liners support the growth of yeasts such as *Candida albicans* and may cause tissue irritation that requires antifungal therapy. Cleaning soft liners on a daily basis in benzalkonium chloride will reduce the growth of yeasts.

Short-Term Soft Liners (Tissue Conditioners)
Short-term soft liners are referred to as *tissue conditioners* or *treatment liners* and are usually placed at chairside. They are supplied as a powder composed of poly (ethyl methacrylate) and softeners or plasticizers of aromatic oils and ethanol (Figure 13-7). The powder and liquid are mixed thoroughly following manufacturer's directions and flowed onto the tissue-bearing surface of the denture that was previously cleaned with soap and water. The denture is reseated in the patient's mouth, and the patient is instructed to gently close into the normal occlusion until the material cures. These liners are capable of readapting to the patient's tissues as they heal, because they have a high degree of flow. As the plasticizers leach out, the resin becomes stiffer. The plasticizers leach out more quickly in the short-term liners than the long-term liners and therefore need frequent replacement. Some short-term liners last only 1 week; others last 2 to 4 weeks. Use of appropriate denture soaks can prolong the useful life of soft liners, so manufacturer's recommendations are important. The dental assistant and hygienist must

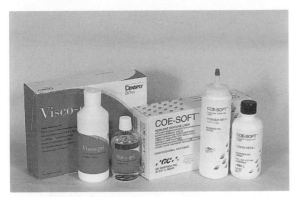

FIGURE 13-7 ■ Short-term soft liners are called tissue conditioners, because they flow and adapt to the tissues as they heal. Seen are components of two tissue conditioners.
(Courtesy Dr. Mark Dellinges, School of Dentistry, University of California, San Francisco.)

be familiar with the materials and procedures for the placement of the liners at chairside and for the home care of both chairside and laboratory-processed liners.

HARD LINING MATERIALS

Dentures become loose over time as the alveolar bone of the ridges resorbs. Immediate dentures are those placed immediately after the extraction of the teeth. They become loose rapidly as the extraction sites heal and the bone resorbs. These loose dentures can often be made to fit well again by placement of a lining material to fill in the spaces. The most common material used for this purpose is an acrylic resin similar to the original denture base material. This hard liner is placed either directly in the patient's mouth at chairside or indirectly in the dental laboratory.

Chairside Reline   With the chairside technique, a chemical-cured acrylic resin is used. First, an acrylic bur is used to remove a thin layer of the tissue-bearing surface of the denture base so that a fresh, clean surface is available for chemical bonding of the lining material to the denture. A lubricant such as petroleum jelly is applied to the denture teeth and non–tissue-bearing surfaces where the liner should not adhere. The freshened surface is primed with some of the liquid (monomer) to make it ready for the liner. The monomer is a good solvent and will

slightly soften the surface, allowing the liner to bond better. The powder and liquid are mixed thoroughly and applied to the primed denture base. The denture is reseated in the patient's mouth. The lips, cheeks, and tongue are moved through appropriate motions to reestablish the peripheral borders (a process called *border molding*). The patient is asked to close into the normal occlusion. This position is held until the material just begins to harden. It should be removed from the mouth before polymerization is complete, because the chemical reaction is exothermic and the heat generated could burn the tissues. Once completely hardened, the excess material is trimmed away and the denture borders are carefully polished.

Laboratory Reline   The laboratory reline uses an indirect technique in which an impression of the tissues is made inside the existing denture and a cast is made from this impression. The technician uses an indexing instrument called a reline device to establish the relationship between the cast and the denture. The impression material is removed, along with a thin layer of the tissue-bearing denture base surface as with the chairside technique. The lining material is heat- and pressure-processed to the denture base.

INFECTION CONTROL PROCEDURES

Proper infection control procedures should be followed when transporting a denture to the dental laboratory and when receiving it from the laboratory to deliver to the patient (see the boxed text "Disinfecting Prostheses" on page 260).

OVER-THE-COUNTER LINERS

Some patients are "do-it-yourselfers" who purchase reline materials in the drugstore and apply them at home. They do not receive professional advice on the use and care of these liners and often use the liners far beyond their useful life. These materials can stiffen with time and cause damage to the tissues, particularly if the occlusion is not properly reestablished with the new lining in place. They are usually porous and promote the growth of yeasts, and patients can end up with fungal infections of the oral tissues. These over-the-counter products are not recommended.

DISINFECTING PROSTHESES

- Properly disinfect all prostheses before trying in the patient's mouth.
- Disinfect at chairside all prostheses going from the patient to the commercial or office laboratory, and package properly for transport.
- Iodophors and synthetic phenols are suitable disinfectants for most prostheses.
- Immerse prostheses for 15 minutes in one of these disinfectants in a denture cup or plastic bag.

Plastic (Acrylic) Teeth

Both plastic (acrylic resin) and porcelain teeth are used for complete and partial dentures. Each has certain advantages. Plastic teeth are tough and chemically bond to the acrylic base of the denture. They are easy to grind in order to adjust the occlusion or to reshape a tooth to fit the available space. They do not wear the opposing natural or artificial teeth or restorations. Their main disadvantage is that they are softer and wear more readily than porcelain teeth. Plastic teeth are made in layers to simulate the colors and translucencies of natural teeth. The gingival portion of the teeth is manufactured so that the acrylic has minimal cross-linking. The bond of the acrylic tooth to the denture base is better without cross-linking. Cross-linking in the other portions of the denture teeth makes them tougher and better able to hold up under function. Plastic teeth are used more than porcelain teeth, because they are somewhat resilient and are thought not to stress the underlying ridges as much as porcelain teeth.

In contrast, porcelain teeth are brittle, hard, and very resistant to wear. They do not bond to the acrylic of the denture base and must have mechanical retention such as metal pins or retention holes to keep them in the denture base acrylic. They have a good esthetic appearance until the surface glaze is lost from wear or abrasive polishing. Porcelain teeth cannot be easily repolished as with plastic teeth. They are highly stain resistant, whereas some plastic teeth will stain over time. They are not indicated for use against natural dentition or most restorative materials because they are very abrasive. They also

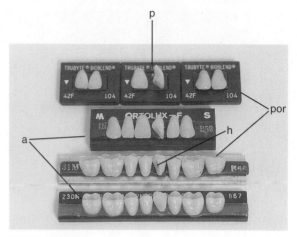

FIGURE 13-8 ■ Plastic and porcelain denture teeth. Porcelain teeth (*por*) do not chemically bond to the denture base, as do plastic teeth (*a*); therefore they have metal pins (*p*) or retention holes (*h*) to lock into the acrylic.

transmit heavier occlusal forces to the ridge and as such may be a factor in patient discomfort, denture sores, and accelerated ridge resorption. Some patients prefer the porcelain teeth because they sense a better ability to chew harder or more fibrous foods (Figure 13-8).

Characterization of Dentures

Dentures can be given individual characteristics to make them seem more lifelike. Denture teeth can be arranged in the standard "ideal" arch alignment, or teeth can be arranged to re-create spaces (diastemas) (Figure 13-9) or overlapping or crooked teeth the patient had with the natural teeth. The denture teeth can be all one shade or can be selected to simulate the lighter and darker teeth most people have in their mouths (e.g., canines are usually darker than the incisors). Some patients request that restorations be placed in the denture teeth to simulate restorations they had in their natural teeth. The denture base acrylic itself is made in several shades, and these can be selected to replicate the color of the patient's mucosa and gingiva. The dental technician can do custom shading with pigmented resins to simulate racial pigmentation in the denture base, because the pigmentation is not always uniformly distributed in the tissues.

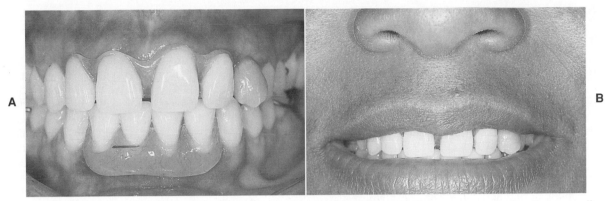

FIGURE 13-9 ■ Characterized temporary partial denture (stayplate) to create a lifelike appearance. Patient had naturally occurring diastemas between her maxillary incisors and wanted to have diastemas in the prosthesis. **A,** Stayplate with diastemas between the incisors. **B,** Natural-looking smile.

(Courtesy Dr. Arun Sharma, School of Dentistry, University of California, San Francisco.)

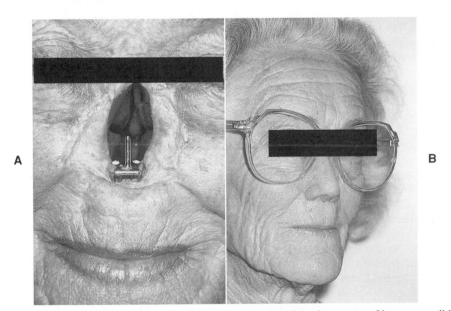

FIGURE 13-10 ■ Flexible acrylic prosthesis for nose lost to cancer. **A,** Metal implant at site of lost nose will hold the prosthesis in place. **B,** Lifelike prosthesis made of silicone rubber replaces the nose.

(Courtesy Dr. Arun Sharma, School of Dentistry, University of California, San Francisco.)

Plastics for Maxillofacial Prostheses

A specialized aspect of a prosthodontic practice may include the fabrication of maxillofacial prostheses to replace lost facial tissues due to trauma, disease, surgery, or birth defect. These prostheses must have specialized characteristics so that they can be colored to match the surrounding skin, must be tear resistant in thin layers, must be resistant to staining, must be very flexible, and must be able to be attached to the surrounding skin with adhesives (Figure 13-10). The best material currently available for these prostheses is silicone rubber, but acrylics and vinyls with plasticizers are also used.

Denture Repair

Acrylic complete and partial dentures can be repaired rather easily when they are broken. The repair of a partial denture with a metal framework is more complex depending on the location of the break. If the break is through the framework or the clasp, it can sometimes be repaired by welding in the dental laboratory. However, many times such a break means that a new partial denture must be made.

CHEMICAL-CURED ACRYLIC REPAIR MATERIAL

The broken prosthesis should be disinfected at chairside before it is transported to the laboratory. To repair an all-acrylic denture or partial denture, the broken parts are pieced together and held with sticky wax. Plaster or stone is poured in the prosthesis to create a cast on which to stabilize the parts while they are being repaired. Sometimes an impression of the patient's mouth must be taken in order to assemble the broken pieces. After the plaster has set, the fracture line is cut with an acrylic bur to create room for a sufficient bulk of repair material, and the adjacent surfaces are ground to expose a fresh surface for bonding. A coating of the liquid monomer is placed on the roughened surface to wet and prime it as with the chairside reline procedure. Often the repair material is the same as the chairside reline material. The repair material is applied to the fracture either in bulk or by the "salt and pepper" technique. With the salt and pepper technique a small quantity of powder is sprinkled onto the wet fracture site and is wet with more liquid. This process of alternately adding powder and liquid continues until the fracture site is slightly overfilled. The prosthesis on the cast is then placed in a pressure pot with warm (not hot) water and about 20 pounds of pressure until cured (at least 20 minutes). Once the repair acrylic has cured, the prosthesis is removed, and excess material is cut back and polished. The prosthesis is disinfected and returned to chairside to try in the patient's mouth to confirm the fit and comfort.

LIGHT-CURED REPAIR MATERIAL

Light-cured dimethacrylates have a number of useful applications, including repair of broken acrylic prostheses. Dimethacrylate is an acrylic resin that con-

tains a chemical activated by light in the blue wave range, as well as an accelerator, inorganic fillers, and pigments to simulate tissue colors. When used for denture repair, the prosthesis is prepared in the same manner as for the chemical-cured material except that a different liquid is painted on the fractured pieces before application of the repair material. The repair material is removed from its lightproof package and is placed in the prepared fracture site. The repair material is coated with a liquid to prevent an oxygen-inhibited layer of uncured material from occurring on the surface (see Chapter 6). Uncured material at the surface makes it more difficult to polish. The prosthesis on the cast is placed into a chamber with intense blue light (Triad light-curing unit) for about 10 minutes, and it rotates on a turntable while the light polymerizes the repair material. After curing it is shaped and polished and delivered to the patient. This technique is somewhat faster than the chemical-cured method. Both methods are safe and effective.

Custom Impression Trays and Record Bases

Chemical-cured and light-cured acrylic resins can be used to construct custom impression trays and the record bases on which wax rims are placed during the process of making dentures. The acrylics contain a high proportion of filler particles to impart strength to the material.

CHEMICAL-CURED TRAY AND RECORD BASE MATERIAL

Similar to the other chemical-cured acrylics, the tray materials are supplied as a powder and liquid. The powder and liquid are mixed, and when the mixture reaches the dough stage the material is adapted over the tissue portion of the cast by hand to a uniform thickness. Before application of the acrylic, the cast has adapted to it a spacer made from one layer of baseplate wax. Before the spacer is applied the cast is usually treated in one of three ways to keep wax and acrylic from sticking to it. It can be soaked in cold water, coated with a separating material, or lightly coated with petroleum jelly. Some clinicians place three or four 2-mm-diameter holes in the wax spacer in the anterior and posterior ridge regions. As the tray material is adapted over the wax, the material presses into the holes and creates elevations inside the tray once the wax is removed. These elevations create stops against the tissues when the impression is taken. The spacer creates a uniform thickness for impression material, and tissue stops keep the tray from being seated too heavily and compressing large areas of tissue during impression taking. After the tray material is adapted to the cast, excess material is cut away with a knife and used to make a handle for the tray. The polymerization reaction is exothermic and the material gets quite hot. Just before the final set when the tray material is firm and warm, it should be carefully pried off the cast and the wax spacer removed. It should be reseated on the cast until polymerization is complete. The tray is trimmed to the appropriate length with acrylic burs or abrasive bands on a lathe (see Procedure 13-1).

Record bases are rigid bases that correspond roughly to the denture base. They are used in the construction stage of the denture and have wax rims added to them over the ridge areas. They are used initially to establish the proper dimension between upper and lower arches, as well as the position of the centric occlusion. Later, the denture teeth are set in the wax rims and the record bases serve to stabilize the wax rims during the try-in appointment. The record bases are also constructed from the same materials as the trays. The difference in their construction is that wax spacers, tissue stops, or handles are not used. If significant tissue undercuts are present on the cast, they are blocked out with wax before construction of the record bases.

LIGHT-CURED TRAY AND RECORD BASE MATERIAL

The light-cured dimethacrylates can be used for construction of custom trays and record bases (see Procedure 13-2). The technique is the same as for the chemical-cured materials except instead of mixing powder and liquid, a sheet of the preformed material is removed from its lightproof package and adapted over the cast or wax spacer. After trimming excess material (and forming a handle if a tray), tray or record base on the cast is placed in the light-curing unit as described previously for light-cured repair materials. The light-cured material does not generate as much heat during polymerization and is much easier to use because no mixing is required. It eliminates the concern of inhaling and handling the monomer associated with the chemical-cured material.

Care of Acrylic Resin Dentures

HOME CARE

The patient needs to be instructed on how to care for the acrylic prosthesis. The patient should clean the tissue surfaces and the teeth and outer surfaces of the denture with a denture brush. Many of the denture brushes have medium or hard bristles. The stiffness of the bristles is not as critical to the abrasion of the acrylic as the cleaner used on the brush. Liquid soap, a mild hand soap, or a nonabrasive denture cleaning paste can be used to remove surface debris. Some commercial denture cleaning pastes are too abrasive and will wear the denture base and plastic teeth.

If the patient cannot brush the prosthesis after meals, it should be rinsed thoroughly. The prosthesis must be cleaned to remove bacterial plaque and debris before putting it in a denture soak. Commercial denture cleaning tablets are used to make a solution in which to soak the denture. They are effective when used on a regular basis. Calculus that accumulates on the denture can be softened and more easily removed by soaking the denture in a solution of white vinegar diluted 1:1 with water. Dentures are soaked overnight in commercial or homemade soaks. The bleach is an effective organic solvent and eliminates yeasts. However, undiluted household bleach should not be used as an overnight soak for complete or partial dentures. It will fade the color from the acrylic and attack the metal framework and clasps of a partial denture and cause them to darken and corrode. Partial dentures with metal components should be soaked in commercial products that do not contain bleach. Clasps on partial dentures can be cleaned with the pointed brush on the end of the denture brush if the two-headed variety is used. The tissue-bearing surfaces of dentures with soft liners should be cleaned gently with a soft toothbrush. Liquid soap can also be used (Figure 13-11). The long- and short-term soft liners may be adversely affected by some of the commercial soaks. Use only the cleaners recommended by the manufacturer.

IN-OFFICE CARE

Patients will accumulate calculus on the denture around the surfaces of the maxillary molars and the mandibular anteriors just as they did with their

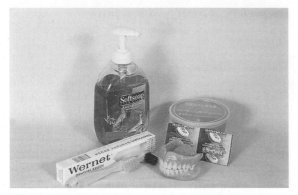

FIGURE 13-11 ■ Home care products for cleaning dentures: brush, liquid soap, denture cleaner tablets, denture cup.

natural dentition. The dental hygienist can provide a service by removing the calculus before returning the prosthesis to the patient. Calculus can be removed by placing the prosthesis in a denture cleaning solution inside a zippered bag placed into an ultrasonic cleaner. It can also be carefully scaled off with hand instruments and the area polished with flour of pumice, then tin oxide or acrylic polishing compounds. Care must be taken so as not to wear down the teeth and acrylic base during the polishing process.

STORAGE OF DENTURES

Acrylic resin prostheses absorb water and are sensitive to water loss. The patient should be instructed to

---

PRECAUTIONS FOR PATIENTS WITH PARTIAL OR COMPLETE DENTURES

- Store dentures in water to prevent warping from loss of moisture.
- Do not clean dentures in hot water because they may warp.
- Avoid soaking dentures in chlorine bleach because it will remove color from the resin and attack metal components of partial dentures.
- Clean dentures over a sink partially filled with water to avoid breaking if dropped.
- Avoid abrasive toothpastes or household cleaners because they will scratch or wear the plastic.

---

keep the prosthesis wet during periods of storage. This will prevent dimensional changes and distortion that can affect the fit. The prosthesis should be kept wet during the dental appointment. It can be stored in a denture cup to which water and a little mouthwash has been added to freshen it. Prostheses with soft liners should not be placed in mouthwash containing alcohol because the alcohol may adversely affect the properties of the soft liner. Instructions for care of complete and partial dentures should be given to nursing home staff and to caregivers for homebound or incapacitated individuals.

SUMMARY

Acrylic resins are vitally important to the success of prosthetic dentistry. They are versatile materials that can be used to replace missing oral structures. The ability of these resins to chemically bond to one another is important when linking plastic teeth to the denture base or when relining or repairing them. When properly handled they are strong and durable. They can readily be relined to improve the fit as the alveolar bone resorbs over time. Lining materials can be similar to the denture base material or can be modified with plasticizers to create soft liners for tissue conditioning or long-term cushioning for patients who cannot tolerate hard liners. Many of the relining procedures can be accomplished in the office at chairside so that the patient does not have to be without the prosthesis for any length of time. Simple fractures of the resin also can readily be repaired in the dental office. The acrylic resins can be colored with pigments to simulate racial pigmentation so the denture can be customized to match the tissue coloration of the patient.

Other resins chemically similar to the methyl methacrylate resins are also used in prosthetic dentistry. The addition of photo initiators and amine activators produces light-cured materials that are easy to use, require no mixing, and eliminate the volatile monomer that is potentially hazardous. The light-cured resins have application for fabrication of custom trays and record bases and for denture repairs. Acrylic and vinyl resins to which plasticizers have been added to soften them are often used in maxillofacial prosthodontics for replacement of facial tissues following trauma or cancer surgery. Noses, cheeks, ears, and other structures can be made from these materials and colored to match the surrounding skin.

The allied oral health provider plays an important role in delivering care to individuals who require prostheses. She or he may be called on to mix, place, remove, or repair any number of these materials. Therefore an intimate knowledge of the properties and handling characteristics of these materials is very important. Additionally, patients need instructions in the proper home care of the prostheses to maintain them and to prevent injury to the oral tissues. Knowledge of the proper cleaning agents and methods is also necessary.

CHAPTER REVIEW

Select the one correct response for each of the following multiple-choice questions:

1. **A polymer is formed by**
   a. Breaking down complex, high-molecular-weight molecules by heating them
   b. Linking nitrogen atoms together with hydrogen bonds
   c. Joining monomer molecules together in a long chain through carbon bonds
   d. Fusing acrylic powder beads together at high temperature

2. **Cross-linking of polymers**
   a. Is used to improve the physical properties of the final resin product
   b. Occurs when long-chain polymers are mixed together, and the chains physically wrap around each other
   c. Usually results in a weaker material, the greater the degree of cross-linking
   d. Occurs when long chains link end-to-end

3. **Addition polymerization**
   a. Results in porosity in the final material
   b. Is the least common method of polymerization used in dentistry
   c. Is an endothermic reaction (absorbs heat)
   d. Is initiated by a free radical that opens the bond between the carbon atoms of the monomer

4. **The stages of the addition polymerization reaction are**
   a. Sandy, stringy, and doughy
   b. Wet, flexible, and stiff
   c. Sol, gel, and solid
   d. Initiation, propagation, and termination

5. **A heat-processed denture differs from a chemical-cured denture. Which one of the following is NOT true for the heat-processed denture?**
   a. It is stronger.
   b. It is more porous.
   c. It is harder.
   d. It has less dimensional change during the first 24 hours after curing.

6. **High-impact resins are created by**
   a. Removal of free monomer
   b. Addition of plasticizers
   c. Heat treating the resin after it has polymerized
   d. Addition of rubber to the acrylic

7. **Which stage of polymerization of acrylic resins is longer for heat-cured resins because of the absence of a tertiary amine?**
   a. Sandy
   b. Stringy
   c. Dough
   d. Exothermic

8. **What is the effect on a denture if it is left on the nightstand overnight?**
   a. It will lose water and shrink.
   b. It will expand.
   c. It will crack.
   d. It will oxidize and lose color.

9. **What is the effect on a partial denture framework if soaked in a chlorine-containing cleaner?**
   a. Nothing will happen.
   b. The metal will clean rapidly and become shiny.
   c. The metal will dissolve and fracture.
   d. The metal will darken and corrode.

10. **The effect porosity has on an acrylic denture can be seen as all of the following EXCEPT:**
    a. It contributes to staining.
    b. It contributes to growth of microorganisms.
    c. It weakens the acrylic.
    d. It decreases the thermal conductivity of the acrylic.

11. **The purpose of the use of a pressure pot during polymerization of a chemical-cured acrylic resin is**
    a. To increase the strength of the acrylic
    b. To decrease the porosity
    c. To decrease the shrinkage
    d. All of the above

12. **Which type of hard liner has the best physical properties?**
    a. Chairside chemical-cured liner
    b. Laboratory chemical-cured liner
    c. Laboratory heat-cured liner
    d. None (they are all the same)

13. **At which stage of polymerization is the heat-cured acrylic resin packed into the denture flask to form the denture base?**
    a. Stringy
    b. Sandy
    c. Ropy
    d. Dough

14. **Long-term soft liners are indicated for all of the following reasons EXCEPT:**
    a. Chronic soreness with hard acrylic denture bases
    b. Severe soft tissue undercuts
    c. Sharp, knife-edge ridges
    d. Soft tissues with chronic fungal infections

15. **Acrylic resins can be made soft and pliable by the**
    a. Use of less monomer in the mix
    b. Use of less powder in the mix
    c. Addition of aromatic esters
    d. Addition of benzoyl peroxide

16. **All of the following statements about short-term soft liners are true EXCEPT:**
    a. They are also called tissue conditioners.
    b. They can readapt to the tissues as healing takes place, because they have a high degree of flow.
    c. They do not need frequent replacement because they absorb water and get softer over time.
    d. They are adversely affected by some commercial denture soaks.

17. **Over-the-counter denture liners have which of the following shortcomings?**
    a. May not reestablish proper occlusion
    b. Are generally porous
    c. Promote growth of yeasts
    d. All of the above

18. **All of the following are advantages of acrylic denture teeth over porcelain teeth EXCEPT:**
    a. They are more wear resistant.
    b. They chemically bond to the denture base.
    c. They are kind to the opposing teeth or ridges.
    d. They can easily be ground and shaped to fit the available space.

19. **When repairing a denture with a chemical-cured acrylic resin, all of the following procedures are performed EXCEPT:**
    a. The pieces are reassembled and held with sticky wax while a cast is poured inside the denture.
    b. A layer of the old resin is removed surrounding the fracture site.
    c. The resin surrounding the fracture site is wet with monomer to enhance the chemical bond with the repair acrylic.
    d. The repair acrylic is mixed, applied to the fracture site, and allowed to cure at room temperature on the laboratory bench for the best results.

20. **Which one of the following statements regarding construction of custom acrylic trays is FALSE?**
    a. Tray acrylic is usually chemical-cured but can also be light-cured.
    b. Tray acrylic is mixed and adapted directly to the cast.
    c. During polymerization the material gets hot.
    d. A wax spacer is used inside the tray to develop a consistent thickness of impression material.

21. **Which one of the following statements is FALSE regarding the care of dentures by the patient?**
    a. Dentures should be stored in water to prevent warping.
    b. Dentures should be cleaned over a sink filled with water or over a towel to prevent fracture if dropped.
    c. Abrasive pastes or cleaners should not be used or they will scratch the acrylic.
    d. The denture should be cleaned in hot water periodically to kill microorganisms.

CASE-BASED DISCUSSION TOPICS

■ A thin, frail 76-year-old widow had complete dentures made about 3 years ago. She comes to the dental office with a chief complaint of "my lower denture hurts me when I eat." In the 3 years since her dentures were made she has had the lower denture relined twice with hard acrylic. This has not improved her comfort. Her lower ridge is sharp and thin. *Can you suggest a process that might make her more comfortable? Is the procedure best done in the office or in a commercial dental laboratory? What kinds of materials are often used?*

◉ A 62-year-old retired janitor comes to the dental office to get his teeth cleaned. He wears an upper complete denture and a lower partial denture with a metal framework that replaces teeth numbers 22 to 26. In addition to calculus on his teeth, he has calculus on his denture and partial denture. *Describe a method of removing the calculus without scratching the acrylic. What home care measures can you recommend for care of his prostheses? What type of cleaner should he avoid on his partial denture? What types of brushes should he use to clean his prostheses?*

◉ A 57-year-old truck driver comes to the dental office with a broken maxillary denture. It is broken in two pieces through the midline of the palatal portion of the denture base. The pieces fit together easily. He said he dropped it in the sink while cleaning it. *What steps should be taken to prepare the denture for repair in the office? What materials could be used for the repair? What is the function of the pressure pot? What advice can be given to the patient to avoid a similar mishap in the future?*

◉ A 71-year-old retired teacher had an upper denture made 6 months ago. She returns to the office complaining that the denture has stained heavily in the palatal portion of the denture base and has developed a foul odor. When you inspect the denture, you confirm a dark stain in the midpalate but also notice numerous small porosities in the acrylic. *Cite causes of porosity during processing of the denture. Why has the denture stained and developed a foul odor? What effect does porosity have on the physical properties of the acrylic?*

REFERENCES

Bird D, Robinson D: Removable prosthodontics. In *Torres and Erhlich modern dental assisting,* ed 6, Philadelphia, 1999, WB Saunders.

Craig RG, editor: Polymers and polymerization. In *Restorative dental materials,* ed 7, St Louis, 1985, Mosby.

Craig RG, Powers JM, Wataha JC: Plastics in prosthetics. In *Dental materials: properties and manipulation,* ed 7, Philadelphia, 2000, Mosby.

Erhlich A, Torres HO, Bird D: Complete and partial dentures. In *Essentials of dental assisting,* ed 2, Philadelphia, 1996, WB Saunders.

Farah JW, Powers JM, editors: Denture resins/liners, *Dental Advisor* 5(4):1, 1988.

Gladwin MA, Bagby MD: Removable prostheses and acrylic resins. In *Clinical aspects of dental materials,* Philadelphia, 2000, Lippincott Williams & Wilkins.

Leinfelder KF, Lemons JE: Dental polymers. In *Clinical restorative materials and techniques,* Philadelphia, 1988, Lea & Febiger.

Phillips RW, Moore BK: Dental polymers. In *Elements of dental materials for dental hygienists and dental assistants,* ed 5, Philadelphia, 1994, WB Saunders.

PROCEDURE 13-1 (see p. 347 for competency sheet)

Fabrication of Custom Acrylic Impression Tray

NOTE: Figures 13-12 through 13-19 Courtesy Dr. Mark Dellinges, School of Dentistry, University of California, San Francisco, Calif.

EQUIPMENT/SUPPLIES

- Maxillary or mandibular edentulous cast
- Sheet of baseplate wax, Bunsen burner, laboratory knife
- Tray powder and liquid, tongue blade or cement spatula, waxed paper cup
- Laboratory handpiece and acrylic bur, sandpaper drum (arbor band), and dental lathe
- Cast-separating medium, disposable brush, petroleum jelly

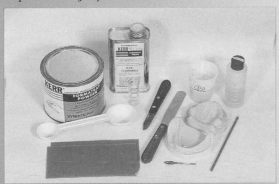

FIGURE 13-12

PROCEDURE STEPS

1 Coat the cast with separating medium using the disposable brush and allow it to dry.

NOTE: The separating medium keeps the tray material and wax from sticking to the cast.

2 Warm a sheet of baseplate wax over the Bunsen burner and place it on the cast. Adapt it to the cast over the edentulous ridges and into the vestibular folds. Use the laboratory knife to trim excess wax away until it is about 2 mm from the depth of the folds.

NOTE: The wax will be removed after the tray is fabricated and will create an even space within the tray for the impression material. It is called a wax spacer.

3 Cut three 2 × 2 mm square holes in the wax over the ridges for the maxillary and mandibular casts, two in the molar area, and one in the incisor area.

NOTE: As tray material is adapted into these holes, resin squares will appear inside the tray. When the impression is taken, these squares will contact the tissues over the ridges and act as stops. The stops will create an even thickness of impression material within the tray (except for the very small area of the square) and will prevent an uneven seating of the tray (Figure 13-13). Some clinicians do not use these stops.

4 Mix powder and liquid of the tray material in wax cup in proportions recommended by the manufacturer. Stir with a tongue blade or cement spatula until thoroughly mixed (Figure 13-14).

NOTE: The mix will be too wet to handle at this stage.

5 Apply petroleum jelly to the gloved hands. When the mixture is doughy, form it into a thick, wide rope that is long enough to fit around the entire ridge (Figure 13-15).

NOTE: Petroleum jelly keeps the tray material from sticking to the gloves.

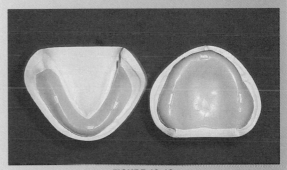

FIGURE 13-13

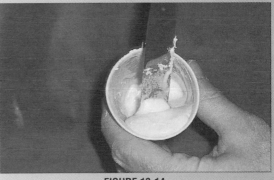

FIGURE 13-14

Continued on following page

PROCEDURE 13-1 (Continued)

6 Adapt the resin over the wax, into the holes in the wax, and into the depth of the vestibular folds. Tray should be 1 to 2 mm thick (Figure 13-16).

NOTE: If the tray is too thin, it might be too flexible to keep the impression from distorting.

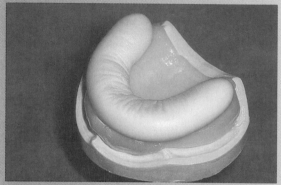

FIGURE 13-15

7 Cut away excess tray material with the laboratory knife and quickly adapt it into the shape of a handle. Wet the tray end of the handle with monomer and place it on the tray. Smooth it into place with the fingers. The handle should be positioned so that it will not be in the way of the lips when seated in the patient's mouth.

NOTE: Wetting the end of the tray with monomer (liquid) dissolves some material at the surface and allows it to stick to the polymerizing tray material.

8 Readapt tray material to the cast continually as polymerization takes place.

NOTE: The tray material shrinks as it polymerizes and tends to pull away from the cast.

9 Remove tray from cast once heat of reaction has cooled. Remove wax from inside the tray. If difficult to remove, heat wax in warm water (Figure 13-17).

NOTE: Residual wax must be removed, or it might prevent the impression material from adhering to the tray.

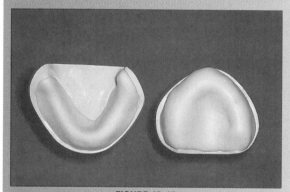

FIGURE 13-16

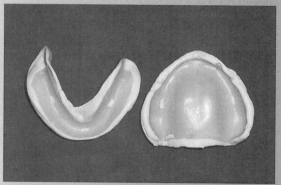

FIGURE 13-17

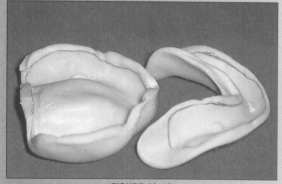

FIGURE 13-18

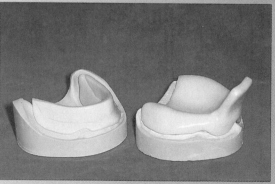

FIGURE 13-19

Continued on following page

PROCEDURE 13-1 (Continued)

10 Trim tray with acrylic bur or arbor band to remove excess material and smooth rough edges. The completed tray should extend 2 mm short of the vestibular folds. Confirm fit of tray on cast (Figures 13-18 and 13-19).

NOTE: The tray must be smooth to the touch or it will be uncomfortable in the patient's mouth. The tray is left short of the depth of the folds to allow room for

compound to be added for border molding. Border molding uses softened compound to shape the location for the borders of the denture as the patient's cheeks and tongue are manipulated through simulated functional movements.

11 Disinfect tray by immersion in appropriate disinfectant and store in sealed bag labeled with patient's name until ready for use.

PROCEDURE 13-2 (see p. 348 for competency sheet)

Fabrication of Record Bases with Light-Cured Acrylic Resin

NOTE: Figures 13-20 through 13-26 Courtesy Dr. Mark Dellinges, School of Dentistry, University of California, San Francisco, Calif.

EQUIPMENT/SUPPLIES (Figure 13-20)

- Edentulous casts (maxillary, mandibular, or both)
- Light-cured record base material (Triad VLC)
- Model releasing agent
- Light-curing unit (Triad VLC)
- Disposable scalpel blade and handle
- 2 × 2 gauze soaked with alcohol
- Low-speed handpiece with acrylic bur
- Laboratory lathe with sandpaper drum (arbor band), rag wheel, and pumice

PROCEDURE STEPS

1 Apply a thin layer of model releasing agent to the surface of the edentulous casts with a disposable brush, and let it dry (Figure 13-21).

2 Remove a sheet of the Triad VLC material from the protective packaging and place it over the cast.

NOTE: The packaging prevents light from polymerizing the material.

3 Press the material gently on the cast, being careful not to trap air between the cast and the material (Figure 13-22).

4 Press the material into the vestibule areas of the cast using the blunt end of the disposable scalpel.

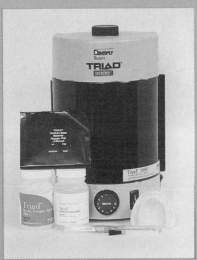

FIGURE 13-20

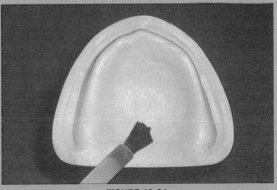

FIGURE 13-21

Continued on following page

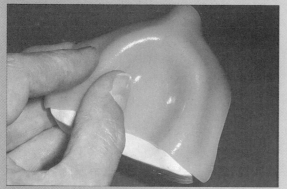

FIGURE 13-22

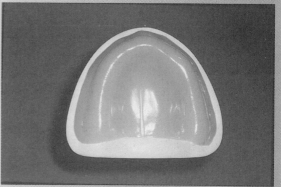

FIGURE 13-23

5 Trim away the excess material that extends beyond the depth of the vestibule with the scalpel blade. Smooth the edges with fingers.

6 Cut a 2-cm-long slit in the back of the palate of the maxillary record base material to allow for the curing shrinkage.

NOTE: Resins shrink when polymerized. Because there is a large volume of material, the shrinkage will be greater. Too much shrinkage will cause the record base to fit poorly. The slit allows shrinkage to occur without lifting material away from the palate (Figure 13-23).

7 Place the cast and record base in the light-curing unit on the turntable according to manufacturer's directions. Activate the turntable and cure for 2 to 4 minutes (Figure 13-24).

8 Place a small amount of the excess uncured base over the slit and press with your fingers. Cure again.
NOTE: This step seals the slit; the majority of the polymerization shrinkage has already occurred.

9 Remove record base from the cast, invert the record base, and cure again.

NOTE: Record base is inverted to cure the internal surface and ensure complete polymerization. The material is opaque and light does not penetrate enough to cure entirely through it from the outside.

10 Wipe the record base after curing with the alcohol 2 × 2s to remove the slippery film on the surface.

NOTE: Resins will have a thin layer of unpolymerized resin on surfaces in contact with air. Oxygen inhibits the polymerization of the resin at the surface. This same phenomenon is seen on the surface of composites and sealants.

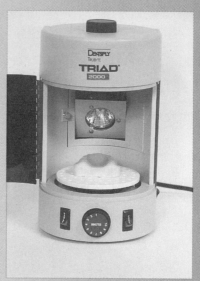

FIGURE 13-24

11 Mark with a pencil the excess acrylic that extends beyond the border of the vestibule. Grind the excess with an acrylic bur or sandpaper drum on a lathe in the laboratory to the correct thickness and length as directed by the dentist (Figure 13-25).

12 Thin the area over the ridges with the sandpaper drum or acrylic bur. Leave it approximately 0.5 mm thick.

NOTE: If the material is too thick over the ridges, it will interfere with the placement of denture teeth when they are set for the wax try-in appointment.

Continued on following page

PROCEDURE 13-2 (Continued)

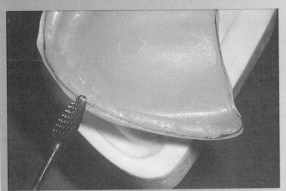

FIGURE 13-25

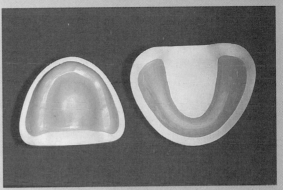

FIGURE 13-26

13 Smooth the periphery with pumice on a rag wheel.

NOTE: This is for the patient's comfort.

14 Confirm the fit on the cast. The record base is now ready for the application of wax rims (Figure 13-26).

PROVISIONAL
RESTORATIONS

OBJECTIVES

On completion of this chapter the student will be able to:

1. State the purpose of provisional coverage.
2. List examples of circumstances that may require provisional coverage.
3. Identify the criteria necessary for a high-quality provisional restoration.
4. List the properties of provisional materials.
5. Distinguish among properties that are important for posterior coverage, for anterior coverage, and for both anterior and posterior coverage.
6. Distinguish between intracoronal and extracoronal restorations.
7. List the advantages and disadvantages of preformed and custom crowns.
8. Differentiate between direct and indirect fabrication techniques.
9. List the advantages and disadvantages of acrylic and composite provisional materials.
10. Describe the technique for fabrication of metal, polycarbonate, custom, and cement provisional restorations.
11. List patient education and home care instructions.
12. Fabricate and cement a metal provisional crown.
13. Fabricate and cement a polycarbonate crown.

14. Fabricate and cement a custom provisional crown.
15. Place an intracoronal cement temporary restoration.

KEY TERMS

Provisional coverage—A restoration that temporarily occupies the place of a permanent restoration, typically for up to 2 to 3 weeks. In the case of implant and complex prosthodontic and periodontally involved cases, provisional restorations may be required to last for extended periods of time. These restorations are also commonly referred to as temporaries.

Finish line—The continuous margin that borders the preparation to which the restoration is fit or finished. For a cast or porcelain restoration, the circumference of the tooth at the finish line must be larger than the occlusal/incisal circumference.

Extracoronal restoration—A restoration that covers all or part of the external surface of the tooth and may extend over the cusp tips on facial or lingual surfaces or include the removal of cusps, such as onlays, three-quarter crowns, full crowns, and veneers.

Indirect fabrication—Provisional restorations made on a cast outside the patient's mouth.

Intracoronal restoration—A restoration within the crown of the tooth, such as an inlay.

Direct fabrication—Provisional restorations made directly inside the patient's mouth.

The increased demand for retention of natural teeth and new technology in restoring and replacing tooth structure has increased the need for high-quality fixed prosthodontic, pedodontic, and endodontic procedures. Fabricating provisional coverage is an important aspect in these treatments. Once the tooth has been prepared, the exposed dentin must be protected from the thermal, chemical, mechanical, and bacterial effects of the oral environment. The adjacent tissues must be protected and the position of the tooth must be maintained. All of this must be accomplished with the provisional coverage with the additional considerations of esthetics, function, and patient comfort.

The dental assistant and dental hygienist may be called on to fabricate, repair, remove, or maintain and give home care instructions for the provisional restoration for various periods of time during which temporary coverage is necessary.

Dental Procedures That May Require Provisional Coverage

Provisional coverage may be required in general, pedodontic, endodontic, and prosthodontic cases. Whenever a situation arises where a permanent restorative material cannot be placed at the time of preparation, a temporary or provisional material may be chosen (Table 14-1).

Criteria for Provisional Coverage

The criteria for a properly placed provisional restoration include the maintenance of tooth position, protection of hard and soft oral structures, and the establishment of function and esthetics. If these criteria are not met, pulpal and periodontal irritation, tooth migration, and patient dissatisfaction will very likely occur.

MAINTAIN PREPARED TOOTH POSITION TO ADJACENT AND OPPOSING TEETH

When a tooth has been prepared to receive a crown, sufficient tooth material has been removed to create a space between both the adjacent tooth and the opposing teeth. A prepared tooth without occlusal/incisal and proximal contact may migrate laterally or occlusally/incisally within a few days. The restoration, which was designed to fit the tooth in its original position, may now be too high because of occlusal/incisal

TABLE 14-1

Dental Procedures Requiring Provisional Coverage

Procedure	Type of Provisional Coverage
Endodontic access preparations	Closes endodontic access preparations between appointments
Vitality of the tooth is in question	Allows the pulp to respond to therapeutic agents or recover from the trauma of preparation
Emergency care	Prevents additional damage and improves esthetics and function while awaiting a permanent solution
Awaiting permanent restoration	Allows time for the laboratory fabrication of cast and porcelain restorations
Restoration of implants	For long-term provisional coverage while the implant site is allowed to heal
Restoration of primary teeth	Placed on primary teeth because of extensive caries, pulpotomies, or pulpectomies until permanent teeth erupt

migration or not seat properly as a result of lateral migration of the prepared tooth. If the provisional restoration itself is too high, the results may be those associated with trauma from occlusion, and if it does not contact adjacent teeth, gingival irritation from food impaction is likely. It is important that precise occlusal/incisal and proximal contacts be provided for. The provisional restoration should share the forces of the adjacent and opposing teeth.

PROTECT THE EXPOSED TOOTH SURFACES AND MARGINS

When the tooth is prepared, the dentinal tubules are exposed to potentially harmful thermal, chemical, mechanical, and bacterial effects of the oral cavity. These opened tubules leave the pulp vulnerable to the effects of temperature and the chemical irritants of the material placed. Provisional materials placed near the pulp must have no adverse chemical effect and be sufficiently insulating to protect the pulp from thermal assaults.

The margins, or **finish line,** of the preparation are particularly susceptible to fracture if not adequately supported. Well-adapted provisional restorations protect the finish line from fracture and from the marginal leakage of oral fluids and bacteria. If the finish line is damaged, the permanent restoration will no longer fit precisely, leaving space for future leakage of oral fluids. The process of caries may even begin during the time the provisional restoration is in place. Because temporary luting agents are highly soluble and may wash out from under the provisional restoration, they cannot be expected to make up for marginal deficiencies.

PROTECT THE GINGIVAL TISSUES

Most crown preparations extend subgingivally, making the margins and the overall contour of the provisional restoration critical to periodontal health. Periodontal tissues are susceptible to irritation from overcontoured, overextended, or overhanging margins; trauma from food impaction; and buildup of plaque. Margins must be flush with the preparation. If a margin is overextended, the resultant tissue irritation may result in gingival recession, adversely affecting the cosmetic effect of the permanent restoration. All surfaces of the provisional restoration must be properly contoured and maintain contacts with adjacent teeth. If surfaces are undercontoured or contacts weak or nonexistent, the process of chewing will excessively force food directly onto the gingiva rather than deflecting it facially and lingually. An overcontured restoration may trap plaque by not allowing for any self-cleansing or gingival stimulation from the chewing process. Both scenarios may lead to irritation, inflammation, and recession (Figure 14-1).

PROVIDE FUNCTION AND ESTHETICS

The provisional restoration should restore ideal occlusal/incisal and surface anatomy. As previously mentioned, deficiencies in contour or contact of the provisional restoration may lead to problems that compromise or prevent the ideal placement of a permanent restoration. Patients must be able to chew, speak, and clean the provisional restoration as they would function with a permanent one. In addition, it is important to consider the importance of esthetics in collaboration with concerns for function. Provisional

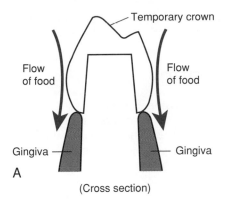

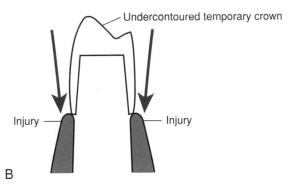

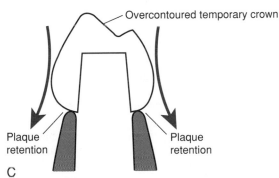

FIGURE 14-1 ■ **A,** Properly contoured provisional crown. **B,** Undercontoured provisional crown. **C,** Overcontoured provisional crown.

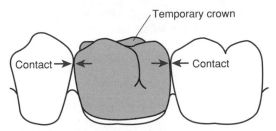

FIGURE 14-2 ■ The provisional crown duplicates natural tooth contour, contact, and occlusion.

CRITERIA FOR PROVISIONAL COVERAGE

Provisional coverage must:
- Reproduce proper interproximal contacts and occlusal alignment
- Contact the tooth at the finish line
- Be contoured to reproduce natural tooth structure
- Remain stable, be functional, and be esthetic

Properties of Provisional Materials

Materials used to fabricate provisional restorations must have properties that comply with the specific requirement of the situation and area in which they are placed. Although most provisional restorations are in place for up to 2 to 3 weeks, provisional coverage may be required for extended periods of time. Strength and hardness are important for posterior and **extracoronal restorations.** Tissue conditions in many areas will not impede the construction of provisional restorations with the direct technique. However, when conditions warrant the compatibility of tissues and the chemical reaction during fabrication must be a consideration. Esthetic concerns are important for many applications; provisional restorations are no exception. In addition, considerations of handling are of special concern in areas difficult to access.

STRENGTH

Materials must have sufficient compressive and tensile strength to resist the forces of mastication. Materials that are used for temporary bridges must

restorations must look like natural tooth structures whenever esthetics is important. Matching shades and customizing provisional materials to duplicate the natural teeth will greatly enhance patient acceptance and thus the success of the provisional restoration (Figure 14-2).

also have sufficient flexural strength to resist deformation from flexing during mastication. Brittle materials such as composite resins do not hold up well when used for long span bridges or with patients who are bruxers.

HARDNESS

The surface hardness must be sufficient to resist abrasion and wear for the period through which the provisional restoration is to be worn. The material should also be able to be polished to a smooth surface and should retain that surface throughout its use.

TISSUE COMPATIBILITY

The material should not produce any additional irritation to pulpal or gingival tissues either during or after setting reactions. Materials that have adverse setting reactions must be carefully considered and may be more appropriate if using the **indirect fabrication** technique. In addition, for patient comfort, materials should not absorb or give off odors or taste.

ESTHETICS

Materials used in areas of esthetic concern must match tooth structures and have good color stability and stain resistance.

HANDLING

Materials must be fast and easy to use, reliable, and inexpensive. The material should have sufficient working time and simplified technique to allow for fabrication. For many customized provisional materials, the working time must also allow for removal from the mouth while still elastic for trimming before reinsertion. For these materials, *tear strength,* the ability of the material to resist tearing or distortion on removal from the mouth or model, is a consideration. The setting time must be fast and accommodate difficult to access areas when using light-activated materials. Materials should be repairable to account for defects and to modify fit. Adding provisional material directly to the margins for repair will help provide good marginal integrity, and relining the provisional with a new mix of material will ensure a good fit. Materials must be eco-nomical to use; provisional coverage must not be excessive in cost of materials or time of fabrication.

Provisional Materials

The choice of provisional material is generally dependent on the type of preparation, area of the mouth, and operator preference. Provisional materials include metals, polycarbonate, acrylics, composites, and cements. These materials may be used alone or in combination such as an aluminum shell crown lined with acrylic. Provisional restorations may be preformed, such as stainless steel or polycarbonate crowns, or made specifically for individual procedures, such as custom acrylic or composite crowns and **intracoronal restorations.**

Provisional cements, acrylic, or composite materials are mixed and placed in a plastic state and allowed to harden either directly in the preparation or on a stone model. Cements are limited to intracoronal placement; provisional acrylic and composites can be used for extracoronal coverage as well.

Preformed crowns have the advantage of convenience, in that they are already premade in a variety of sizes and anatomic forms. This saves time because it eliminates the need for a crown template and is particularly useful in emergency situations and for badly broken down teeth. Even though they come in different sizes, time must be spent establishing contact, contour, occlusion, and marginal integrity.

Customized crowns are more versatile and more consistently meet the criteria for successful provisional restorations. They do, however, require the additional step of obtaining a template or matrix for the final product. This template is a reproduction of the tooth structures as they exist before the preparation. This additional step can be further complicated if the original tooth is badly broken down or fractured.

Temporary luting cements are used to cement provisional crowns in place.

PREFORMED CROWNS

The process of temporization using preformed crowns includes the use of stainless steel and aluminum crowns, polycarbonate, and celluloid crown forms lined with acrylic or composite materials (Figure 14-3). As previously mentioned, this method

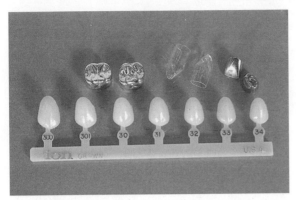

FIGURE 14-3 ■ Aluminum shell, celluloid crown, stainless steel, and polycarbonate crown forms.

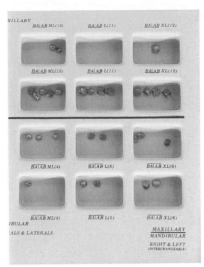

FIGURE 14-4 ■ A selection of pedodontic stainless steel crowns.

may be time saving, particularly in emergency situations when the patient has a fractured tooth, but does not consistently produce successful temporization when less than ideal situations exist. A crown with exact interproximal and length dimensions may require considerable adjustments of the preformed crown. Because the prepared tooth is much smaller than this preformed shell, a reline of acrylic or composite material is generally required. Metal crowns are generally used only in posterior cases with polycarbonate and celluloid forms used on anterior teeth. Preformed crowns may be used for single crowns only and are not appropriate for temporary bridges.

STAINLESS STEEL CROWNS

The stainless steel crown is the most durable of the preformed crowns, providing provisional coverage lasting months and even years (Figure 14-4). The stainless steel crown has been traditionally used to restore primary teeth. These durable and economical restorations are now being considered for older adults where financial and health concerns would otherwise result in the recommendation of extractions. The primary advantage of these crowns is their malleability, which provides for good contact, occlusion, and marginal integrity. The crown is cut with crown and bridge scissors and crimped and contoured at the contact and margins with crimping and contouring pliers. If the stainless steel crown is replacing the use of a cast restoration for prolonged periods of time, minimal reduction of the tooth is ideal to preserve natural strength and protect the pulp. With the marginal seal and occlusion intact,

these crowns may be a solution to long-term provisional coverage of posterior teeth. Margins of stainless steel crowns are never a replacement for cast restorations.

ALUMINUM SHELL CROWNS

Aluminum shell crowns are used for provisional coverage of posterior teeth. Lined with acrylics or composites and cemented with temporary cement, a well-fitted aluminum shell crown can last for several weeks. The softness of the metal allows for easy manipulation of the contact, occlusion, and margins because the metal can be stretched and burnished without wrinkling. These crowns are easily trimmed with crown and bridge scissors to adjust their length. Because of their softness, these crowns wear easily and must be checked for occlusal integrity.

POLYCARBONATE AND CELLULOID CROWN FORMS

Preformed polycarbonate crowns, like their metal partners, come in several sizes and shapes. Unlike metal, they are rigid and may need to be adapted with acrylic burs and disks or may be carefully cut with sharp crown scissors. The primary advantage is their esthetics for replacement of anterior teeth and the compatibility with acrylic resins to further customize the fit and margins.

Performed celluloid forms are filled with acrylic resins or composites, which are matched to tooth shade, and then inserted onto the prepared tooth in much the same way a template is used in the **direct fabrication** technique. The form must first be cut to fit the tooth, which can easily be accomplished with scissors. Usually one or two small holes are placed in the occlusal portion of the crown form to allow excess resin or composite material to flow out when the crown form is seated. This prevents trapping air and creation of voids in the material.

CUSTOMIZED PROVISIONALS

The use of acrylics and composites, both self-cured and light-cured, to produce high-quality custom provisional restoration for inlays, crowns, and bridges has gained the market share of provisional materials (Figure 14-5). Whether fabricated directly in the mouth or indirectly on a stone cast or poly-vinyl siloxane (PVS) die, these custom provisionals more consistently meet the criteria for a successful provisional restoration. A customized provisional for individual situations allows for better function and fit. The superior esthetics improves patient acceptability, and the ability to fabricate multiunit temporary bridges for replacement of missing teeth makes these materials extremely popular.

A matrix or template creates the external contours and anatomy, and the prepared tooth or stone model creates the internal dimensions. Matrix or template materials include thermoplastic wax, alginate, silicone impression materials, and vacuum-formed plastic. Alginate and wax are the easiest and least expensive templates and are used extensively for single-unit, direct-technique provisionals. Vacuum-formed plastic is the most common choice for multiunit and indirect provisional techniques (Figure 14-6).

Direct Technique   Using the direct technique for provisional coverage, the provisional is fabricated directly on the prepared tooth. A template of the tooth before preparation is obtained using wax or an impression material directly in the mouth. After the tooth is prepared, the template is filled with a provisional material and reinserted into the mouth. This technique is faster and provides a provisional restoration that duplicates the original tooth. Problems with access and damage to inflamed tissues must be evaluated before using this technique.

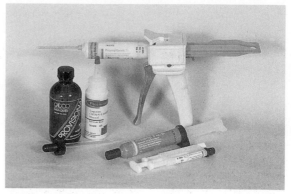

FIGURE 14-5 ■ Acrylic and composite provisional crown materials in hand mix and automix.

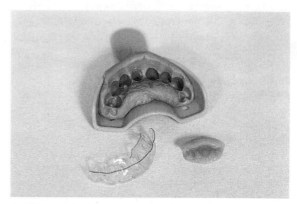

FIGURE 14-6 ■ Silicone putty, thermoplastic wax, and vacuum-formed plastic templates.

Indirect Technique   Using the indirect technique, an impression of the area is made and poured in stone; the template is then made on this model. If it is necessary to account for missing tooth structure caused by caries or trauma, the defect can be corrected on the model with wax or other materials. The template can be used directly in the mouth, or the process can continue indirectly with fabrication of the provisional on the model and then relined before it is placed on the preparation. Some operators prefer to prepare the stone model by cutting the replica tooth to closely duplicate the final preparation, thus further customizing the provisional and eliminating excessive relining. The process of producing indirect provisional restorations is similar to the indirect composite procedure discussed in Chapter 6. The indirect technique allows for superior access and the time and convenience for making multiunit bridges or crowns in difficult to access areas. Although the indirect technique requires the additional time to fabricate a stone model or PVS die, this technique may well end up saving time in complicated cases and may be required if hard or soft tissue conditions would be further traumatized by direct fabrication.

ACRYLIC PROVISIONAL MATERIALS

Acrylic materials in the form of methacrylates have been used for many years as custom temporaries. Their good esthetics, ease of manipulation, and low cost made them a popular choice over preformed crowns. The high shrinkage and heat released during polymerization and patient complaints regarding the acrylic odor and taste are distinct disadvantages. Care must be taken in their fabrication to "pump" them on and off the preparation after initial polymerization to prevent them from locking on the tooth and protect the tooth from heat generated during polymerization. If these materials are allowed to polymerize outside the preparation, the amount of shrinkage may be sufficient to inhibit their seat. Their low cost, variety of shades available, and color stability make them an appropriate choice in many situations (Figure 14-7).

> **CAUTION**
> *Heat generated during the polymerization of chemical-cured acrylic can potentially damage the pulp or burn soft tissues, especially when used in a large volume such as a bridge pontic.*

COMPOSITE PROVISIONAL MATERIALS

Composite provisional materials were developed to offset the disadvantages of the acrylic materials. Low shrinkage and heat release during curing, good strength, less wear, and biocompatibility are distinct advantages. These advantages come with a noticeable increase in cost, and some of these materials are too brittle for long span bridges, especially when used on bruxers. Light-cured, self-cured, and dual-cured versions of these materials are available. Automixed and hand-mixed self-cured materials may be used with any matrix. Light-cured materials

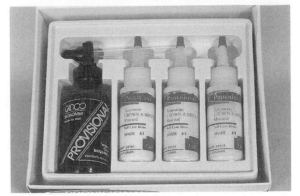

FIGURE 14-7 ■ Acrylic provisional material: liquid and three shades of powder.

TABLE 14-2

Properties of Acrylic and Composite Provisional Materials

Acrylic	Composite
High heat during polymerization	Low heat during curing
High shrinkage during polymerization	Low shrinkage during curing
Possible tissue irritation	Good tissue biocompatibility
Poor taste and smell	Good hardness and flexural strength
Variety of color shades	Color shades are limited
Inexpensive	Expensive

require clear plastic templates and are difficult to cure in deep areas. The dual-cured materials require additional time to light-cure after the chemical cure, but allow for removal from undercut areas while still puttylike and are then trimmed and replaced for final curing (Table 14-2).

Intracoronal Cement Provisionals

Patients requiring less extensive provisional coverage, such as in the case of endodontic procedures, inlays, and less extensive emergency care, may benefit from cement provisionals. In addition, because cement provisionals are most frequently fabricated with zinc oxide eugenol cement, the additional palliative

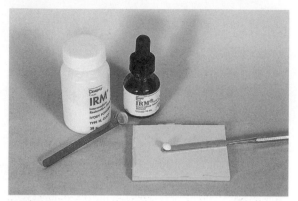

FIGURE 14-8 ■ Provisional cement used for intracoronal provisional coverage.

benefits of the cement may be helpful to sensitive or traumatized teeth (Figure 14-8). It should be noted that zinc oxide eugenol provisionals should not be used if a permanent restoration is to be cemented with a resin luting agent, because eugenol-containing cements inhibit polymerization of the resin cement.

Cements are placed directly into the cavity preparation with the aid of matrix and wedge when appropriate. The cement is carved and contoured and allowed to set. Final check of occlusion is done with articulating paper followed by additional carving as necessary. These materials are highly soluble, have low strength, and have an unpleasant taste, limiting them to short-term and protected intracoronal placement.

> **CAUTION**
> *Eugenol-containing provisional restorations or luting agents should not be used if the final restoration will be bonded or cemented with a resin cement. Eugenol inhibits the set of resins.*

Patient Education

Scheduled appointment time for fabricating provisional coverage must be adequate to instruct and demonstrate appropriate home care techniques, educate patients as to the limitations and expectations of the coverage, and address patient concerns. Patients should appreciate that provisional coverage, although functional and frequently esthetic, does not give the same results as permanent coverage.

Because of limitations in the provisional materials, patients must be instructed not to eat sticky or hard foods in that area and instructed that there may be a possible increase in temperature sensitivity and taste associated with the provisional material. To avoid costly appointment time resulting from tooth movement or loss of tooth structure, patients must be told to immediately call the office if the provisional is dislodged or lost. Strict adherence to appointment intervals is extremely important. Patients must return to the office at the appropriate time for the placement of the permanent restoration. Limitations in esthetics may include imperfections in color matching, anatomic contour, and smoothness. To avoid dissatisfaction, patients must be reminded that temporary restorations are not the same as permanent ones.

> **CLINICAL TIP** If a provisional crown comes off during a time that the dental office is closed, the patient can be instructed to replace it after cleaning the interior of the crown and placing a small amount of denture adhesive into the crown.

Home care instructions include brushing the restoration (as any other tooth) and flossing, but removing the floss by pulling it out to the side under the contact rather than back in an occlusal/incisal direction. Removing the floss back through the contact in an occlusal/incisal direction might dislodge the provisional coverage because it is usually cemented with a weak provisional cement. If the provisional coverage includes a pontic, the additional use of floss threaders or end-tufted brushes must be stressed for cleaning the tissue-contacting surface and the proximal embrasures. The maintenance of healthy tissue during provisional coverage is crucial to the success of the permanent restoration.

SUMMARY

Provisional coverage provides protection of tooth and periodontal structures for a variety of dental procedures. Regardless of the material and technique selected, a high-quality provisional restoration must have proper contact, contour, and occlusion and be functional and acceptable to the patient. If these criteria are not met, pulpal and periodontal irritation, tooth migration, and patient dissatisfaction will likely occur.

CHAPTER REVIEW

Select the one correct response for each of the following multiple-choice questions:

1. **Intracoronal provisional restorations must**
   a. Contact adjacent teeth and be crimped with crimping pliers to fit snugly
   b. Contact adjacent teeth, be crimped with crimping pliers to fit snugly, and be sealed at the margins
   c. Contact adjacent teeth and be sealed at the margins
   d. Contact adjacent teeth, be crimped with crimping pliers to fit snugly, be sealed at the margins, and be made of metal for strength on posterior teeth

2. **Polycarbonate crowns are primarily used**
   a. On posterior teeth
   b. On anterior teeth
   c. For multiunit bridges
   d. For inlays

3. **If provisional coverage does not fit the tooth properly**
   a. Food impaction may occur and periodontal irritation may occur
   b. Periodontal irritation may occur and tooth migration may occur
   c. Food impaction may occur, periodontal irritation may occur, and hypersensitivity of the prepared tooth may occur
   d. Food impaction may occur, periodontal irritation may occur, hypersensitivity of the prepared tooth may occur, and tooth migration may occur

4. **Properties of provisional materials used for posterior teeth include all of the following EXCEPT:**
   a. Strength
   b. Tissue compatibility
   c. Esthetics
   d. Ease of handling

5. **All of the following are appropriate choices for extracoronal provisional coverage EXCEPT:**
   a. Cements
   b. Provisional composite material
   c. Polycarbonate crowns
   d. Provisional acrylic material

6. **You will need to obtain a prepreparation template of the tooth before fabricating**
   a. Intracoronal provisional restorations
   b. Aluminum crown provisionals
   c. Polycarbonate crown provisionals
   d. Custom provisional restorations

7. **The first step in fabricating a stainless steel crown is**
   a. Determining occlusal/incisal to gingival dimensions
   b. Determining mesial/distal dimensions
   c. Determining contour of finish line
   d. Determining occlusal height

8. **To customize the internal fit of a preformed crown**
   a. Composite provisional material is used
   b. Zinc phosphate cement is used
   c. Acrylic provisional material is used
   d. Composite and acrylic provisional materials are used

9. **When placing cement temporary restorations**
    a. Wipe the cement toward the margin
    b. Wipe the cement away from the margin
    c. Wipe the cement toward the matrix band
    d. Allow the cement to harden before sealing the margins

10. **Criteria for a cement temporary includes all of the following EXCEPT:**
    a. Marginal ridges at the same height as adjacent teeth
    b. Sufficient contact with adjacent teeth
    c. Detailed occlusal anatomy
    d. Reproduction of gingival embrasure

CASE-BASED DISCUSSION TOPICS

◉ How would each of the following situations be best handled? *(1) A patient has a badly fractured central incisor. Which provisional material and technique would be most appropriate? (2) A custom composite provisional is deficient at the gingival margin of the facial surface. How would you correct this problem? (3) Your patient is concerned about the color match and smoothness of the provisional crown. Which provisional material and technique would be most appropriate? (4) A three-unit posterior bridge is appointed. The patient has very limited opening due to temporomandibular joint pain. Which provisional material and technique would be most appropriate?*

REFERENCES

Albers HF: *Temporary crown and bridge fabrication,* ed 4, Cotati, CA, 1985, Alto Books.
Anglis L: Provisional restorations and patient satisfaction, *General Dentistry* 46(2):197, 1998.
Berry T, Troendle K: Provisional restorations: guidelines for proper selection, placement, *Dental Teamwork* p 25, Nov/Dec 1995.
Berry T, Troendle K: Provisional restorations: guidelines for custom fit, oral hygiene care, *Dental Teamwork* p 23, Jan/Feb 1996.
Christensen G: Provisional restorations for fixed prosthodontics, *J Am Dent Assoc* 127:150, 1996.
Ettinger R et al: An in vitro evaluation of the integrity of stainless steel crown margins cemented with different luting agents, *SCD Special Care in Dentistry* 18(2):78, 1998.
Gottlieb M: Using an old technique with modern materials to fabricate esthetic temporary restorations, *J Am Dent Assoc* 130(1):99, 1999.
Hester R: Fabricating high-quality provisional restorations for indirect inlays, onlays or crown preparations, *J Am Dent Assoc* 130(7):1093, 1999.
Higginbottom F: Quality provisional restorations: a must for successful restorative dentistry, *Compendium* 16(5):442, 1995.
Lepe X et al: Retention of provisional crowns fabricated from two materials with the use of four temporary cements, *J Prosthet Dent* 81(4):469, 1999.
Miller M, editor: *Reality,* vol 13, *Provisional crowns,* Houston 1999, Reality Publishing.
Provisional materials, *Dental Advisor* 12(3):1, 1995.
Yannikakis S et al: Color stability of provisional resin materials, *J Prosthet Dent* 80(5):533, 1998.

PROCEDURE 14-1 (See p. 349 for competency sheet)

Metal Provisional Crown

EQUIPMENT/SUPPLIES (Figure 14-9)

- Mirror and explorer
- Selection of metal crowns
- Crown and bridge scissors
- Contouring pliers
- Ball burnisher
- Articulating paper
- Dental floss
- Isolation materials
- Cement and armamentarium
- Sandpaper disk and rubber wheel

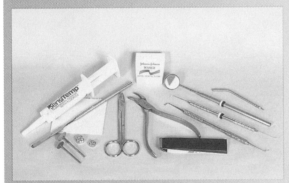

FIGURE 14-9

PROCEDURE STEPS

1 Measure the mesiodistal width of the space between adjacent teeth.

2 Choose a crown that has a mesiodistal width equal to that of the original tooth.

NOTE: If the crown does not fit, it may be sterilized and replaced in the kit.

3 Try in the crown, noting the occlusal relationship to adjacent and opposing dentition.

NOTE: The crown will be considerably higher than the adjacent teeth (Figure 14-10).

4 Scribe a line on the facial and lingual crown surfaces to match the contour of the gingiva, and approximate the amount of crown length that must be trimmed.

NOTE: The crown is longer on the facial and lingual surfaces and shorter on the mesial and distal, forming a waving line.

5 Trim to within 1 mm of the scribed line using curved crown and bridge scissors.

NOTE: Try to blend your cutting junctions to avoid producing burs of metal that will irritate the tissues (Figure 14-11).

6 Contour the trimmed areas using contouring pliers. Advance the pliers around the crown periphery as you continually squeeze the pliers with the ball portion of the pliers inside the crown and the curved beak on the outside of the crown.

NOTE: This inverts the crown edge, adapting the circumference to the finish line (Figure 14-12).

7 Retry crown to confirm fit.

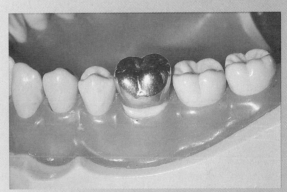

FIGURE 14-10

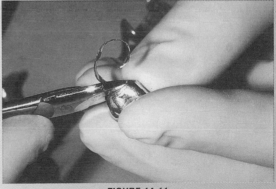

FIGURE 14-11

Continued on following page

PROCEDURE 14-1 (Continued)

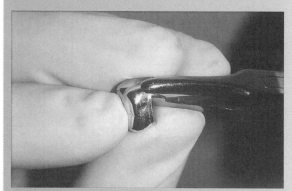

FIGURE 14-12

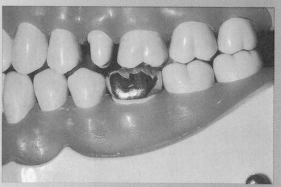

FIGURE 14-13

8 Check occlusion with articulating paper; make sure the crown is occluding properly when the patient's teeth are in occlusion.

NOTE: If the crown is interfering with occlusion, further reduction will be necessary, either by trimming the margins or by reducing the occlusal height on the occlusal surface. Only minor adjustments will be able to be made on the occlusal surface before perforating the surface (Figure 14-13).

9 Check the contacts using dental floss to determine if contacts are present and in the proper location.

NOTE: If contact points must be established, use the ball burnisher or contouring pliers with the ball portion inside and curved beak outside and gently squeeze to establish the contact at the appropriate location.

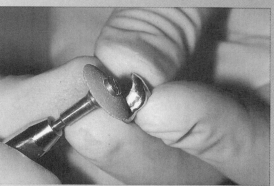

FIGURE 14-14

10 Trim and polish the crown margins with disks and a rubber wheel to make the crown smooth and prevent tissue irritation (Figure 14-14).

11 Isolate the area and cement following the manufacturer's directions for mixing the appropriate cement.

NOTE: Completely coat the inside surfaces of the crown to avoid trapping air.

12 Seat the crown onto the preparation and have the patient bite on a cotton roll or wooden stick in a mesiodistal direction to improve force distribution.

NOTE: Make sure the patient is *not* biting only on the crown rather than the adjacent teeth in the quadrant because this may force the crown too far in a gingival direction (Figure 14-15).

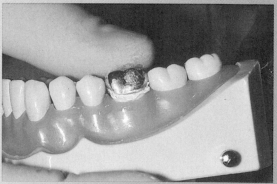

FIGURE 14-15

13 When appropriate, remove excess facial and lingual cement. Remove interproximal cement by drawing dental floss through the contact (Figure 14-16).

Continued on following page

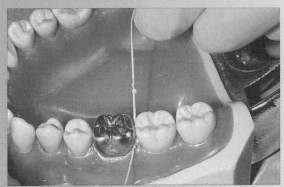

FIGURE 14-16

OPTIONAL STEPS

NOTE: The crown may be lined with an acrylic or composite provisional material to further customize the internal fit.

1 Mix the acrylic or composite provisional material according to the manufacturer's directions.

2 Place the material in the prepared crown, making sure to line the crown to avoid trapping air.

3 Place the crown back on the preparation and have the patient bite in occlusion.

4 After the material has reached the desired consistency, remove the crown and remove the excess.

NOTE: Material should be removed while still elastic to avoid trapping the crown in undercuts.

5 Polish the crown and proceed with steps 11 through 13.

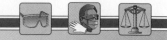

PROCEDURE 14-2 (See p. 350 for competency sheet)

Polycarbonate Provisional Crown

EQUIPMENT/SUPPLIES (Figure 14-17)

- Mirror and explorer
- Selection of polycarbonate crowns
- Articulating paper
- Dental floss
- Acrylic stones and sandpaper disks
- Pumice and rag wheel
- Isolation materials
- Cement and armamentarium

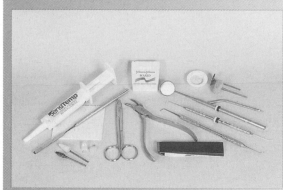

FIGURE 14-17

PROCEDURE STEPS

1 Measure the mesiodistal width of the space between adjacent teeth.

2 Choose a crown that has a mesiodistal width equal to that of the original tooth.

NOTE: Choose a crown that is slightly larger if an exact size cannot be found.

3 Try in the crown, noting the occlusal relationship to adjacent and opposing dentition.

NOTE: The crown will be considerably higher than the adjacent teeth. If the crown does not fit, it may be sterilized and replaced in the kit (Figure 14-18).

4 Scribe a line on the facial and lingual crown surfaces to match the contour of the gingiva, and approximate the amount of crown length that must be trimmed.

NOTE: The crown is longer on the facial and lingual surfaces and shorter on the mesial and distal, forming a waving line.

5 Trim to within 1 mm of the scribed line with scissors or an acrylic stone on a slow-speed handpiece.

NOTE: Trim a small amount at a time, continuing to try and retry the crown until the desired amount is removed. If the crown was slightly larger than the space, it may be necessary to trim the proximal surfaces to establish a good seat (Figure 14-19).

6 Check occlusion with articulating paper; make sure the crown is occluding properly when the patient's teeth are in occlusion.

NOTE: If the crown is interfering with occlusion, further reduction will be necessary, either by trimming the margins or by reducing the occlusal height on the occlusal surface. Only minor adjustments will be able to be made on the occlusal surface before perforating the surface.

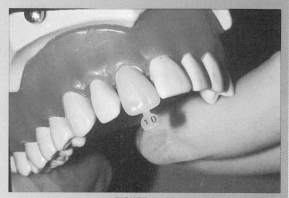

FIGURE 14-18

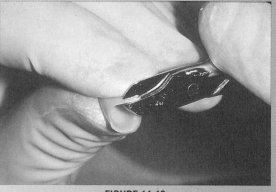

FIGURE 14-19

Continued on following page

PROCEDURE 14-2 (Continued)

7 Check the contacts using dental floss to determine if contacts are present and in the proper location.

NOTE: If contact points are too tight or not at appropriate location, you will need to trim the proximal surface of the crown to establish correct location. If contact points are not present, you may need to add to the proximal surface with acrylic.

8 Trim and polish the crown margins with disks and pumice on a rag wheel to make the crown smooth and prevent tissue irritation.

9 Isolate the area and cement following the manufacturer's directions for mixing the appropriate cement.

NOTE: Completely coat the inside surfaces of the crown to avoid trapping air.

10 Seat the crown onto the preparation and have the patient bite on a cotton roll or wooden stick in a mesiodistal direction to improve force distribution.

NOTE: Make sure the patient is *not* biting only on the crown rather than the adjacent teeth in the quadrant because this may force the crown too far in a gingival direction (Figure 14-20).

11 When appropriate, remove excess facial and lingual cement. Remove interproximal cement by drawing dental floss through the contact.

OPTIONAL STEPS

NOTE: The crown may be lined with an acrylic or composite provisional material to further customize the internal fit.

1 Mix the provisional material according to the manufacturer's directions (Figure 14-21).

2 Place the material in the prepared crown, making sure to line the crown to avoid trapping air (Figure 14-22).

3 Place the crown back on the preparation and have the patient bite in occlusion (Figure 14-23).

4 After the material has reached the desired consistency, remove the crown and remove the excess.

NOTE: Material should be removed while still elastic to avoid trapping the crown in undercuts (Figure 14-24).

5 Polish the crown and proceed with steps 8 through 11 (Figures 14-25 and 14-26).

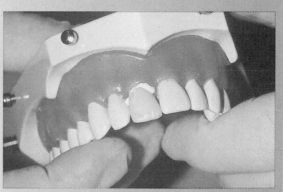

FIGURE 14-20

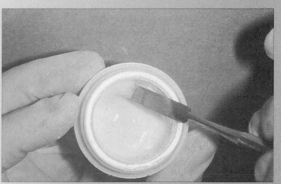

FIGURE 14-21

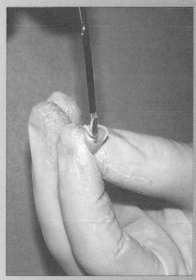

FIGURE 14-22

Continued on following page

PROCEDURE 14-2 (Continued)

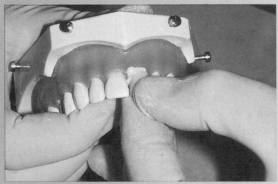

FIGURE 14-23

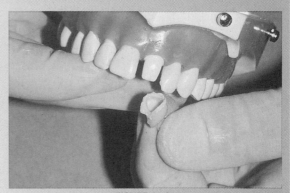

FIGURE 14-24

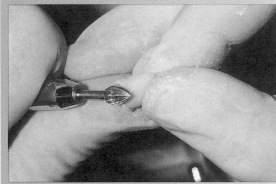

FIGURE 14-25

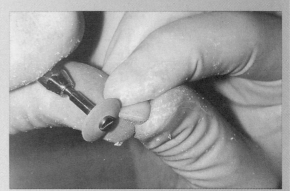

FIGURE 14-26

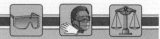

PROCEDURE 14-3 (See p. 351 for competency sheet)

Custom Provisional Coverage: Direct Technique

EQUIPMENT/SUPPLIES (Figure 14-27)

- Mirror and explorer
- Template of the tooth before preparation
- Acrylic or composite provisional material
- Separating medium
- Dispensing syringe
- Acrylic stones and sandpaper disks
- Pumice and rag wheel
- Isolation materials
- Cement and armamentarium

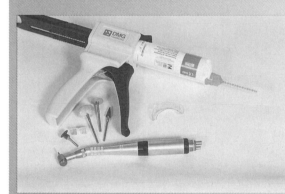

FIGURE 14-27

PROCEDURE STEPS: PREPARING THE TEMPLATE

1 Before preparing the tooth, prepare the template by taking an alginate impression or using a thermoplastic button.

NOTE: Alginate impressions should be kept moist until used.

2 Trim the alginate impression or thermoplastic button to relieve undercuts.

OR

1 Before preparing the tooth, obtain an alginate impression and pour in stone.

2 Using a vacuum former and an acrylic template sheet, fabricate a custom acrylic template of the quadrant.

3 Trim the template to relieve undercuts.

PROCEDURE STEPS: PREPARING THE PROVISIONAL COVERAGE

1 Coat the prepared tooth with separating medium.

NOTE: This will aid in separating the material from the preparation while in a doughy stage (Figure 14-28).

2 Thoroughly dry the template.

NOTE: This is not necessary if using a vacuum-formed template.

3 Prepare the acrylic or composite provisional material according to the manufacturer's directions.

NOTE: Custom shading must be considered at this time, matching adjacent teeth.

4 Dispense the provisional material directly into the template, making sure not to trap air.

NOTE: A delivery syringe is useful to extrude material directly into the template beginning at the bottom (Figure 14-29).

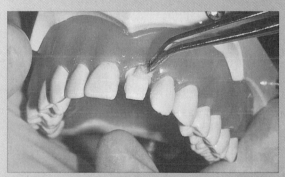

FIGURE 14-28

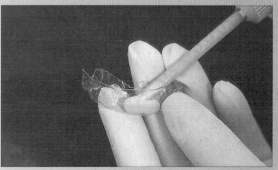

FIGURE 14-29

Continued on following page

PROCEDURE 14-3 (Continued)

5 Place the template back into the patient's mouth, aligning it precisely on the prepared tooth.

NOTE: A notch cut in the template at a visually accessible location will help facilitate replacing the template in the mouth (Figure 14-30).

6 Check the initial set of the material in the patient's mouth; initial set occurs within 1 to 3 minutes.

NOTE: Check material in the patient's mouth, because heat and moisture will accelerate the set; use the material that has extruded from the location notch.

7 Remove the template with provisional material in place when a firm/elastic consistency is reached.

NOTE: If the material is too soft it will tear or stretch; if too hard it may be difficult to remove it from undercut areas.

8 Remove the provisional material from the template and allow it to reach its final set.

NOTE: If acrylic materials are used, you must immediately replace the provisional back onto the preparation to avoid polymerization shrinkage. If composite materials are used, you should allow the material to reach its final set outside the mouth.

9 Trim excess material with acrylic stones and disks.

NOTE: If composite material is used, you will first have to remove the greasy air-inhibited layer of unset resin with alcohol.

10 Reinsert the provisional and check occlusion and contact, adjusting as necessary.

NOTE: If slight air voids are present, they may be repaired with freshly mixed material (Figures 14-31 and 14-32).

11 Finish polishing with pumice or whiting on a rag wheel.

12 Cement with appropriate luting agent and remove excess.

NOTE: The custom provisional may be completely fabricated on a stone model and then tried into the mouth and adjusted as necessary.

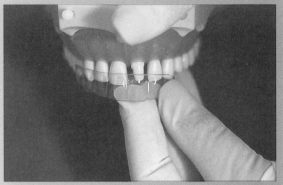

FIGURE 14-30

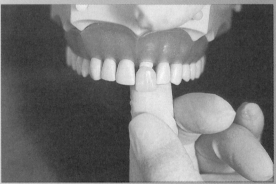

FIGURE 14-31

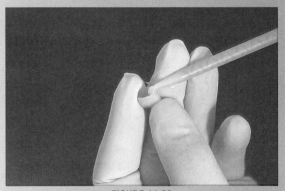

FIGURE 14-32

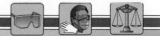

PROCEDURE 14-4 (See p. 352 for competency sheet)

Intracoronal Cement Temporary Restoration

EQUIPMENT/SUPPLIES (Figure 14-33)

- Mouth mirror and explorer
- Isolation materials
- Matrix band and wedges
- Matrix retainer
- Cotton pliers
- Burnisher
- Temporary cement (powder/liquid)
- Paper mixing pad
- Cement spatula
- Plastic instrument
- Condenser
- Occlusal carver
- Interproximal carver
- Articulating paper
- Dental floss

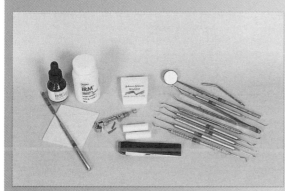

FIGURE 14-33

PROCEDURE STEPS

1 Isolate tooth and note size and class of cavity.

NOTE: This will determine the amount of cement necessary and the size of matrix for placement.

2 Place matrix and wedge.

NOTE: Be sure to obtain contact with adjacent teeth; use a burnisher to press the band to the adjacent tooth at the contact area.

3 Prepare a mix of the temporary cement to a puttylike consistency.

NOTE: The mix should be lightly coated in powder and not stick to your gloved fingers (Figure 14-34).

4 Roll the mix into a small ball and place a portion into proximal area.

NOTE: Begin by filling the proximal areas, then across the pulpal floor (Figure 14-35).

5 Use the condenser to condense into the preparation, packing the cement firmly to avoid trapping air.

NOTE: Tap the end of the condenser into remaining loose powder to prevent it from sticking to the cement.

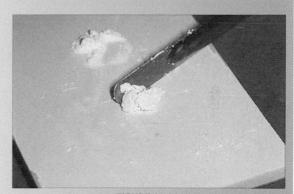

FIGURE 14-34

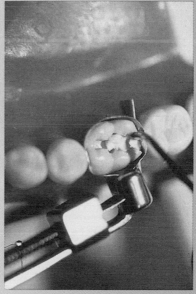

FIGURE 14-35

Continued on following page

6 Place and pack cement into rest of cavity with the condenser.

7 Do not overfill; pack cement only slightly higher than the cavosurface margin of the preparation.

8 Using the blade of the plastic instrument, wipe material toward margin to ensure good seal.

NOTE: Always wipe toward the margins; wiping away from the margins will pull material away from this important area (Figure 14-36).

9 Remove excess material around matrix in proximal areas and at occlusal margins.

NOTE: Remove excess carefully because material has not set. Material must be set enough so it is not pulled from the preparation margins.

10 Remove wedges, retainer, and matrix.

NOTE: Be careful not to pull material away with the band.

11 Seal any open proximal margins by wiping still-malleable cement toward them.

12 Remove proximal and gingival excess with interproximal carver, then from marginal ridge.

NOTE: The marginal ridge should be at the same height as that of the adjacent tooth.

13 Create embrasure.

14 Remove excess from occlusal surface and carve anatomic form with an occlusal carver.

NOTE: The occlusal anatomy should approximate the original tooth form; it is not necessary to carve detailed anatomy (Figure 14-37).

15 Carve from tooth to filling material, keeping half the instrument on the tooth and half on the filling.

NOTE: This prevents breaking the material from the margins or ditching the margins of the material.

16 Check the occlusion with articulating paper; adjust as necessary.

17 Check contacts with dental floss.

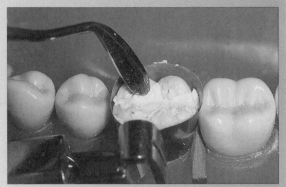

FIGURE 14-36

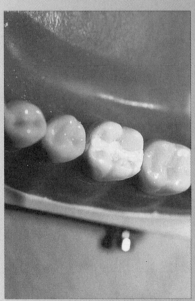

FIGURE 14-37

DENTAL WAXES

CHAPTER OUTLINE

Composition and Properties
Melting range
Flow
Excess residue
Dimensional change

Classification of Waxes
Pattern waxes
Processing waxes
Impression waxes

Manipulation

Lost Wax Technique

Summary

Chapter Review

Case-Based Discussion Topics

References

Procedure
Wax bite registration

OBJECTIVES

On completion of this chapter the student will be able to:

1. Identify the common components of dental waxes.
2. Identify the properties of waxes.
3. Describe the clinical/laboratory significance of each of the properties.
4. Identify the three classifications of waxes.
5. Differentiate between direct and indirect waxings and identify which property of dental waxes is most important in their difference.
6. Describe the usual color, form, and use of inlay, casting, baseplate, boxing, utility, and sticky waxes.
7. Obtain a bite registration using bite registration or utility wax.

KEY TERMS

Wax pattern—A duplicate of the restoration carved in wax.
Melting range—A range of melting points of the individual components of the wax.
Flow—The movement of the wax as it approaches the melting range.
Excess residue—A wax film remaining on an object after the wax is removed.
Lost wax technique—The procedure for fabricating a metal restoration by encasing the wax pattern in stone and then vaporizing the wax under high temperatures to leave an empty impression space once occupied by the wax. Molten wax is then cast into the space and takes the shape of the pattern.

Dental waxes are used in a wide variety of clinical and laboratory dental procedures. Clinically they may be used to fabricate direct waxings for cast restorations, alterations and adaptations for impression trays, and wax bite registrations. In the laboratory they may be used to box an impression before pouring a gypsum product, as baseplates for full and partial dentures, to hold components together before articulation, and to provide indirect patterns for casting.

The dental assistant and hygienist typically will not fabricate the actual direct or indirect wax pattern for a dental casting, but they do need an appreciation for the many steps in the procedure known as the lost wax technique (described later in this chapter). The assistant and hygienist, either assisting or acting as the operator, will frequently manipulate waxes in the taking of alginate impressions, pouring the impression, and taking a wax bite registration for articulation of the models.

Composition and Properties

Dental waxes are composed of a mixture of components from natural and synthetic sources. Natural waxes are produced from plants, used in carnauba wax; insects, used in beeswax; and minerals, used in paraffin wax. These natural waxes contribute properties to the wax, but are rarely used in their pure form. They are combined or mixed with synthetic waxes, gums, fats, oils, resins, and coloring agents. Each component is added to obtain the physical properties desirable for the wax application.

Properties that contribute to the **melting range, flow, thermal expansion,** and **excess residue** are important considerations for dental wax. The operator must regard these properties when making a wax selection, as well as during the manipulation of the wax.

MELTING RANGE

Dental waxes have a **melting range,** a range of temperatures at which each component of the wax will start to soften and then flow. The components with lower melting points will soften first; then, as the temperature is increased, more components soften and the wax will eventually flow. Controlling the temperature of the wax allows operator control of

the viscosity of the wax. In many cases the operator does not want the wax to flow but only soften. A flame source is needed if a flowable state is desired.

FLOW

Flow is the movement of the wax as molecules slip over each other. As the temperature of the wax increases, the viscosity of the wax decreases until the wax becomes a liquid. Control of the flow and the melting range, which produces a flowable material, is important in manipulating the wax. If a wax were capable of flowing at room temperature it would be very difficult to control. However, even at mouth temperature there is a point at which flow is undesirable. If you were using a wax for a wax bite registration, you would not want it to flow at mouth temperature, causing distortion of the wax. It is important that the wax does not require temperatures much greater than mouth temperature to soften or it would be uncomfortable when placed in the mouth of the patient. A melting range that is only slightly higher than mouth temperature is desirable for this wax application. For laboratory purposes, waxes may have a much higher melting range. However, even for laboratory purposes, high melting ranges may be undesirable. If you wanted to use a wax in the boxing of an impression, for example, it is much more desirable to mold the wax using the heat of your hands or warm water rather than having to use a flame.

EXCESS RESIDUE

It is important that all of the wax is removed from the object it is melted onto. If **excess residue** remains after the wax is removed, it may result in inaccuracies in the object being produced. This is especially important in the lost wax technique when the wax pattern is melted out of the investment mold.

DIMENSIONAL CHANGE

Waxes expand when heated and contract when cooled; the thermal expansion and contraction of waxes is greater than any other dental material. This is a property especially important for pattern waxes. If a wax is heated too far above the melting range or heated unevenly, expansion above acceptable standards will result. Manufacturers provide temperature and handling guidelines for pattern waxes to prevent inaccuracies in the final casting. In addition, if waxes are allowed to stand, dimensional changes occur from the release of residual stress. Wax patterns should be invested within 30 minutes of carving. (See Chapter 12 for more on investments.)

Classification of Waxes

Waxes are grouped into three classifications: pattern waxes, processing waxes, and impression waxes. Manufacturers produce these waxes in several forms. Sticks, sheets, blocks, and tins are used. Waxes have unique coloring to distinguish them in use (Figure 15-1).

PATTERN WAXES

Pattern waxes are used in the construction of metal castings and bases for dentures.

Inlay Waxes   Inlay waxes are used to produce patterns for metal casting using the lost wax technique. They may be used directly in the mouth (type I), placed onto the prepared tooth in the direct waxing technique, or more frequently melted onto a die outside the mouth in the indirect technique (type II) (Figure 15-2). Type I wax, used directly in the mouth, has a much lower melting range for the comfort of the patient and the accuracy of the wax on removal. Because direct waxing is done in the patient's mouth, all the limitations of the mouth must be considered. Because of these limitations, most dentists prefer to use the indirect waxing technique and have a dental laboratory technician produce the wax pattern and casting. These waxes are supplied in sticks, pellets, and tins, generally in dark colors of blue or green. They are labeled hard, medium, and soft, which refers to their melting ranges. American Dental Association (ADA) specification number 4 sets standards for pattern waxes; low thermal expansion, complete removal of excess residue, and appropriate melting ranges are important properties.

Casting Waxes   Casting waxes are used to construct the metal framework of partial and complete dentures. These waxes come in sheets and preformed shapes. The physical properties of casting waxes are similar to inlay waxes with the exception of melting range. Because these waxes are not softened in the mouth, the melting range is only important for laboratory procedures.

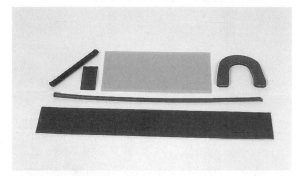

FIGURE 15-1 ■ Various forms of wax: sheets, ropes, and sticks.

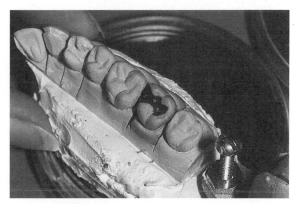

FIGURE 15-2 ■ Inlay waxing on a die.

Baseplate Wax   Baseplate waxes are sheets of wax generally pink in color. These sheets are usually layered to produce the form on which denture teeth are set (Figure 15-3). This initial form is then tried into the mouth to establish denture dimensions. The wax must not distort at mouth temperatures.

PROCESSING WAXES

Processing waxes are used primarily to aid in dental procedures both clinically and in the laboratory.

Boxing Wax   Boxing wax is used to form the base portion of a gypsum model. The 1.5-inch-wide, red strip of boxing wax is wrapped around the impression to produce a form into which the gypsum is poured. This wax is easily manipulated at room temperature; it is also slightly tacky at room temperature, allowing it to adhere to itself to secure the boxed form (See Chapter 12 for more on gypsum products.)

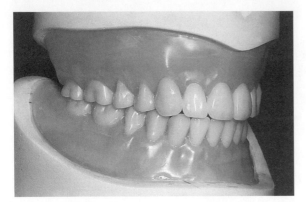

FIGURE 15-3 ■ Denture setup on baseplates.

Utility Wax   Also called periphery wax, this wax comes in ropes that are easily manipulated at room temperature. The wax rope is used to adapt the periphery of the impression tray to customize the tray and aid in patient comfort. The wax provides a better fit into the vestibule and control of the movement of the impression material. Utility wax ropes are given to orthodontic patients to cover sharp brackets and wires. Utility wax sheets may be layered to form a horseshoe shape and used for wax bite registrations. These waxes come in various colors of pink, white, and red.

Sticky Wax   Sticky wax comes in orange sticks that at room temperature are hard and brittle, but when heated under flame become soft and sticky. Sticky wax is used to adhere components of metal, gypsum, or resin together temporarily during fabrication and repair. Because of its brittle nature at room temperature, even the slightest torque will fracture the wax. This is an important characteristic, because it alerts the operator that distortion has occurred during manipulation.

IMPRESSION WAXES

Impression waxes are used to obtain impressions of the oral structures.

Corrective Impression Wax   Corrective impression wax is used in conjunction with other impression materials in the process of taking edentulous impressions. This wax flows at mouth temperature and is used within another impression material to correct undercut areas.

Bite Registration Wax   Bite registration wax is used to produce wax bite registrations for articulation of models. The preformed horseshoe shapes are often reinforced with metal particles to provide stability. However, like corrective impression wax, this wax is susceptible to distortion at temperatures only slightly higher than mouth temperature and must be carefully monitored. For fabrication of a wax bite registration, see Procedure 15-1.

Manipulation

Wax should be softened evenly in dry heat, with warm hands, or by flame. If a wax is softened by flame it should be rotated above the flame until it evenly softens or flows. Melted wax should be added in layers onto an object. As previously mentioned, because of changes by relaxation of residual stress, wax patterns should be invested within 30 minutes of carving. Waxes such as boxing and utility wax are slightly tacky at room temperature to help them adhere to themselves. They must remain dry to take advantage of this characteristic.

To avoid distortion of waxes, they should be stored at or slightly below room temperature.

Lost Wax Technique

Artisans have used the **lost wax technique** for several hundred years. In the 1500s artisans, in conjunction with medical practitioners, invented a method for casting gold for dental restorations in molds; today's techniques are much the same (Figure 15-4). The primary steps in the lost wax procedure are as follows:
1. An impression of the preparation must first be obtained and poured into a high-strength die stone forming the die.
2. A wax pattern of the restoration is carved on the die.
3. A wax or plastic sprue is attached to the pattern to form the channel into which the molten metal will be forced.
4. The pattern and attached sprue are encased in an investment ring into which investment gypsum is poured.
5. Once hardened, the investment enclosed pattern and sprue are heated in a burnout oven at high temperatures, causing the wax and sprue to

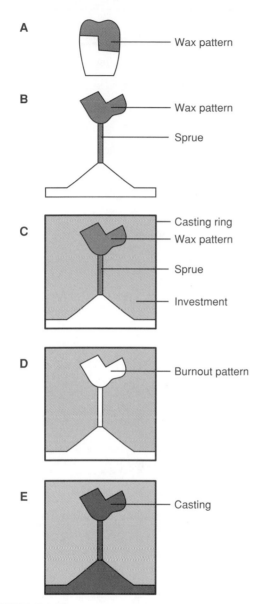

FIGURE 15-4 ■ Lost wax technique. **A,** Wax pattern on a die. **B,** Wax pattern with sprue on a die. **C,** Wax and sprue in investment ring. **D,** Wax pattern vaporized from investment. **E,** Metal casting of wax pattern.

vaporize (lost wax), leaving an impression of the wax pattern in the now-empty space.

6. The molten metal is forced through the empty channel formed by the sprue and into the empty wax pattern space.

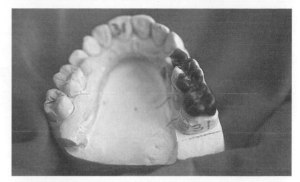

FIGURE 15-5 ■ Waxing of inlays and crown.

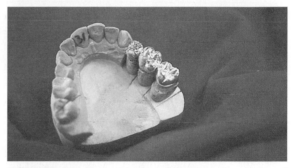

FIGURE 15-6 ■ Cleaned and polished metal castings of inlays and crowns.

7. The metal cools, the sprue is removed, and the casting is cleaned and polished. It is now ready to be cemented onto the tooth (Figures 15-5 and 15-6).

The lost wax procedure takes several steps, each of which can cause inaccuracies in the final product. Properties of expansion and contraction in the impression material, die stone, wax, investment material, and metal must all be controlled to achieve a final casting that will have intimate contact with the tooth preparation.

SUMMARY

The dental assistant and hygienist may have occasion to use dental waxes in a variety of clinical and laboratory procedures. Although waxes have inherent disadvantages in dimensional stability and control of flow, they are successfully used. The operator must keep in mind the limitations of each wax to use it to its best advantage.

CHAPTER REVIEW

Select the one correct response for each of the following multiple-choice questions:

1. **The melting range can best be described as**
   a. The point at which the wax flows
   b. The point at which the wax softens
   c. The temperature of the heat source required
   d. A combination of melting points

2. **A direct wax pattern is fabricated in the mouth. Which property of the inlay wax is the most important?**
   a. Flow
   b. Residual stress
   c. Melting range
   d. Excess residue

3. **A wax pattern is invested and burned out in the lost wax procedure. Which property of the inlay wax is the most important?**
   a. Melting range
   b. Flow
   c. Residual stress
   d. Excess residue

4. **The wax used to form a base to pour a gypsum model is**
   a. Boxing wax
   b. Sticky wax
   c. Pattern wax
   d. Baseplate wax

5. **Utility wax ropes are used to**
   a. Hold components together for repair
   b. Make forms for wax bite registrations
   c. Make corrections in undercut areas of impressions
   d. Adapt the periphery of impression trays

6. **The sprue is used in the lost wax procedure to**
   a. Make the channel into which molten metal is forced
   b. Account for delayed expansion and contraction in the final casting
   c. Hold the wax pattern in the investment
   d. Aid in lowering the melting range of the wax

7. **If it is necessary to store a wax pattern or bite registration, it should be stored**
   a. At room temperature
   b. Wrapped with gauze
   c. In a cool, dry place
   d. Refrigerated

CASE-BASED DISCUSSION TOPICS

◉ A gypsum model is articulated with a wax bite registration and left in the dental laboratory over a hot weekend. When the assistant comes in on Monday, she discovers that the model is no longer in the correct occlusion. **What property of the dental wax most likely caused the problem? What could have been done to avoid this problem?**

◉ A gypsum model is being poured using boxing wax. The wax is formed around the impression but will not hold in place. **What can the assistant do to the wax to help it adhere to itself and the tray?**

◉ After correcting the preceding problem, the impression is poured. When the hygienist separates the boxed model, he finds that there is a thin layer of wax on the base portion. *What property of the wax most likely caused this and what property of the gypsum product contributed to this problem?*

◉ A final impression for an edentulous case is corrected with corrective impression wax; the impression is then sent to the dental laboratory. *What precautions must be considered when sending the impression?*

REFERENCES

Anusavice K: Inlay casting wax. In *Phillips' science of dental materials,* ed 10, Philadelphia, 1996, WB Saunders.

Kotsiomite E, McCabe JF: Waxes for functional impressions, *J Oral Rehabil* 23:114, 1996.

Kotsiomite E, McCabe JF: Improvements in dental wax, *J Oral Rehabil* 24:517, 1997.

McCrorie JW: Some physical properties of dental modelling waxes and of their main constituents, *J Oral Rehabil* 1:29, 1974.

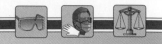

Wax Bite Registration

EQUIPMENT/SUPPLIES (Figure 15-7)

- Bite registration wax or utility wax
- Heat source
- Laboratory knife

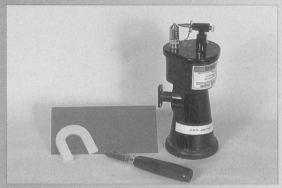

FIGURE 15-7

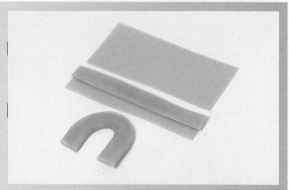

FIGURE 15-8

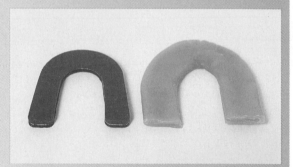

FIGURE 15-9

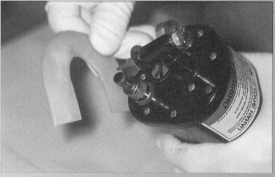

FIGURE 15-10

PROCEDURE STEPS

1 Heat utility wax sheets until pliable and fold several times to get four layers of wax.

NOTE: You will need 3 to 4 mm of thickness to avoid distortion when removing.

2 Form wax into horseshoe shape (Figure 15-8).

NOTE: You may need to continue heating the wax to keep it pliable.

3 Try the wax into the mouth, cutting the ends to fit only to the middle of the last tooth in the arch.

NOTE: If you are using preformed wax bite registration blocks, you will only need to trim them for length (Figure 15-9).

4 Seat the patient in the upright position and give instruction on closing.

NOTE: Patients in the supine position who have had their mouth open for a long period of time or are numb may close in an abnormal position.

5 Heat the wax again until softened.

NOTE: If using a flame source, assure the patient that the wax will not burn (Figure 15-10).

6 Place the wax horseshoe onto the occlusal surfaces of the maxillary teeth (Figure 15-11).

7 Instruct the patient to bite gently yet firmly into the wax.

NOTE: If the patient bites too firmly, the wax may distort or tear; if not firmly enough, an impression of the occlusal/incisal surfaces may be difficult to read (Figure 15-12).

Continued on following page

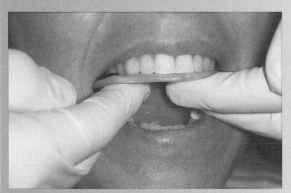

FIGURE 15-11

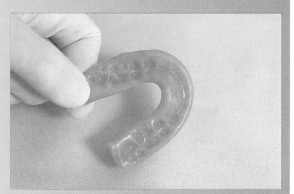

FIGURE 15-13

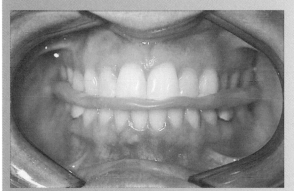

FIGURE 15-12

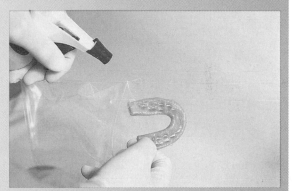

FIGURE 15-14

8 Allow wax to cool in the patient's mouth for 1 to 2 minutes.

NOTE: Use air syringe to hasten cooling by gently spraying the area around the wax.

9 Have the patient open with a straight snap to avoid distortion of the wax.

10 Remove the wax bite registration carefully, being sure not to break or distort the wax (Figure 15-13).

11 Disinfect the wax bite and store it in a bag labeled with the patient's name.

NOTE: Follow the manufacturer's recommendations for use on this material; some disinfecting agents may break down the wax.

12 Store the wax at room temperature or slightly lower (Figure 15-14).

NOTE: You should try to use the wax as soon as possible to articulate the models to avoid relaxation of residual stress.

RESOURCES

THE INTERNET

The Internet is a worldwide network of computers that allows any connected computer to communicate with any other. A wealth of information can be obtained on any conceivable topic on the Internet. For our purposes in dentistry, we can obtain useful information regarding health care organizations, professional societies and associations and their meetings, dental manufacturers and their products, dental hygiene and dental assisting schools, and research organizations and their publications. The Internet is also a valuable source of educational materials. If an individual does not have a computer or Internet connection, many schools and libraries have these resources available free or for a small fee.

Basically, one gains access to the Internet (also called the *World Wide Web* and designated as *www* in an Internet address) through a service provider (ISP) such as America On Line (AOL), Microsoft Network (MSN), or another provider. These providers supply software that runs on your computer and connects it to the service. Once connected to the Internet, one uses a program called a *web browser* to navigate the Internet. Two common web browsers are Microsoft Internet Explorer and Netscape Communicator. If the address of a specific web site is known, that address can be entered and the browser will connect to it. If a general topic is known rather than a specific site, a search can be conducted to find web sites related to that topic. Key words about the subject are entered into a program called a *search engine* that searches the Internet for web sites that have those words or related subjects. It takes some practice to define the search so that a list of thousands of web sites or more is not generated. Many search engines have helpful suggestions for narrowing a search. Before long, you can be successfully "surfing" the net (visiting web sites on the World Wide Web). Some of the search engines used for general searches are the following:

- **www.altavista.com**
- **www.excite.com**
- **www.google.com**
- **www.hotbot.com**
- **www.webcrawler.com**
- **www.yahoo.com**

There are numerous web sites of particular interest to professionals in the dental health field. For example, ADA Online at **www.ada.org** provides:

- Information about the ADA and Dental Societies
- Events, meetings, and continuing education
- Online publications: JADA, ADA News Daily, and ADA news
- Research and clinical issues
- ADA library services

- Dental practice, education, and technological advances
- ADA member directory
- Information on licensure, legislative, and regulatory actions
- Patient education materials

Another useful site is ADHA Online at **www.adha.org**, which provides:

- Oral health information
- Career information
- Continuing education including a new online course
- Professional interests and health care issues
- Student information, membership, and job searching
- Membership information, licensing information, and legislative activity
- Annual session information
- Publications
- Answers to frequently asked questions

The Dental Site at **www.dentalsite.com** provides information for dental assistants, dental hygienists, dentists, and the public. Resources for dental assistants include the following:

- Lists of American and international schools
- Student sites
- Publications
- Assisting topics
- Directories

Resources for dental hygienists are as follows:

- Dental Hygiene Schools
- Student sites
- Publications
- Hygiene board reviews
- Seminars and courses
- Dental Hygienists' Guide to the Internet
- National Center for Dental Hygiene Research
- Periodontics Online
- Hygiene listserves (mailing list of hygienists), chat and bulletin boards

Proctor & Gamble Crest Dental Resource Net, an excellent commercial web site at **www.dentalcare.com**, provides:

- Continuing education (CE) courses online at no cost, some of which are available for dental hygiene and dental assisting.
- Patient education information that can be printed out in six different languages
- Access to MEDLINE (a library database of published clinical and research articles in medi-

cine, dentistry, pharmacy, nursing, and allied health fields)

- Product information and technique guides
- Faculty resources, including a slide library, a lecture series, handouts, case studies, and a faculty resource center.
- Student resources: covers principles on how to approach patient case studies as well as a series of cases.
- Online Journal of Contemporary Dental Practice

CONTINUING DENTAL EDUCATION VIA THE INTERNET

The Internet has made continuing education (CE) very convenient. Courses can be accessed when convenient for the student and can be completed at his or her own pace. Some sites provide free CE courses and some charge a fee for each course.

UNIVERSITY-BASED ONLINE CE COURSES:

Baylor College of Dentistry
Clinically related courses and case studies
www.tambcd.edu/dentalce/Distance_Learning/ distance_learning.html

Marquette University
Online dental hygiene continuing education
www.dental.mu.edu

Medical University of South Carolina, College of Dental Medicine
Common drugs
www2.musc.edu/dentistry/top40/Headers/ main6.htm

Temple University School of Dentistry
Internet basics and medical library search
www.temple.edu/dentistry/di/ce

University of California, Los Angeles
Case studies in radiology, oral pathology and removable prosthodontics
www.dent.ucla.edu/ce

University of Illinois at Chicago
Free updates on a variety of topics
www.dentistry.uic.edu

University of Kentucky College of Dentistry
Independent Dental Education for Assistants Program: 275 lessons (15 units) reviewed by ADAA. Not all courses are available online
www.rxce.org/cde

University of Michigan, School of Dentistry
Managed care
www.dent.umich.edu/cdeunit/

University of Texas HSC at San Antonio, Dental School
Nitrous oxide conscious sedation
www.smile.uthscsa.edu/
Note that many schools are developing online CE courses, so search the web for new listings or see the ADA site listed below.

COMMERCIALLY AVAILABLE ONLINE CE COURSES/MATERIALS

Dentalxchange
Over 50 online courses on dental assisting, many approved by ADAA
www.dentalxchange.com/ce/

Dentsply
A variety of CE materials
www.dentsply.com

Direct Dental Courses
A variety of online courses
www.dentalcours.com

dentrek.com
A variety of online courses
www.dentrek.com

goDENT.com
A variety of online courses/journals
www.goDENT.com

Medical Specialists' Network
Dental news and research
www.MDLinx.com

Proctor & Gamble
A variety of online courses/journals
www.dentalcare.com

rdental.com
A variety of online courses
www.rdental.com

3M
A variety of CE materials
www.3M.com/dental
Many dental manufacturers' web sites contain CE courses or materials that can be accessed free of charge by dental professionals. In addition, the ADA has a web-based CE course listing that can be accessed by members free of charge at **www.ada.org/prof/ed/ce/**.
The ADHA has CE listings on their site at **www.adha.org**.
Online and offline courses also can be found at listings by:
- Dental Products Report: This free site lists CE courses searchable by location, date, and topic at www.dentalproducts.net.
- dentalcourses.com: A free site for dental professionals to locate courses by date, state, subject, or course title at **www.dentalcourses.com**.

THE JOY OF DISCOVERY

You may discover other continuing education sites while surfing the net. For example, if you visit Dental Globe at **www.dentalglobe.com** to view their list of dental manufacturers you will find in their index a category entitled "Dental Auxiliaries." Clicking on that category will take you to a dental auxiliary index that includes information relevant to dental hygienists, dental assistants and continuing education. Clicking on the Continuing Education listing links you with university and commercial continuing education available for dentists and dental hygienists. Clicking on the Dental Hygiene Education listing links you to a web site developed by Margaret Fehrenbach, RDH, MS, that has links to many sites of interest to dental hygienists. Among those links is a link to Student Cases that in turn provides links to free continuing education of interest to dental hygienists and dental assistants on the following topics:
- Basic science and oral biology
- Community dentistry and public health
- Dental materials and restorative studies
- General case studies in dentistry
- General information on board review
- Legal and ethical concerns
- Nutrition
- Pathology and periodontology
- Pharmacology
- Radiology
- Review questions and terminology

PATIENT EDUCATION MATERIALS

Patient Education materials are also available at many manufacturers' web sites as well as the ADA, ADHA, and many state association web sites. Some of these materials are available for downloading and printing. Some are available in brochure form for a fee.

ONLINE LIBRARY SEARCH (MEDLINE) FOR DENTAL JOURNAL ARTICLES

The National Library of Medicine maintains a database of 4,300 international biomedical journals dating back to 1966 that contains more than 11 million citations. It adds about 400,000 new journal articles each year. The database, called MEDLINE, is available online, free to the public. Information can be searched for by subject, title of the article, or author's name. When the search is conducted by subject, the information provided is a listing of articles on that topic published within the time frame specified. Usually, an abstract is available that summarizes the article as well as author information and journal citation. Medline can be accessed at any of the following addresses:

- www.nlm.nih.gov/medlineplus/
- www.igm.nlm.nih.gov/
- www.healthy.net/library/search/medline.htm

Temple University offers a 3-unit CE course on how to use library databases like MEDLINE.

JOURNALS OF INTEREST FOR DENTAL MATERIALS OR CLINICAL TECHNIQUES

Access
American Dental Hygienists' Association
444 N Michigan Avenue
Chicago, IL 60611
(312) 440-8900
  www.adha.org

Compendium of Continuing Education in Dentistry
Dental Learning Systems
241 Forsgate Dr.
Jamesburg, NJ 08831
(800) 926-7636
  www.dentallearning.com

Dental Materials
Academy of Dental Materials
P.O. Box 660677
Dallas, TX 75266
(214) 828-8378
  www.elsevier.nl/locate/dental

Dental Update
George Warman Publications (UK) Ltd.
Warman House
20 Leas Road
Guildford
Surrey, GU1 4QT
UNITED KINGDOM
0483-304944
  www.gwarman.co.uk/dupdate

Dentistry Today
26 Park St.
Montclair, NJ 07042
(973) 783-3935
  www.dentistrytoday.com

Journal of the American Dental Association
ADA
211 E. Chicago Ave.
Chicago, IL 60611
(312) 440-2790
  www.ada.org

Journal of the Canadian Dental Association
1815 Alta Vista Dr.
Ottawa, ON K1G-3Y6
CANADA
(613) 523-1770
  www.cda-adc.ca

Journal of Dental Hygiene
American Dental Hygienists' Association
444 N Michigan Avenue
Chicago, IL 60611
(312) 440-8900
  www.adha.org

Journal of Dental Research
IADR/AADR
1619 Duke St.
Alexandria, VA 22314-3406
(703) 548-0066
  www.dentalresearch.org

Journal of Esthetic Dentistry
B.C. Decker
P.O. Box 620 L.C.D.1
Hamilton, ON L8N 3K7
CANADA
(800) 568-7281
www.bcdecker.com

Journal of Practical Hygiene
Montage Media Corp.
1000 Wyckoff Ave.
Mahwah, NJ 07430
(800) 899-5350
www.montagemedia.com

Oral Health
1450 Don Mills Rd.
Don Mills, ON M3B 2X7
CANADA
(800) 387-0273

The Dental Assistant
American Dental Assistants' Association
203 N LaSalle Street, Suite 1320
Chicago, IL 60601
(312) 541-1550
www.dentalassistant.org

PUBLICATIONS EVALUATING DENTAL MATERIALS

CRA Newsletter
Clinical Research Associates: Clinician's Guide to
Dental Products and Techniques
(801) 226-2121
www.cranews.com

Reality
Evaluates dental materials, clinical techniques and
research articles relating to dental materials and
has many other useful features.
(800) 544-5999
www.realityesthetics.com

The Dental Advisor
Resource for product and equipment selection
based upon its evaluations.
(800) 347-1330
www.dentaladvisor.com

DENTAL AND RELATED HEALTH/ REGULATORY AGENCIES

Students may need to contact these organizations to
gain information on a variety of topics. The web sites
are very informative.

American Dental Association (ADA)
(800) 621-8099
www.ada.org

American Dental Assistants' Association (ADAA)
(800) SEE-ADAA
www.dentalassistant.org

American Dental Hygienists' Association (ADHA)
(312) 440-8900
www.adha.org

American Dental Education Association (ADEA)
(202) 667-9433
www.aads.jhu.edu

American National Standards Institute (ANSI)
(212) 642-4900
www.ansi.org

American Society for Testing and Materials (ASTM)
(610) 832-9500
www.astm.org

Canadian Dental Association (CDA)
(613) 523-1770
www.eda-adc.ca/

Centers for Disease Control and Prevention (CDC)
(404) 639-3311
www.cdc.gov

Dental Assisting National Board (DANB)
(312) 642-3368
www.danb.org

Dental Manufacturers' of America, Inc. (DMA)
(215) 731-9975
www.dmanews.org

Food and Drug Administration (FDA)
(800) 638-2041
www.fda.gov/cdrh

International and American Associations for Dental
Research (IADR and AADR)
(703) 548-0066
www.iadr.com

International Healthcare Worker Safety Center (IHCWS)
(804) 924-5159
www.med.virginia.edu/~epinet

Latex Allergy Information Service (LAIS)
(860) 482-6869
www.latexallergyhelp.com

National Association of Dental Laboratories (NADL)
(800) 950-1150
www.nadl.org

National Institute of Dental and Craniofacial Research (NIDCR)
(301) 496-4261
www.nidr.nih.gov

National Institutes of Health (NIH)
(301) 496-4000
www.nih.gov

Oral Health America (OHA)
(312) 787-6270
www.oralhealthamerica.org

Organization for Safety and Asepsis Procedures (OSAP)
(800) 298-6727
www.osap.org

United States Occupational Safety and Health Administration (OSHA)
(202) 219-7125
www.osha.gov

INDEX OF MANUFACTURERS OF DENTAL MATERIALS

Most dental manufacturers have web sites, but these vary in the amount and type of information available. Some provide limited information that pertains mostly to a description of products and how to order the products over the Internet (online). Other web sites are very elaborate and include detailed information about the products, technical guides on use, patient education information, continuing education opportunities, online journals, and links to other interesting sites. The listing below includes manufacturers of many of the dental materials discussed in this book as well as products related to the clinical or laboratory use of the materials. Toll-free telephone numbers and web sites are included when available so the reader can easily contact the manufacturers to obtain more information regarding their products. So the reader does not have to know which manufacturer produces a particular type of product, the listing is categorized by the type of product. Some manufacturers will be found under more than one heading because they provide products in several categories.

ABRASIVES AND STONES

American Diamond Instruments
American Eagle Instruments, Inc.
(800) 551-5172
www.ameagle.com

Axis Dental Corporation
(888) 654-2947
www.axisdental.com

Brasseler
(800) 841-4522
www.brasselerusa.com

Danville Materials
(800) 822-9294
www.danvillematerials.com

Dedeco International, Inc.
(800) 431-3022
www.dedeco.com

Dentatus USA
(800) 323-3136
www.dentatus.com

DENTSPLY Trubyte
(800) 877-0020
www.dentsply.com

E.C. Moore
(800) 331-3548
www.ecmoore.com

GC America, Inc.
(800) 322-7063
www.gcamerica.com

G. Hartzell & Son
(800) 950-2206
www.ghartzellandson.com

Heraeus Kulzer, Inc.
(800) 343-5336
www.kulzer.com

Hu-Friedy Manufacturing Company, Inc.
(800) 483-7433
www.hu-friedy.com

Lasco Diamond Products, Inc.
(800) 621-4726
www.lascodiamond.com

Pfingst & Company
(800) 221-1268
www.pfingst.co@rcn.com

Premier Dental Products Co.
(888) 773-6872
www.premusa.com

Shofu Dental Corporation
(800) 775-0503
www.shofu.com

3M Dental Products Division
(800) 634-2249
www.3m.com/dental

Whip Mix Corporation
(800) 626-5651
www.whipmix.com

ACRYLIC RESINS

American Tooth Industries
(800) 235-4639
www.americantooth.com

Astron Dental Corporation
(800) 323-4144
no web site

DENTSPLY Trubyte
(800) 877-0020
www.dentsply.com

GC America, Inc.
(800) 322-7063
www.gcamerica.com

Harry J. Bosworth Company
(800) 323-4352
www.bosworth.com

Lang Dental Manufacturing Company, Inc.
(800) 222-5264
www.langdental.com

Tokuyama America, Inc.
(800) 275-2867
www.tokuyamaamerica.com

ALGINATES

American Tooth Industries
(800) 235-4639
www.americantooth.com

Cadco Dental Products, Inc.
(800) 833-8267
www.cadco.com

DENTSPLY Caulk
(800) 532-2855
www.dentsply.com

Discus Dental
(800) 442-9448
www.discusdental.com

GC America, Inc.
(800) 322-7063
www.gcamerica.com

Harry J. Bosworth Company
(800) 323-4352
www.bosworth.com

Heraeus Kulzer, Inc.
(800) 343-5336
www.kulzer.com

J. Morita USA, Inc.
(800) 752-9729
www.jmoritausa.com

ALLOYS AND AMALGAM

Austenal, Inc.
(800) 621-0381
www.austenal.com

Degussa-Ney Dental
(800) 221-0168
www.neydental.com

Dentaurum, Inc.
(800) 323-3136
www.dentaurum.com

DENTSPLY Caulk
(800) 532-2855
www.dentsply.com

DENTSPLY Ceramco
(800) 487-0100
www.dentsply.com

GC America, Inc.
(800) 322-7063
www.gcamerica.com

Ivoclar North America
(800) 533-6825
www.ivoclarna.com

Jelenko Dental Health Products
(800) 431-1785
www.jelenko.com

Kerr Corporation
(800) 537-7123
www.kerrdental.com

Pentron Corporation
(800) 551-0283
www.pentron.com

Sterngold
(800) 243-9942
www.sterngold.com

World Alloys & Refining, Inc.
(800) 535-5536
www.worldalloys.com

Wykle Research, Inc.
(800) 859-6641
www.wykledirect.com

Zenith Dental/DMG
(800) 662-6383
www.zenithdmg.com

CEMENTS

Bisco, Inc.
(800) 247-3368
www.bisco.com

Cadco Dental Products, Inc.
(800) 833-8267
www.cadco.com

DENTSPLY Caulk
(800) 532-2855
www.dentsply.com

Essential Dental Systems
(800) 223-5394
www.edsdental.com

GC America, Inc.
(800) 322-7063
www.gcamerica.com

Harry J. Bosworth Company
(800) 323-4352
www.bosworth.com

Heraeus Kulzer, Inc.
(800) 343-5336
www.kulzer.com

Ivoclar North America
(800) 533-6825
www.ivoclarna.com

J. Morita USA, Inc.
(800) 831-3222
www.jmoritausa.com

Kuraray America, Inc.
(800) 879-1676
www.kurarayamerica.com

Mirage Dental Systems
(800) 366-0001
www.miragecdp.com

Parkell
(800) 243-7446
www.parkell.com

Pentron Corporation
(800) 551-0283
www.pentron.com

Premier Dental Products Co.
(888) 773-6872
www.premusa.com

Roydent Dental Products, Inc.
(800) 992-7767
www.roydent.com

Scientific Pharmaceuticals
(800) 634-3047
www.scipharm.com

Septodont, Inc.
(800) 872-8305
www.septodontinc.com

Shofu Dental Corporation
(800) 775-0503
www.shofu.com

Sultan Chemists, Inc.
(800) 637-8582
www.sultanintl.com

Temrex Corporation
(800) 645-1226
www.temrex.com

3M Dental Products Division
(800) 634-2249
www.3m.com/dental

Tokuyama America, Inc.
(800) 275-2867
   www.tokuyamaamerica.com

Zenith Dental
(800) 662-6383
   www.zenithdmg.com

COMPOSITES AND BONDING AGENTS

Bisco, Inc.
(800) 247-3368
   www.bisco.com

Centrix
(800) 235-5862
   www.centrixdental.com

Coltene/Whaledent
(800) 221-3046
   www.coltenewhaledent.com

Cosmedent, Inc.
(800) 621-6729
   www.cosmedent.com

Danville Materials
(800) 822-9294
   www.danvillematerials.com

Den-Mat
(800) 433-6628
   www.denmat.com

Dentatus USA Ltd.
(800) 323-3136
   www.dentatus.com

DENTSPLY Caulk
(800) 532-2855
   www.dentsply.com

Discus Dental
(800) 422-9448
   www.discusdental.com

Essential Dental Systems
(800) 223-5394
   www.edsdental.com

GC America, Inc.
(800) 322-7063
   www.gcamerica.com

George Taub Products & Fusion Company, Inc.
(800) 828-2634
no web site

Global Dental Products, Inc.
(516) 221-8844
   www.tubulicid.com

Heraeus Kulzer, Inc.
(800) 343-5336
   www.kulzer.com

Ivoclar/Vivadent
(800) 533-6825
   www.ivoclarna.com

J. Morita USA, Inc.
(800) 831-3222
   www.jmoritausa.com

Kerr Corporation
(800) 537-7123
   www.kerrdental.com

Kuraray America, Inc.
(800) 879-1676
   www.kurarayamerica.com

Mirage Dental Systems
(800) 366-0001
   www.miragecdp.com

Parkell
(800) 243-7446
   www.parkell.com

Pentron Corporation
(800) 551-0283
   www.pentron.com

Premier Dental Products Co.
(800) 773-6872
   www.premusa.com

Protech Professional Products, Inc.
(800) 872-8898
   www.dentallabproducts.com

Scientific Pharmaceuticals
(800) 634-3047
   www.scipharm.com

Septodont, Inc.
(800) 872-8305
   www.septodontinc.com

Shofu Dental Corporation
(800) 775-0503
   www.shofu.com

Southern Dental Industries, Inc.
(800) 228-5166
www.sdi.com.au

Temrex Corporation
(800) 645-1226
www.temrex.com

3M Dental Products Division
(800) 634-2249
www.3m.com/dental

Tokuyama America, Inc.
(800) 275-2867
www.tokuyamaamerica.com

Ultradent Products, Inc.
(800) 552-5512
www.ultradent.com

Zenith Dental/DMG
(800) 662-6383
www.zenithdmg.com

DENTURE ACRYLICS FOR BASE, RELINE, AND REPAIR

Astron Dental Corp.
(800) 323-4144
no web site

DENTSPLY Trubyte
(800) 877-0020
www.dentsply.com

GC America, Inc.
(800) 322-7063
www.gcamerica.com

GC Lab Technologies, Inc.
(800) 323-7063
www.gcamerica.com

Harry J. Bosworth Company
(800) 323-4352
www.bosworth.com

Ivoclar North America
(800) 533-6825
www.ivoclarna.com

J. Morita USA, Inc.
(800) 831-3222
www.jmoritausa.com

Lang Dental Manufacturing Company, Inc.
(800) 222-5264
www.langdental.com

Micro Select
(800) 840-2650
www.msproducts.com

Moyco Union Broach
(800) 221-1344
www.moycotech.com/moyco

Pascal Company, Inc.
(800) 426-8051
www.pascaldental.com

Protech Professional Products, Inc.
(800) 872-8898
www.dentallabproducts.com

Temrex Corporation
(800) 645-1226
www.temrex.com

Tokuyama America, Inc.
(800) 275-2867
www.tokuyamaamerica.com

FLUORIDES AND PREVENTIVE MATERIALS

Almore International, Inc.
(800) 547-1511
www.almore.com

Biotrol International
(800) 822-8550
www.biotrol.com

Block Drug Corporation
(800) 652-5625
www.blockdrug.com

Colgate-Palmolive
(800) 265-4283
www.colgate.com

Crescent Dental Manufacturing Company
(800) 989-8085
www.cresentproducts.com/dental.htm

Denovo
(800) 854-7949
www.denovodental.com

Dentatus USA Ltd.
(800) 323-3136
www.dentatus.com

Dentsply Preventive Care
(800) 877-0020
www.prevent.dentsply.com

Discus Dental
(800) 422-9448
  www.discusdental.com

E-Z Floss
(800) 227-0208
  www.e-zfloss.com

Glide Products By Gore
(800) 645-4337
  www.glidefloss.com

Ivoclar North America, Inc.
(800) 533-6825
  www.ivoclarna.com

John O. Butler Company
(800) 228-4890
  www.jbutler.com

Johnson & Johnson
(800) 325-9821
  www.johnsonandjohnson.com

Jordco, Inc.
(800) 752-2818
  www.jordco.com

Laclede Professional Products, Inc.
(800) 922-5856
  www.laclede.com

Omnii Products
(800) 445-3386
  www.omniiproducts.com

Oral-B Laboratories USA
(800) 446-7252
  www.oralb.com

Pascal Company, Inc.
(800) 426-8051
  www.pascaldental.com

Pharmascience
(800) 207-4477
  www.pharmascience.com

POH (Oral Health Products, Inc.)
(918) 664-4949
  www.oralhealthproducts.com

Procter & Gamble
(800) 543-2577
  www.dentalcare.com

Pro-Dentec/Rotadent
(800) 228-5595
  www.prodentec.com

SDI Laboratories, Inc.
(800) 227-8507
  www.sdilabs.com

Sultan Dental Products
(800) 238-6739
  www.sultandental.com

Wykle Research, Inc.
(800) 859-6641
  www.wykledirect.com

GYPSUM PRODUCTS

DENTSPLY Trubyte
(800) 877-0020
  www.dentsply.com

Heraeus Kulzer, Inc
(800) 343-5336
  www.kulzer.com

Kerr Company
(800) 322-6666
  www.kerrdental.com

Whip Mix
(800) 626-5651
  www.whipmix.com

IMPRESSION AND BITE REGISTRATION MATERIALS

Aluwax
(616) 895-4385
  www.aluwaxdental.com

Cadco Dental Products, Inc.
(800) 833-8267
  www.cadco.com

Centrix
(800) 235-5862
  www.centrixdental.com

Coltene/Whaledent
(800) 221-3046
  www.coltenewhaledent.com

DENTSPLY Caulk
(800) 532-2855
  www.dentsply.com

Gingi-Pak
(800) 437-1514
www.gingi-pak.com

Heraeus Kulzer, Inc.
(800) 343-5336
www.kulzer.com

Kerr Corporation
(800) 537-7123
www.kerrdental.com

Parkell
(800) 243-7446
www.parkell.com

Pentron Corporation
(800) 551-0283
www.pentron.com

Roydent Dental Products, Inc.
(800) 992-7767
www.roydent.com

3M Dental Products Division
(800) 634-2249
www.3m.com/dental

Van R Dental Products
(800) 833-8267
www.vanr.com

PADS AND SLABS FOR MIXING

Bisco, Inc.
(800) 247-3368
www.bisco.com

Cadco Dental Products, Inc.
(800) 833-8267
www.cadco.com

Clive Craig
(800) 833-8267
www.clivecraig.com

Coltene/Whaledent
(800) 221-3046
www.coltenewhaledent.com

Confi-Dental Products Company
(800) 383-5158
www.confics@aol.com

Dental Disposables International, Inc.
(800) 825-5727
www.dentaldisposables.com

DENTSPLY Caulk
(800) 532-2855
www.dentsply.com

Harry J. Bosworth Company
(800) 323-4352
www.bosworth.com

Heraeus Kulzer, Inc.
(800) 343-5336
www.kulzer.com

Moyco Union Broach
(800) 221-1344
www.moycotech.com/moyco

Pentron Corporation
(800) 551-0283
www.pentron.com

Temrex Corporation
(800) 645-1226
www.temrex.com

PERIODONTAL THERAPY MATERIALS

Cadco Dental Products, Inc.
(800) 833-8267
www.cadco.com

Dentatus USA
(800) 323-3136
www.dentatus.com

DENTSPLY Caulk
(800) 532-2855
www.dentsply.com

G. Hartzell & Son
(800) 950-2206
www.ghartzellandson.com

John O. Butler Company
(800) 228-4890
www.jbutler.com

Omnii Products
(800) 445-3386
www.omniiproducts.com

Thornton International, Inc.
(800) 445-3567
www.thorntonfloss.com

PINS AND POSTS

Bisco, Inc.
(800) 247-3368
www.bisco.com

Coltene/Whaledent
(800) 221-3046
www.coltenewhaledent.com

Dentatus USA
(800) 323-3136
www.dentatus.com

Essential Dental Systems
(800) 223-5394
www.edsdental.com

Ivoclar North America
(800) 533-6825
www.ivoclarna.com

J. Morita USA, Inc.
(800) 831-3222
www.jmoritausa.com

Pentron Corporation
(800) 551-0283
www.pentron.com

Premier Dental Products Co.
(888) 773-6872
www.premusa.com

Roydent Dental Products, Inc.
(800) 992-7767
www.roydent.com

Wykle Research, Inc.
(800) 859-6641
www.wykledirect.com

POLISHES

Dental Disposables International, Inc.
(800) 825-5727
www.dentaldisposables.com

George Taub Products & Fusion Company, Inc.
(800) 828-2634
no web site

Ivoclar North America
(800) 533-6825
www.ivoclarna.com

Preventive Technologies, Inc.
(800) 474-8681
www.preventech.com

Protech Professional Products, Inc.
(800) 872-8898
www.dentallabproducts.com

Scientific Pharmaceuticals
(800) 634-3047
www.scipharm.com

Shofu Dental Corporation
(800) 775-0503
www.shofu.com

PROPHY BRUSHES, CUPS, AND PASTES

Dental Resource, Inc.
(800) 328-1276
www.dentalresourceinc.com

Denticator
(800) 227-3321
www.denticator.com

DENTSPLY Caulk
(800) 532-2855
www.dentsply.com

Discus Dental
(800) 422-9448
www.discusdental.com

Heraeus Kulzer, Inc.
(800) 343-5336
www.kulzer.com

John O. Butler Company
(800) 228-4890
www.jbutler.com

Medidenta International, Inc.
(800) 221-0750
www.medidenta.com

Moyco Union Broach
(800) 221-1344
www.moycotech.com/moyco

Omnii Products
(800) 445-3386
www.omniiproducts.com

Premier Dental Products Co.
(888) 773-6872
   www.premusa.com

Preventive Technologies, Inc.
(800) 474-8681
   www.preventech.com

Sultan Dental Products
(800) 238-6739
   www.sultandental.com

3M Dental Products Division
(800) 634-2249
   www.3m.com/dental

Waterpik Technologies
(800) 525-2020
   www.waterpik.com

Whip Mix Corporation
(800) 626-5651
   www.whipmix.com

Young Dental Manufacturing
(800) 325-1881
   www.youngdental.com

PROVISIONAL MATERIALS

Almore International, Inc.
(800) 547-1511
   www.almore.com

American Tooth Industries
(800) 235-4639
   www.americantooth.com

Astron Dental Corporation
(800) 3234114
no web site

Danville Materials
(800) 827-7940
   www.danvillematerials.com

Denovo
(800) 854-7949
   www.denovodental.com

DENTSPLY Caulk
(800) 532-2855
   www.dentsply.com

GC America, Inc.
(800) 323-7063
   www.gcamerica.com

Gramm Technologies
(800) 752-8846
   www.grammtechnikdc.com

Harry J. Bosworth Company
(800) 323-4352
   www.bosworth.com

Ivoclar/Vivadent
(800) 533-6825
   www.ivoclarna.com

JS Dental Manufacturing, Inc.
(800) 284-3368
   www.jsdental.com

Kerr Corporation
(800) 537-7123
   www.kerrdental.com

Lang Dental Manufacturing Company, Inc.
(800) 222-5864
   www.langdental.com

Masel Enterprises
(800) 423-8227
   www.maselortho.com

Pentron Corporation
(800) 551-0283
   www.pentron.com

Precision Ceramics Dental Laboratory
(800) 223-6322
   www.pcdl-usa.com

SciCan USA
(800) 572-1211
   www.scican.com

Sterngold
(800) 243-9942
   www.sterngold.com

3M Dental Products Division ESPE
(888) 364-3577
   www.3m.com/dental

Vita Zahnfabrik (Vident in USA)
(800) 828-3839
   www.vident.com

World Alloys & Refining, Inc.
(800) 535-5536
www.worldalloys.com

Zenith Dental/DMG
(800) 662-6383
www.zenithdmg.com

SEALERS, DENTIN, AND FISSURE

Bisco, Inc.
(800) 247-3368
www.bisco.com

Den-Mat
(800) 433-6628
www.denmat.com

DENTSPLY Preventive Care
(800) 532-2855
www.prevent.dentsply.com

Ivoclar/Vivadent
(800) 533-6825
www.ivoclarna.com

J. Morita USA, Inc.
(800) 831-3222
www.jmoritausa.com

Kerr
(800) 537-7634
www.kerrdental.com

Lang Dental Manufacturing Company, Inc.
(800) 222-5264
www.langdental.com

Pentron Corporation
(800) 551-0283
www.pentron.com

Scientific Pharmaceuticals
(800) 634-3047
www.scipharm.com

Septodont, Inc.
(800) 872-8305
www.septodontinc.com

Southern Dental Industries, Inc.
(800) 228-5166
www.sdi.com.au

3M Dental Products Division
(800) 634-2249
www.3m.com/dental

Zenith Dental
(800) 662-6383
www.zenithdmg.com

TEETH, PLASTIC AND PORCELAIN

American Tooth Industries
(800) 235-4639
www.americantooth.com

DENTSPLY Trubyte
(800) 877-0020
www.dentsply.com

Ivoclar/Vivadent
(800) 533-6825
www.ivoclarna.com

Lang Dental Manufacturing Company, Inc.
(800) 222-5264
www.langdental.com

Vita Zahnfabrik (Vident in USA)
(800) 828-3839
www.vident.com

TOOTH WHITENING AND BLEACHING

Den-Mat
(800) 433-6628
www.rembrandt.com

Discus Dental
(800) 422-9448
www.discusdental.com

Ivoclar North America
(800) 533-6825
www.ivoclarna.com

Kerr
(800) 537-7634
www.kerrdental.com

Omnii Products
(800) 445-3386
www.omniiproducts.com

Premier Dental Products Co.
(888) 773-6872
www.premusa.com

Southern Dental Industries, Inc.
(800) 228-5166
www.sdi.com.au

Temrex Corporation
(800) 645-1226
 www.temrex.com

3M Dental Products Division
(800) 634-2249
 www.3m.com/dental

Ultradent Products, Inc.
(800) 552-5512
 www.ultradent.com

TRAYS, IMPRESSION AND ACCESSORIES

Affordable Dental Products, Inc.
(800) 666-9008
 www.fixdecay.com

American Tooth Industries
(800) 235-4639
 www.americantooth.com

Astron Dental Corporation
(800) 323-4144
no web site

Banta Healthcare Group
(800) 225-8434
 www.bantahealthcare.com

Cadco Dental Products, Inc.
(800) 833-8267
 www.cadco.com

Clive Craig
(800) 833-8267
 www.clivecraig.com

Coltene/Whaledent
(800) 221-3046
 www.coltenewhaledent.com

Confi-Dental Products Company
(800) 383-5158
 www.confics@aol.com

Denovo
(800) 854-7949
 www.denovodental.com

DENTSPLY Caulk
(800) 532-2855
 www.dentsply.com

DENTSPLY Trubyte
(800) 877-0020
 www.dentsply.com

Discus Dental
(800) 442-9448
 www.discusdental.com

GC America, Inc.
(800) 322-7063
 www.gcamerica.com

Gingi-Pak
(800) 437-1514
 www.gingi-pak.com

Harry J. Bosworth Company
(800) 3234352
 www.bosworth.com

J. Morita USA, Inc.
(800) 831-3222
 www.jmoritausa.com

Kerr
(800) 537-7634
 www.kerrdental.com

Lang Dental Manufacturing Company, Inc.
(800) 222-5264
 www.langdental.com

Mirage Dental Systems
(800) 336-0001
 www.miragecdp.com

Premier Dental Products Co.
(888) 773-6872
 www.premusa.com

Sultan Dental Products
(800) 238-6739
 www.sultandental.com

Temrex Corporation
(800) 645-1226
 www.temrex.com

Van R Dental Products
(800) 833-8267
 www.vanr.com

Young Dental Manufacturing
(800) 325-1881
 www.youngdental.com

VARNISHES

Cetylite Industries, Inc.
(800) 257-7740
www.cetylite.com

Challenge Products, Inc.
(800) 322-9800
www.challengeproducts.com

Global Dental Products, Inc.
(516) 221-8844
www.tubulicid.com

Harry J. Bosworth Company
(800) 323-4352
www.bosworth.com

Medicom
(800) 435-9267
www.medicom.ca

Scientific Pharmaceuticals
(800) 634-3047
www.scipharm.com

WAXES

Almore International, Inc.
(800) 547-1511
www.almore.com

Aluwax Dental Products
(616) 895-4385
www.aluwaxdental.com

American Tooth Industries
(800) 235-4639
www.americantooth.com

Coltene/Whaledent
(800) 221-3046
www.coltenewhaledent.com

DENTSPLY Trubyte
(800) 877-0020
www.dentsply.com

Harry J. Bosworth Company
(800) 323-4352
www.bosworth.com

Heraeus Kulzer, Inc.
(800) 343-5336
www.kulzer.com

Moyco Union Broach
(800) 221-1344
www.moycotech.com/moyco

Whip Mix Corporation
(800) 626-5651
www.whipmix.com

WEB SITES WITH LISTINGS OF A BROAD SCOPE OF DENTAL MANUFACTURERS

The following web sites have product information databases that can be searched by material type or by manufacturer:

- Dental Equipment & Materials: **www.dental equipment.net**
- Dental Globe: **www.dentalglobe.com**
- Dental Products Report: **www.dentalproducts. net**
- net32.com: **www.net32.com**
- Online Dental Product Showcase: **www. rdental.com**
- Vertical Net: **www.e-dental.com**

B COMPETENCIES

COMPETENCY 5-1: ENAMEL AND DENTIN BONDING

PERFORMANCE OBJECTIVE: The student should be able to demonstrate the procedures for bonding to enamel and dentin.

PROCEDURE	SELF-EVALUATION	INSTRUCTOR EVALUATION
1 Set up appropriate instruments and supplies		
2 Established isolation of the field		
3 Etched enamel and dentin for appropriate time		
4 Rinsed acid and left dentin moist		
5 Applied bonding agent appropriately		
6 Light-cured bonding agent for appropriate time		
7 Maintained infection control throughout procedure		

Time allowed: _____ Time started: _____ Time finished: _____

Instructor comments: _____

Instructor signature: _____

COMPETENCY 5-2: PREPARING PORCELAIN SURFACES FOR BONDING

PERFORMANCE OBJECTIVE: The student will demonstrate the procedures to prepare porcelain for bonding.

PROCEDURE	SELF-EVALUATION	INSTRUCTOR EVALUATION
1 Set up appropriate instruments and supplies		
2 Isolated field and cleaned tooth with pumice		
3 Cleaned surface of porcelain		
4 Etched porcelain for 1 minute with hydrofluoric acid		
5 Rinsed, dried, and applied silane		
6 Applied bonding agent to porcelain (uncured)		
7 Prepared tooth for bonding (see Competency 5-1)		
8 Mixed and applied resin cement to restoration		
9 Seated restoration, removed excess cement, light-cured		
10 Maintained infection control throughout procedure		

Time allowed: _____ Time started: _____ Time finished: _____

Instructor comments: _____

Instructor signature: _____

COMPETENCY 5-3: BONDING OF ORTHODONTIC BRACKETS

OBJECTIVE: The student will prepare the teeth and bond (or assist with placement by the dentist) orthodontic brackets.

PROCEDURE	SELF-EVALUATION	INSTRUCTOR EVALUATION
1 Set up appropriate instruments and supplies		
2 Explained procedure to the patient and cleaned enamel surfaces for bonding		
3 Obtained good isolation of the teeth		
4 Etched appropriate portion of the enamel for bonding		
5 Applied bonding resin primer to the enamel and light-cured it		
6 Applied bonding adhesive resin to the back of the bracket and placed bracket or transferred it to the dentist with bracket pliers		
7 Used or transferred scaler for positioning of bracket and removed excess resin		
8 Light-cured adhesive resin for appropriate time		
9 Maintained infection control throughout the procedure		

Time allowed: _____ Time started: _____ Time finished: _____

Instructor comments: _____

Instructor signature: _____

COMPETENCY 6-1: ASSIST WITH PLACEMENT OF CLASS II COMPOSITE RESIN RESTORATION

PERFORMANCE OBJECTIVE: The student will perform steps in the placement of a class II composite resin restoration as permitted by state law.

PROCEDURE	SELF-EVALUATION	INSTRUCTOR EVALUATION
1 Set up appropriate instruments and supplies		
2 Applied topical anesthetic and took shade		
3 Applied rubber dam		
4 Applied sectional matrix, wedge, and spring ring to prepared tooth		
5 Etched enamel and dentin for appropriate length of time		
6 Applied and light-cured bonding agent		
7 Applied composite resin in small increments and light-cured		
8 Finished and polished composite		
9 Removed rubber dam		
10 Checked occlusion		
11 Maintained infection control throughout the procedure		

Time allowed: _____ Time started: _____ Time finished: _____

Instructor comments: _____

Instructor signature: _____

COMPETENCY 7-1: APPLYING TOPICAL FLUORIDE

PERFORMANCE OBJECTIVE: The student will apply a topical fluoride foam/gel to a patient in disposable stock trays.

PROCEDURE	SELF-EVALUATION	INSTRUCTOR EVALUATION
1 Set up appropriate instruments and supplies		
2 Seated and informed patient regarding procedure		
3 Selected appropriate trays		
4 Loaded and placed trays		
5 Managed salivary flow and excess fluoride		
6 Applied fluoride for appropriate length of time		
7 Removed trays, residual foam/gel		
8 Provided posttreatment instructions		
9 Maintained infection control throughout the procedure		

Time allowed: _____ Time started: _____ Time finished: _____

Instructor comments: _____

Instructor signature: _____

COMPETENCY 7-2: APPLYING DENTAL SEALANTS

PERFORMANCE OBJECTIVE: The student will apply dental sealants to pits and fissures of teeth as prescribed by the dentist.

PROCEDURE	SELF-EVALUATION	INSTRUCTOR EVALUATION
1 Set up appropriate instruments and supplies		
2 Cleaned teeth with pumice		
3 Established and maintained isolation		
4 Etched enamel for appropriate time		
5 Applied sealant and adequately covered pits and fissures		
6 Cured sealant material for appropriate length of time		
7 Checked sealants for retention and porosity		
8 Checked occlusion		
9 Checked contacts with floss		
10 Informed patient or parent of importance of periodic maintenance visits		
11 Maintained infection control throughout the procedure		

Time allowed: _____ Time started: _____ Time finished: _____

Instructor comments: _____

Instructor signature: _____

COMPETENCY 7-3: IN-OFFICE BLEACHING

PERFORMANCE OBJECTIVE: The student will apply in-office bleaching material to a patient's teeth (or assist if procedure is not permitted by the state dental practice act).

PROCEDURE	SELF-EVALUATION	INSTRUCTOR EVALUATION
1 Set up appropriate instruments and supplies		
2 Obtained informed consent		
3 Cleaned teeth with pumice		
4 Took and recorded pretreatment shade		
5 Isolated teeth with dam and protected gingiva and other soft tissues		
6 Applied bleach and light/heat source as appropriate		
7 Checked for desired result; repeated application of bleach as needed		
8 Rinsed off bleach, removed dam, and inspected tissues for chemical burns (reported to dentist and patient, if present)		
9 Gave home care and follow-up instructions		
10 Maintained infection control throughout the procedure		

Time allowed: _____ Time started: _____ Time finished: _____

Instructor comments: _____

Instructor signature: _____

COMPETENCY 7-4: CLINICAL PROCEDURES FOR HOME BLEACHING

PERFORMANCE OBJECTIVE: The student will prepare the patient for home bleaching in two appointments to include shade taking, alginate impressions, fitting of custom trays, and home care instructions.

PROCEDURE	SELF-EVALUATION	INSTRUCTOR EVALUATION
1 Set up appropriate instruments and supplies for each visit		
First Visit		
2 Discussed procedures and obtained consent		
3 Took and recorded pretreatment shade		
4 Selected appropriate impression trays		
5 Made and disinfected alginate impressions		
6 Poured alginate impressions in dental stone (fabrication of custom trays assessed separately)		
Second Visit		
7 Tried in custom trays for fit and comfort		
8 Demonstrated loading of trays, tray insertion, removal of excess bleaching gel, and cleaning of trays		
9 Gave verbal and written instructions and reviewed potential adverse effects		
10 Scheduled follow-up visits		
11 Maintained infection control throughout each visit		

Time allowed: _____ Time started: _____ Time finished: _____

Instructor comments: _____

Instructor signature: _____

COMPETENCY 7-5: FABRICATION OF CUSTOM BLEACHING TRAYS

PERFORMANCE OBJECTIVE: The student will fabricate custom bleaching trays from stone casts using thermoplastic vinyl material.

PROCEDURE	SELF-EVALUATION	INSTRUCTOR EVALUATION
1 Set up appropriate instruments and supplies		
2 Trimmed casts appropriately		
3 Applied reservoir for bleach to cast		
4 Softened and adapted thermoplastic polyvinyl sheet to cast		
5 Trimmed tray with scalloped border to follow gingival crest		
6 Cleaned and disinfected tray		
7 Stored tray in sealed container labeled with patient's name		

Time allowed: _____ Time started: _____ Time finished: _____

Instructor comments: _____

Instructor signature: _____

COMPETENCY 7-6: FABRICATION OF A SPORTS MOUTH PROTECTOR

PERFORMANCE OBJECTIVE: The student will fabricate a sports mouth protector from a stone cast using thermoplastic vinyl sports guard material.

PROCEDURE	SELF-EVALUATION	INSTRUCTOR EVALUATION
1 Set up appropriate instruments and supplies		
2 Prepared and trimmed casts appropriately for the procedure		
3 Softened and adapted thermoplastic polyvinyl material to maxillary cast		
4 Trimmed excess material to leave proper extensions for guard		
5 Mounted upper and lower casts on articulator in proper relationship		
6 Corrected bite on the guard using the articulated casts		
7 Removed excess vinyl material created on the occlusal surface of the guard during bite correction		
8 Flamed and smoothed occlusal surface and borders		
9 Attached face guard strap (optional)		
10 Washed and disinfected guard		
11 Stored guard in sealed container labeled with patient's name		

Time allowed: _____ Time started: _____ Time finished: _____

Instructor comments: _____

Instructor signature: _____

COMPETENCY 8-1: MIX AND PLACE AMALGAM FOR CLASS II CAVITY PREPARATION

PERFORMANCE OBJECTIVE: The student will properly mix and place amalgam in a class II cavity preparation.

PROCEDURE	SELF-EVALUATION	INSTRUCTOR EVALUATION
1 Set up appropriate instruments and supplies		
2 Matrix band, retainer, and wedge properly applied		
3 Base, liner, or dentin sealer properly placed		
4 Amalgam capsule activated and mixed for recommended time and speed; satisfactory mix achieved		
5 Amalgam carried to and placed in cavity preparation in proper increments and delivered to locations appropriate for the sequence		
6 Followed correct sequence for removal of the matrix retainer, wedge, and band after removal of gross excess amalgam		
7 Checked contact with dental floss and demonstrated good judgment as to clinical acceptability of contact relationship		
8 Gave patient appropriate instructions regarding amount of biting pressure to use and marked occlusal contacts on restoration with articulating paper		
9 Gave appropriate postoperative instructions regarding when patient may chew on the restoration		
10 Maintained infection control throughout the procedure		

Time allowed: _____ Time started: _____ Time finished: _____

Instructor comments: _____

Instructor signature: _____

COMPETENCY 9-1: FINISHING AND POLISHING A PREEXISTING AMALGAM RESTORATION

PERFORMANCE OBJECTIVE: The student will demonstrate the procedure for finishing and polishing a preexisting amalgam restoration.

PROCEDURE	SELF-EVALUATION	INSTRUCTOR EVALUATION
1 Set up appropriate instruments and supplies		
2 Used appropriate patient and clinician protection		
3 Examined cavosurface margins for excess material		
4 Removed excess material in appropriate manner		
5 Defined occlusal anatomy in appropriate manner		
6 Finished smooth surface anatomy in appropriate manner		
7 Finished proximal contacts appropriately		
8 Polished in proper sequence—coarse to fine		
9 Polished with pumice and tin oxide		
10 Thoroughly rinsed area between abrasives		
11 Polished proximal surfaces with strip or dental tape		
12 Maintained infection control throughout procedure		

Time allowed: _____ Time started: _____ Time finished: _____

Instructor comments: _____

Instructor signature: _____

COMPETENCY 9-2: FINISHING AND POLISHING A PREEXISTING COMPOSITE RESTORATION

PERFORMANCE OBJECTIVE: The student will demonstrate the procedure for polishing a preexisting composite restoration.

PROCEDURE	SELF-EVALUATION	INSTRUCTOR EVALUATION
1 Set up appropriate instruments and supplies		
2 Used appropriate patient and clinician protection		
3 Examined restoration for staining		
4 Removed cavosurface flash		
5 Used appropriate abrasive with sweeping motion		
6 Finished margins in appropriate manner		
7 Polished in proper sequence—coarse to fine		
8 Thoroughly rinsed between abrasives		
9 Polished proximal surfaces with strip or dental tape		
10 Maintained infection control throughout procedure		

Time allowed: _____ Time started: _____ Time finished: _____

Instructor comments: _____

Instructor signature: _____

COMPETENCY 10-1: ZINC OXIDE EUGENOL CEMENT

PERFORMANCE OBJECTIVE: The student will demonstrate the procedure for mixing zinc oxide eugenol cement.

PROCEDURE	SELF-EVALUATION	INSTRUCTOR EVALUATION
1 Set up appropriate instruments and supplies		
2 Used appropriate patient and clinician protection		
3 Properly dispensed powder and liquid onto mixing surface		
4 Properly mixed cement to gain a homogeneous mix with minimal incorporation of air		
5 Cement mixed for recommended time to gain desired consistency Primary/luting consistency Secondary consistency		
6 Maintained infection control throughout procedure		

Time allowed: _____ Time started: _____ Time finished: _____

Instructor comments: _____

Instructor signature: _____

COMPETENCY 10-2: ZINC PHOSPHATE CEMENT

PERFORMANCE OBJECTIVE: The student will demonstrate the procedure for mixing zinc phosphate cement.

PROCEDURE	SELF-EVALUATION	INSTRUCTOR EVALUATION
1 Set up appropriate instruments and supplies		
2 Used appropriate patient and clinician protection		
3 Properly dispensed powder and liquid onto mixing surface		
4 Properly mixed cement in increments to dissipate heat and gain a homogeneous mix with minimal incorporation of air		
5 Cement mixed for recommended time to gain desired consistency Primary/luting consistency Secondary consistency		
6 Maintained infection control throughout procedure		

Time allowed: _____ Time started: _____ Time finished: _____

Instructor comments: _____

Instructor signature: _____

COMPETENCY 10-3: ZINC POLYCARBOXYLATE CEMENT

PERFORMANCE OBJECTIVE: The student will demonstrate the procedure for mixing zinc polycarboxylate cement.

PROCEDURE	SELF-EVALUATION	INSTRUCTOR EVALUATION
1 Set up appropriate instruments and supplies		
2 Used appropriate patient and clinician protection		
3 Properly dispensed powder and liquid onto mixing surface		
4 Properly mixed cement in increments to gain a homogeneous mix with minimal incorporation of air		
5 Cement mixed for recommended time to gain desired consistency Primary/luting consistency Secondary consistency		
6 Maintained infection control throughout procedure		

Time allowed: _____ Time started: _____ Time finished: _____

Instructor comments: _____

Instructor signature: _____

COMPETENCY 10-4: GLASS IONOMER CEMENT

PERFORMANCE OBJECTIVE: The student will demonstrate the procedure for mixing glass ionomer cement.

PROCEDURE	SELF-EVALUATION	INSTRUCTOR EVALUATION
1 Set up appropriate instruments and supplies		
2 Used appropriate patient and clinician protection		
3 Activated predosed capsule of cement		
4 Seated capsule in amalgamator and set timer of amalgamator for appropriate amount of time		
5 Placed mixed capsule in cement dispenser		
6 Extended capsule applicator and expressed small amount of cement		
7 Properly loaded crown to eliminate air and passed to operator		
8 Maintained infection control throughout procedure		

Time allowed: _____ Time started: _____ Time finished: _____

Instructor comments: _____

Instructor signature: _____

COMPETENCY 10-5: RESIN-BASED CEMENT

PERFORMANCE OBJECTIVE: The student will demonstrate the procedure for mixing resin-based cement.

PROCEDURE	SELF-EVALUATION	INSTRUCTOR EVALUATION
1 Set up appropriate instruments and supplies		
2 Used appropriate patient and clinician protection		
3 Cleaned the preparation with a rubber cup and nonfluoride cleaning paste		
4 Prepared the internal surface of the restoration		
5 Assisted in the application of tooth conditioner		
6 Thoroughly rinsed and blot dried the preparation		
7 Gained isolation of the area		
8 Assisted in the application of the prime/bond adhesive		
9 Dispensed cement for light-cure technique or dual-cure technique		
10 Properly loaded crown to eliminate air and passed to the operator		
11 Assisted in the seating and curing of the restoration		
12 Assisted in the removal of excess cement		
13 Maintained infection control throughout procedure		

Time allowed: _____ Time started: _____ Time finished: _____

Instructor comments: _____

Instructor signature: _____

COMPETENCY 11-1: MAXILLARY AND MANDIBULAR ALGINATE IMPRESSIONS

PERFORMANCE OBJECTIVES:
1. The student will make alginate impressions suitable for diagnostic casts.
2. The student will properly manage the patient during the procedure.

PROCEDURE	SELF-EVALUATION	INSTRUCTOR EVALUATION
1 Prepared operatory and organized all supplies		
2 Seated patient, explained procedure, draped and positioned patient, rinsed mouth, removed prostheses		
3 Selected appropriate tray		
4 Proportioned powder and water; mixed to smooth consistency		
5 Loaded tray		
6 Seated tray and stabilized it until alginate set		
7 Removed tray		
8 Evaluated impression using criteria of acceptability (see Table 11-3); determined acceptability or need to repeat impression		
9 Performed disinfecting and storage procedures		
10 Inspected mouth for retained alginate and removed it		
11 Managed patient, maintained infection control throughout procedure		

Time allowed: _____ Time started: _____ Time finished: _____

Instructor comments: _____

Instructor signature: _____

COMPETENCY 11-2: MAKING A DOUBLE-BITE IMPRESSION FOR A CROWN

PERFORMANCE OBJECTIVE: The student will demonstrate the proper procedures for making an impression for a crown using a double-bite tray.

PROCEDURE	SELF-EVALUATION	INSTRUCTOR EVALUATION
1 Prepared operatory and assembled all supplies		
2 Tried in tray and rehearsed centric closure		
3 Maintained isolation until final tray placement		
4 Removed retraction cord and assessed site before attempting impression		
5 Properly loaded syringe and placed material around the preparation		
6 Properly loaded tray, placed tray, and checked reference teeth		
7 Removed and evaluated impression		
8 Followed proper infection control procedures throughout, including disinfecting impression and placing it in labeled, zippered plastic bag for transport to laboratory		

Time allowed: _____ Time started: _____ Time finished: _____

Instructor comments: _____

Instructor signature: _____

COMPETENCY 11-3: BITE REGISTRATION WITH AN ELASTOMERIC MATERIAL

PERFORMANCE OBJECTIVES:
1. The student will demonstrate proper procedures for taking an accurate registration of the bite using an elastomeric material.
2. The student will demonstrate proper procedures for disinfecting, labeling, and storing the bite registration.

PROCEDURE	SELF-EVALUATION	INSTRUCTOR EVALUATION
1 Prepared operatory and organized all supplies		
2 Seated and draped patient, explained procedure, and rinsed patient's mouth		
3 Prepared and assembled automatic mixing gun with bite registration material and mixing tip		
4 Tried in bite tray		
5 Checked bite relation		
6 Loaded bite tray with material; dried teeth		
7 Positioned and seated tray, closed patient into centric occlusion, and checked for proper bite		
8 Removed tray when material was set		
9 Inspected bite for accuracy		
10 Rinsed and disinfected bite registration		
11 Labeled and stored bite registration		
12 Complied with proper infection control procedures throughout entire procedure		

Time allowed: _____ Time started: _____ Time finished: _____

Instructor comments: _____

Instructor signature: _____

COMPETENCY 11-4: DISINFECT IMPRESSION OR BITE REGISTRATION

PERFORMANCE OBJECTIVE: The student will demonstrate proper procedures for disinfecting, labeling, and storing impressions and bite registration.

PROCEDURE	SELF-EVALUATION	INSTRUCTOR EVALUATION
1 Rinsed impression/bite under running water		
2 Removed pooled water		
3 Sprayed or immersed impression/bite in appropriate disinfectant		
4 Treated material for appropriate length of time		
5 Rinsed off residual disinfectant		
6 Wrapped impression/bite for storage in sealed plastic bag for transport to laboratory		
7 Labeled storage container with patient's name		
8 Maintained proper infection control practices throughout entire procedure		

Time allowed: _____ Time started: _____ Time finished: _____

Instructor comments: _____

Instructor signature: _____

COMPETENCY 12-1: MIXING GYPSUM PRODUCTS

PERFORMANCE OBJECTIVE: The student will demonstrate the procedure for mixing a gypsum product to pour an impression.

PROCEDURE	SELF-EVALUATION	INSTRUCTOR EVALUATION
1 Set up appropriate instruments and supplies		
2 Measured recommended amount of water and gypsum		
3 Sifted the powder gradually into the water		
4 Mixed the material vigorously for 60 seconds until all the material was smooth and incorporated		
5 Vibrated the material to remove all air incorporated while mixing		
6 Mixing procedure completed in no more than 2 minutes		
7 Cleaned all equipment		

Time allowed: _____ Time started: _____ Time finished: _____

Instructor comments: _____

Instructor signature: _____

COMPETENCY 12-2: POURING THE ANATOMIC PORTION OF THE CAST

PERFORMANCE OBJECTIVE: The student will demonstrate the procedure for pouring the anatomic portion of the cast.

PROCEDURE	SELF-EVALUATION	INSTRUCTOR EVALUATION
1 Set up appropriate instruments and supplies		
2 Rinsed impression of all disinfecting solution		
3 Placed a small increment of gypsum in the most posterior area of the impression		
4 Added successive increments and allowed them to flow into individual tooth indentations		
5 Tilted the tray to move the gypsum forward across the anterior portion of the impression		
6 Tilted the tray to allow the gypsum to move to the outer end of the impression		
7 Filled impression slightly higher than the periphery of the impression and tray		
8 Cleaned all equipment		

Time allowed: _____ Time started: _____ Time finished: _____

Instructor comments: _____

Instructor signature: _____

COMPETENCY 12-3: POURING THE ART PORTION OF THE CAST

PERFORMANCE OBJECTIVE: The student will demonstrate the procedure for pouring the art portion of the cast.

PROCEDURE	SELF-EVALUATION	INSTRUCTOR EVALUATION
1 Set up appropriate instruments and supplies		
2 Prepared a mixture of gypsum for the base		
3 Placed the mixture on glass tile; 0.5 inch thick and slightly larger than dimensions of the impression and tray		
4 Inverted the poured impression onto the base		
5 Made sure the poured impression was parallel with the base		
6 Moved the base material up to meet the heels and sides of the impression		
7 Made sure there were no large air pockets and no excessive material was touching the impression tray		
8 Smoothed the tongue area of the mandibular cast		
9 Allowed the gypsum to set completely before separating		

Time allowed: _____ Time started: _____ Time finished: _____

Instructor comments: _____

Instructor signature: _____

COMPETENCY 12-4: TRIMMING DIAGNOSTIC CASTS

PERFORMANCE OBJECTIVE: The student will demonstrate the procedure for trimming diagnostic casts.

PROCEDURE	SELF-EVALUATION	INSTRUCTOR EVALUATION
1 Set up appropriate instruments and supplies		
2 Art portion of casts soaked in water for 5 minutes		
3 Working table of model trimmer secured and at a 90° angle to the trimming wheel		
4 Excess gypsum cut from models to allow articulation		
5 Small bubbles of gypsum removed from occlusal surfaces		
6 Maxillary and mandibular casts measured for height		
7 Base cuts parallel with occlusal surfaces and in the correct proportion		
8 Side and back cuts measured for length and width		
9 Side and back cuts straight and symmetric		
10 Anterior cut of maxillary pointed and mandibular rounded		
11 Heel cuts approximately 0.5 inch long and symmetric		
12 Model finished and labeled		

Time allowed: _____ Time started: _____ Time finished: _____

Instructor comments: _____

Instructor signature: _____

COMPETENCY 13-1: FABRICATE A CUSTOM ACRYLIC IMPRESSION TRAY

PERFORMANCE OBJECTIVE: The student will fabricate a custom impression tray using chemical-cured acrylic tray material and a wax spacer.

PROCEDURE	SELF-EVALUATION	INSTRUCTOR EVALUATION
1 Set up appropriate instruments and supplies		
2 Applied separator to cast		
3 Adapted wax spacer and cut holes for stops in appropriate locations		
4 Mixed and adapted tray material		
5 Trimmed excess material and attached handle in appropriate location		
6 Removed wax spacer		
7 Removed excess material and smoothed borders		
8 Confirmed fit of tray on cast		
9 Disinfected and stored tray in sealed bag labeled with patient's name		

Time allowed: _____ Time started: _____ Time finished: _____

Instructor comments: _____

Instructor signature: _____

COMPETENCY 13-2: FABRICATION OF LIGHT-CURED RECORD BASES

PERFORMANCE OBJECTIVE: The student will construct record bases for complete dentures using light-cured material.

PROCEDURE	SELF-EVALUATION	INSTRUCTOR EVALUATION
1 Set up appropriate instruments and supplies		
2 Prepared cast correctly		
3 Applied and trimmed light-cured record base material		
4 Placed shrinkage relief slit and sealed it after initial polymerization		
5 Light-cured record base on both sides and removed uncured film		
6 Adjusted periphery with acrylic bur or sand drum		
7 Smoothed borders with pumice on a rag wheel		
8 Confirmed fit on the cast.		

Time allowed: _____ Time started: _____ Time finished: _____

Instructor comments: _____

Instructor signature: _____

COMPETENCY 14-1: METAL PROVISIONAL CROWN

PERFORMANCE OBJECTIVE: The student will demonstrate the procedure for fabricating and cementing a metal provisional crown.

PROCEDURE	SELF-EVALUATION	INSTRUCTOR EVALUATION
1 Set up appropriate instruments and supplies		
2 Used appropriate patient and clinician protection		
3 Chose a crown with a mesiodistal width equal to that of the missing space		
4 Trimmed the crown to match the contour of the gingiva and the occlusal relationship of the adjacent dentition		
5 Crown margins meet the preparation		
6 Crown contour resembles the adjacent tooth facially, lingually, interproximally, and occlusally/incisally		
7 Crown fits snugly against the finish line		
8 Crown contacts the adjacent teeth		
9 Crown occlusion replicates that of the adjacent teeth		
10 All crown surfaces are smoothed and polished		
11 Isolated the area and loaded the crown with an appropriate provisional cement		
12 Seated the crown and established appropriate pressure on the crown and adjacent teeth		
13 Restored tooth and surrounding area are free of excess cement		
14 Crown margins are sealed		

Time allowed: _____ Time started: _____ Time finished: _____

Instructor comments: _____

Instructor signature: _____

COMPETENCY 14-2: POLYCARBONATE PROVISIONAL CROWN

PERFORMANCE OBJECTIVE: The student will demonstrate the procedure for fabricating and cementing a polycarbonate provisional crown.

PROCEDURE	SELF-EVALUATION	INSTRUCTOR EVALUATION
1 Set up appropriate instruments and supplies		
2 Used appropriate patient and clinician protection		
3 Chose a crown with a mesiodistal width equal to that of the missing space		
4 Trimmed the crown to match the contour of the gingiva and the occlusal relationship of the adjacent dentition		
5 Crown margins meet the preparation		
6 Crown contour resembles the adjacent tooth facially, lingually, interproximally, and occlusally/incisally		
7 Retried the crown and checked for occlusion		
8 Crown occlusion replicates that of the adjacent teeth		
9 Established the contacts of the adjacent teeth		
10 All crown surfaces are smooth and polished		
11 Isolated the area and loaded the crown with an appropriate provisional cement		
12 Seated the crown and established appropriate pressure on the crown and adjacent teeth		
13 Restored tooth and surrounding area are free of excess cement		
14 Crown margins are sealed		

Time allowed: _____ Time started: _____ Time finished: _____

Instructor comments: _____

Instructor signature: _____

COMPETENCY 14-3: CUSTOM PROVISIONAL CROWN

PERFORMANCE OBJECTIVE: The student will demonstrate the procedure for fabricating and cementing a custom provisional crown.

PROCEDURE	SELF-EVALUATION	INSTRUCTOR EVALUATION
1 Set up appropriate instruments and supplies		
2 Used appropriate patient and clinician protection		
3 Prepared a template of the tooth before crown preparation		
4 Prepared the custom provisional material		
5 Dispensed the provisional material into the template without trapping air		
6 Replaced the template into the patient's mouth in the proper alignment		
7 Removed the material in the appropriate time frame		
8 Trimmed excess material from the crown		
9 Crown occlusion replicates that of the adjacent teeth		
10 Crown contacts the adjacent teeth		
11 All crown surfaces are smooth and polished		
12 Isolated the area and loaded the crown with an appropriate provisional cement		
13 Seated the crown and established appropriate pressure on the crown and adjacent teeth		
14 Restored tooth and surrounding area are free of excess cement		
15 Crown margins are sealed		

Time allowed: _____ Time started: _____ Time finished: _____

Instructor comments: _____

Instructor signature: _____

COMPETENCY 14-4: INTRACORONAL CEMENT PROVISIONAL RESTORATION

PERFORMANCE OBJECTIVE: The student will demonstrate the procedure for fabricating an intracoronal provisional restoration.

PROCEDURE	SELF-EVALUATION	INSTRUCTOR EVALUATION
1 Set up appropriate instruments and supplies		
2 Used appropriate patient and clinician protection		
3 Isolated area and placed matrix and wedge		
4 Prepared an appropriate mix of provisional cement		
5 Condensed the material into the proximal and then occlusal areas without trapping air		
6 Sealed margins with the provisional material		
7 Removed excess material from proximal and occlusal margins		
8 Created embrasure		
9 Established occlusal anatomy and height		
10 Established the contacts		
11 Maintained infection control throughout procedure		

Time allowed: _____ Time started: _____ Time finished: _____

Instructor comments: _____

Instructor signature: _____

COMPETENCY 15-1: WAX BITE REGISTRATION

PERFORMANCE OBJECTIVE: The student will demonstrate the procedure to obtain a legible bite registration.

PROCEDURE	SELF-EVALUATION	INSTRUCTOR EVALUATION
1 Set up appropriate instruments and supplies		
2 Formed utility wax into a horseshoe shape		
3 Customized wax to shape of patient's arch		
4 Gave appropriate patient instructions		
5 Placed wax over occlusal surfaces of maxillary teeth		
6 Gave patient instructions on biting pressure		
7 Removed wax without distortion		
8 Disinfected and stored wax registration		
9 Maintained infection control throughout procedure		

Time allowed: _____ Time started: _____ Time finished: _____

Instructor comments: _____

Instructor signature: _____

CONVERSION TABLES

TEMPERATURE

Celsius ($^\circ$ C) = 5/9 Fahrenheit ($^\circ$ F) – 32
Fahrenheit ($^\circ$F) = 9/5 Celsius ($^\circ$ C) + 32

LINEAR MEASUREMENT

METRIC

1 meter (m) = 100 centimeters (cm)
1 centimeter (cm) = 0.01 meter (m)
1 millimeter (mm) = 0.001 meter (m)
1 micrometer (μm, also called micron) = 0.001 millimeter (mm)
1 nanometer (nm) =0.000001mm
1 Angstrom (Å) = 0.0000001 mm

CONVERTING USA (ENGLISH) MEASUREMENTS TO METRIC

1 inch (in) = 25.4 millimeters (mm) = 2.54 centimeters (cm)
39.37 inches (in) = 1 meter (m)
3.28 feet (ft) = 1 meter
1 yard (yd) = 0.9144 meter (m)

LIQUID MEASUREMENT

METRIC

1 liter (l) = 1000 milliliters (ml) = 1000 cubic centimeters (cc)

CONVERTING USA (ENGLISH) MEASUREMENTS TO METRIC

1 quart (qt) = 0.946 liter (l)
1 ounce (oz) = 29.6 milliliters (ml)

WEIGHT

METRIC

1 kilogram (kg) = 1000 grams (g)
1 gram (g) = 0.001 kilogram (kg) = 1,000,000 micrograms (μg)
1 milligram (mg) = 0.001 gram

CONVERTING METRIC TO USA (ENGLISH) MEASUREMENTS

1 kilogram (kg) = 2.2 pounds (lb)
1 gram (g) = 0.0022 pound (lb) = 0.035 ounce (oz)
28.35 gram (g) = 1 ounce (oz)

COMMON MEASURES OF WEIGHT FOR GOLD

1 troy ounce = 20 pennyweight (dwt)
1 pennyweight = 1.555 grams = 24 grains (gr)
1 grain (gr) = 0.065 gram

MEASURES OF GOLD CONTENT

24 carat = 100% gold = 1000 fine
12 carat = 50% gold = 500 fine

MEASURES OF FORCE (PER AREA)

1 kilogram/square centimeter (kg/cm^2) = 14.223 pounds/square inch (lb/in^2)
1 kg/cm^2 = 0.0981 megapascals (MPa)
1 meganewton/square meter (MN/m^2) = 145 lb/in^2

ANSWERS TO REVIEW QUESTIONS

Chapter 2

1. b
2. c
3. c
4. c
5. b
6. a
7. d
8. c
9. c
10. a

Chapter 3

1. a
2. b
3. c
4. d
5. b
6. a
7. b
8. b
9. c
10. b

Chapter 4

1. d
2. d
3. a
4. c
5. c
6. d
7. c

Chapter 5

1. a
2. a
3. a
4. c
5. e
6. a
7. b
8. c
9. b
10. b
11. c
12. b

Chapter 6

1. c
2. d
3. d
4. a
5. c
6. c
7. b
8. d
9. d
10. c
11. a
12. c
13. a

Chapter 7

1. b
2. b
3. c
4. c
5. d
6. c
7. b
8. c
9. d
10. a
11. b
12. d
13. b
14. b

Chapter 8

1. c
2. c
3. c
4. d
5. c
6. c
7. a
8. d
9. d
10. c
11. a
12. d
13. b
14. a
15. a
16. a
17. b
18. a
19. d
20. c
21. c
22. d
23. d
24. b
25. d
26. a
27. d
28. a
39. d
30. d

Chapter 9

1. d
2. c
3. d
4. d
5. d
6. d
7. c
8. b

Chapter 10

1. b	7. a
2. b	8. d
3. d	9. d
4. c	10. d
5. b	11. b
6. c	12. c

Chapter 11

1. b	11. d
2. a	12. c
3. c	13. b
4. d	14. d
5. c	15. d
6. d	16. c
7. a	17. a
8. d	18. a
9. d	19. d
10. d	20. b

Chapter 12

1. a	6. a
2. c	7. c
3. c	8. d
4. c	9. a
5. c	10. d

Chapter 13

1. c	12. c
2. a	13. d
3. d	14. d
4. d	15. c
5. b	16. c
6. d	17. d
7. c	18. a
8. a	19. d
9. d	20. b
10. d	21. d
11. d	

Chapter 14

1. c	6. d
2. b	7. b
3. d	8. d
4. c	9. a
5. a	10. c

Chapter 15

1. b	5. d
2. a	6. a
3. d	7. c
4. a	

GLOSSARY

Abrasive—a material comprised of particles of sufficient hardness and sharpness to cut or scratch a softer material when drawn across its surface.

Adhesion—the act of sticking two things together. In dentistry it is used to describe the bonding or the cementation process. Chemical adhesion occurs when atoms or molecules of dissimilar substances bond together and differs from cohesion in which attraction among atoms and molecules of like (similar) materials holds them together.

Adhesive—an intermediate material that causes two materials to stick together.

Alginate—a versatile, irreversible hydrocolloid impression material that is the most used in the dental office; however, it lacks the accuracy and fine surface detail needed for impressions for crown and bridge procedures.

Alloy—a mixture of two or more metals.

Alloy, admixed—a mixture of lathe-cut and spherical alloys for amalgam.

Alloy, base metal—an alloy comprised of non-noble metals.

Alloy, high noble—an alloy containing at least 60% noble metals, 40% of which must be gold.

Alloy, lathe-cut—irregular-shaped particles formed by shaving fine particles from an alloy ingot for amalgam.

Alloy, noble—an alloy comprised of metals that do not corrode readily.

Alloy, porcelain bonding—special casting alloy manufactured for its compatibility with porcelain that has been bonded to it at high temperature.

Alloy, spherical—alloy particles produced as small spheres for amalgam.

Alloy, wrought metal—an alloy that has been mechanically changed into another form to improve its properties.

Amalgamation—a reaction that occurs when silver-based alloy is mixed with mercury.

Amalgam, dental—restorative material comprised of silver-based alloy mixed with mercury.

Anneal—to modify physical properties of a metal by heating it.

Antibacterial mouth rinse—a liquid used to rinse the oral cavity to reduce mouth odor and suppress bacteria associated with periodontal disease and dental caries.

Base/high-strength base—a thick layer of cement used in a cavity preparation to protect the pulp from chemical insult or to act as a thermal insulator.

Bio-aerosol—a cloud like mist containing droplets, tooth dust, materials dust, and bacteria of a particle size less that 5 μm in diameter.

Biocompatible—the property of a material that allows it not to impede or adversely affect living tissue.

Bite registration—an impression of the occlusal relationship of opposing teeth in centric occlusion (patient's normal bite).

Bleaching—a cosmetic process that uses chemicals to remove discolorations from teeth or to lighten them.

Bond or **Bonding**—to connect or fasten; to bind (*Webster's New World Dictionary*). Basically, there are two ways that items are joined together at the surface: by mechanical adhesion (physical interlocking) and by chemical adhesion.

Bonding agent—a low-viscosity resin that penetrates porosities and irregularities in the surface of the tooth or restoration created by acid etching for the purpose of facilitating bonding.

Build-up—a restorative material such as amalgam, composite resin, or glass ionomer cement used to replace missing tooth structure in a badly broken-down tooth and act as support for a restoration such as a crown.

Calcium hydroxide—used as a low-strength base and direct pulp-capping material to stimulate secondary dentin formation.

Cariogenic—substances or microorganisms that promote dental caries.

Casts—hard replicas of hard and soft tissue of the patient's oral cavity made from gypsum products. They are also referred to as models in some literature.

Chemical-set materials—materials that set through a timed chemical reaction with the combination of a catalyst and base.

Chroma—the intensity or strength of a color (e.g., a bold yellow has more chroma than a pastel yellow).

Cleansing—the removal of soft deposits from the surface of restorations and tooth structure. Polishing and cleansing are done to remove surface stains and soft deposits from the clinical crowns and exposed root surfaces of teeth after all hard deposits are removed. Aside from abrasives there are also chemical cleansing products that are used primarily for removable prostheses.

Coefficient of thermal expansion (CTE)—the measurement of change of volume or length in relationship to change in temperature.

Compomer—a composite resin that has polyacid, fluoride-releasing groups added.

Composite, dual-cured—composite that contains components of light-cured and self-cured composites. When the two parts are mixed together, it polymerizes by a chemical reaction that can be accelerated with blue light activation.

Composite, flowable—a light-cured, low-viscosity composite resin that contains fewer filler particles.

Composite, hybrid—composite that contains both macro-filler and micro-filler particles to obtain the strength of a macrofill and the polishability of a microfill.

Composite, light-cured—composite that polymerizes when a chemical is activated by light in the blue wave range.

Composite, macrofilled—an early generation of composite that contained filler particles ranging from 10 to 100 μm.

Composite, microfilled—composite that contains very small filler particles averaging 0.04 μm in diameter.

Composite, packable—a light-cured, highly viscous, heavily-filled composite resin for dentists who use a placement technique with composite that is similar to that of amalgam.

Composite resin—tooth-colored material comprised of an organic resin matrix and inorganic filler particles.

Composite, self-cured—composite that polymerizes by a chemical reaction when two resins are mixed together.

Compressive force—force applied to compress an object.

Contamination—contact with a substance that changes the chemical or mechanical properties (e.g., contamination of the etched surface of the tooth with saliva prior to bonding).

Corrosion—deterioration of a metal because of a chemical attack or electrochemical reaction with dissimilar metals in the presence of a solution containing electrolytes (such as saliva).

Corrosive—usually an acid or strong base that can cause damage to skin, clothing, metals, and equipment.

Creep—the gradual change in the shape of a restoration because of compression from occlusion or adjacent teeth.

Cure or **polymerization**—a reaction that links low-molecular-weight resin molecules (monomers) together into high-molecular-weight chains (polymers) that harden or set. The reaction can be initiated by strictly a chemical reaction (self-cure), by light in the blue-wave range (light-cure), by a combination of the two (dual-cure), or by heat.

Custom-made—made specifically to fit one individual.

Demineralization—the action usually caused by acids that removes minerals from the tooth.

Density—the measure of the weight of a material compared to its volume.

Dental caries—a process whereby bacteria in plaque metabolize carbohydrates and produce acids that remove minerals from teeth and permit bacteria to invade.

Dental stone—a stronger, less porous form of gypsum product used in dentistry. (It is stronger than plaster.)

Desensitizing agent— a chemical that seals open dentinal tubules to reduce tooth sensitivity to air, sweets, and temperature changes.

Diagnostic casts—positive replicas of the teeth produced from impressions that create a negative representation of the teeth. They are commonly called *study models,* and generally are made from dental plaster or stone. They are used for patient education, treatment planning and for tracking the progress of treatment (e.g., orthodontic models or for numerous chair-side and laboratory procedures).

Dies—replicas of the prepared teeth that are generally removable from the working cast.

Die stone—the densest form of gypsum product used in dentistry.

Dimensional change—a change in the size of matter. For dental materials, this usually manifests as expansion caused by heating and contraction caused by cooling.

Direct fabrication—provisional restorations made directly inside the patient's mouth.

Direct restorative materials—restorations placed directly into cavity preparation.

Dual-set materials—materials that polymerize by a chemical reaction when the material is mixed with a catalyst or initiated by exposure to a blue light (or by a combination of chemical or light reaction).

Ductility—the ability of an object to be pulled or stretched under tension without rupture.

Edge strength—the strength of a material at fine margins.

Elasticity—the ability of a material to recovers its shape completely after deformation from an applied force.

Erosion—the loss of tooth mineral caused by acids, *not* bacterial metabolism.

Esthetic materials, direct placement—tooth-colored materials that can be placed directly into the cavity preparation without being constructed outside of the mouth first.

Esthetic materials, indirect placement—tooth-colored materials that are used to construct restorations outside of the mouth on replicas of the prepared teeth in the dental laboratory or at chair-side. Later they are cemented to the teeth.

Etching or **Conditioning**—terms used interchangeably to describe the process of preparing the surface of a tooth or a restoration for bonding. The most common etching material (etchant) used is phosphoric acid.

Excess residue—a wax film remaining on an object after the wax is removed.

Exothermic reaction—the production of heat resulting from the reaction of the components of some materials when they are mixed.

Extracoronal restoration—a restoration that covers all or part of the external surface of the tooth and may extend over the cusp tips on facial or lingual surfaces such as onlays, ¾ crown, full crowns, and veneers.

Extrinsic stains—stains occurring on the tooth surface.

Fatigue failure—a fracture resulting from repeated stresses that produce microscopic flaws that grow.

Film thickness—the minimum thickness obtainable by a layer of a material. It is particularly important to dental cements.

Final set time—the time at which the material has reached its ultimate state.

Finish line—the continuous margin that borders the preparation to which the restoration is fit or finished.

Finishing—a procedure used to reduce excess restorative material to develop appropriate occlusion and contour. This usually is done with rotary instruments. Finishing removes surface blemishes and produces a smooth surface.

Flash—featherlike excess of material that extends beyond the cavity margins.

Flash point—The lowest temperature at which the vapor of a volatile substance will ignite with a flash. A low flash point means that a substance can catch fire very easily.

Flexural stress—bending a combination of tension and compression.

Flow—the movement of the wax as it approaches the melting range.

Fluorapatite—a tooth mineral that results when fluoride is incorporated into hydroxyapatite.

Fluoride—a naturally occurring chemical that helps to protect tooth structure from dental caries.

Fluorosis—enamel abnormality caused by consumption of excessive levels of fluoride.

Free radical—a reactive group on one end of a monomer that initiates the joining of adjacent monomer molecules to form a polymer.

Galvanism—an electric current transmitted between two dissimilar metals.

Gamma-2 phase—a chemical reaction between tin in the silver-based alloy and mercury that causes corrosion in the amalgam.

Gauge—a measure of the thickness of a wire. For example, an 8-gauge wire is thicker than a 16-gauge wire.

Gel—a semisolid state in which colloidal particles form a framework that traps liquid (e.g., Jell-O).

Glass ionomer—a self-cured, tooth-colored, fluoride-releasing restorative material that bonds to tooth structure without an additional bonding agent.

Glass ionomer cement—one of the most versatile cements; used as a permanent luting agent and restorative material, and for low- and high-strength base and core buildups.

Grit—the particle size of the abrasive, typically classified as coarse, medium, fine, and superfine.

Gypsum—a material found in nature and composed of the dihydrate of calcium sulfate; used to make dental casts and dies.

Hardness—the resistance of a solid to penetration.

Hazardous chemicals—dangerous chemicals that are poisonous and can cause burns to the skin or cause fire.

Hue—the color of the tooth or restoration. It may include a mixture of colors, such as yellow-brown.

Hybrid (resin-modified) glass ionomer—a glass ionomer to which resin has been added to improve its physical properties.

Hybrid layer—a resin/dentin layer formed by the penetration of the dentin bonding resin through collagen fibrils exposed by acid etching and into the etched dentin surface. It serves as an excellent resin-rich layer onto which the restorative material, such as composite resin, can be bonded.

Hydrocolloid—gluelike material comprised of two or more substances in which one substance does not go into solution but is suspended within another substance. It has at least two phases: (1) a liquid phase called a sol and (2) a semisolid phase called a gel.

Hydrocolloid, irreversible—an impression material that is mixed to a sol state, and as it sets it converts to a gel by a chemical reaction that irreversibly changes its nature.

Hydrocolloid, reversible—an impression material that can be heated to change a gel into a fluid sol state that can flow around the teeth, then cooled to gel again to make an impression of the shapes of the oral structures.

Hydrodynamic theory of tooth sensitivity—pain caused by movement of pulpal fluid in open (unsealed) dentinal tubules. Actions that cause a change in the pressure on the fluid within the dentinal tubules stimulate nerve fibers in the processes of odontoblasts in the pulp to send out a pain response.

Hysteresis—the property of a material to have two different temperatures for melting and solidifying, unlike water, which has one temperature for both.

Ignitable—a material or chemical that can erupt into fire easily.

Imbibition—the act of absorbing moisture.

Implant, endosseous (endosteal)—implant placed into the bone.

Implant, subperiosteal—implant placed on top of the bone and under the periosteum.

Implant, transosteal—implant that penetrates entirely through the bone.

Impression compound—an impression material comprised of resin and wax with fillers added to make it stronger and more stable than wax.

Impression plaster—an impression material comprised of a gypsum product similar to plaster of paris.

Indirect fabrication—construction of provisional or final restorations on a cast outside the patient's mouth.

Indirect restorative materials—materials used to fabricate restorations outside the mouth that are subsequently placed into the mouth.

Initial set time—the time at which the material can no longer be manipulated in the mouth.

Inorganic filler particles—fine particles of quartz, silica, or glass that give strength and wear resistance to the material.

Insulators—materials having low thermal conductivity.

Interface—the space between the walls of the preparation and the restoration.

Intermediate—materials expected to last from a few weeks to a year.

Intracoronal restoration—a restoration within the crown of the tooth, such as an inlay.

Intrinsic stains—stains that are incorporated into the tooth structure usually during the tooth's development.

Light-activated materials—materials that require a blue light source to initiate a reaction.

Liner/low-strength base—a thin layer of material used to protect the tooth from the components of dental materials and microleakage, stimulate reparative dentin, or act as a pulp capping.

Lost wax casting technique—the procedure for fabricating a metal restoration by encasing the wax pattern in stone then vaporizing the wax under high temperatures to leave an empty impression space (pattern) once occupied by the wax. Molten metal is then cast into the space and takes the shape of the pattern.

Luting—to cement two components together such as an indirect restoration cemented on or in a tooth (e.g., inlays, crowns, bridges, veneers, orthodontic bracket and bands, posts and pins).

Malleability—the ability to be compressed and formed into a thin sheet without rupture.

Margination—a procedure for removal of excessive restorative material from margins of restorations.

Material safety data sheet (MSDS)—A printed product report from the manufacturer containing important information about the chemicals, hazards, clean-up, and special personal protective equipment related to a product.

Melting range—a range of melting points of the individual components of the wax.

Microleakage—leakage of fluid and bacteria caused by microscopic gaps that occur at the interface of the tooth and the restoration margins.

Mixing time—the amount of time allotted to bring the components of a material together into a homogenous mix.

Model plaster—the weakest, most porous form of gypsum product used in dentistry.

Monomer—low-molecular-weight molecules that are joined in long chains to form polymers. As used in dentistry monomers are usually liquids.

Mouthguard—a hard or pliable resin that protects teeth from trauma during sports activities or from teeth grinding.

Opaque—optical property in which light is completely absorbed by an object.

Organic resin (polymer) matrix—thick resin liquids made up of two or more organic molecules that form a matrix around filler particles.

Osseointegration—bone growth in into intimate contact with an implant.

Overhang—excessive restorative material present at the cervical cavosurface margin.

Over-the-counter (OTC)—available in retail or drug stores without a doctor's prescription.

Particulate matter—very small particles (e.g., dust from dental plaster or stone).

Percolation—movement of fluid in the microscopic gap of the restoration margin as a result of differences in the expansion and contraction rates of the tooth and the restoration with temperature changes associated with ingestion of cold or hot fluids or foods.

Permanent—lasting indefinitely.

Personal protective equipment (PPE)—equipment for the employee that provides protection during clinical or laboratory procedures.

Pigments—coloring agents that give composites their color.

Plasticizer—liquid added to acrylic resin to soften it and make it more pliable.

Polishing—a procedure that produces a shiny, smooth surface by eliminating fine scratches, minor surface imperfections, and surface stains using mild abrasives frequently found in the form of pastes or compounds.

Poly (methyl methacrylate)—a polymer comprised of numerous methyl methacrylate monomers linked together into a long chain.

Polyether—a rubber impression material with ether functional groups. It has high accuracy and is popular for crown and bridge procedures.

Polymer—a long chain, high-molecular-weight molecule produced by the linking of many low-molecular-weight monomer molecules.

Polymerization—the act of forming polymers.

Polymerization, addition—a common form of polymerization of dental materials. Monomer molecules are added to one another sequentially as the reactive group on one molecule initiates bonding with an adjacent monomer molecule and frees another reactive group to repeat the process.

Polymers, cross-linked—the joining of adjacent long-chain polymers by bonding of short chains along their sides.

Polysulfide—a rubber impression material that has sulfur-containing (mercaptan) functional groups.

Porcelain—a tooth-colored ceramic material comprised of crystals of feldspar, alumina, and silica that are fused together at high temperatures to form a hard, uniform glass-like material.

Porosity—numerous microscopic holes or voids within a material often caused during polymerization of resins when a monomer vaporizes and is lost.

Post—a metal or non-metal dowel placed within the root canal to retain a core build-up.

Post, active—a post that engages the root canal surface like a screw.

Post, custom—a post cast to fit precisely in the root canal space, and it usually has the core attached.

Post, passive—a post that sits in the prepared canal space but does not engage the root surface.

Post, preformed—a factory-made post supplied in several sizes.

Pouring—the process of vibrating the flowable gypsum product into the impression. This process must produce a cast that is the exact replica of the impression.

Precious metal—the classification of metal based upon its high cost.

Prevention/preventive aids—chemicals, devices, or procedures that reduce or eliminate disease or tooth destruction in the oral cavity.

Primary consistency—less-viscous mix of material that flows easily, can be drawn to a 1" string with a spatula when lifted from the center of its mass, and is suitable for luting.

Proportional limit—the greatest stress a structure can withstand without permanent deformation.

Prosthesis—a device used for the replacement of missing tissues. It can serve both cosmetic and functional roles.

Provisional coverage—a restoration that temporarily occupies the place of a permanent restoration, typically for up to 2 to 3 weeks. In the case of implant and complex prosthodontic and periodontally involved cases, provisional restorations may be used to last for extended periods of time. These restorations are also commonly referred to as temporaries.

Reactive—ability of a substance to take part in a chemical reaction resulting in a different end product.

Resilience—the resistance of a material to permanent deformation.

Resin-based cement—modified composite used to bond ceramic indirect restoration, conventional crowns and bridges, and orthodontic brackets.

Restorative agents—materials used to reconstruct tooth structure.

Retention—a material's ability to maintain its position without displacement under stress.

Sealant—a protective coating usually composed of resin that is bonded to enamel to protect pits and fissures from dental caries.

Secondary consistency—thick, putty-like, condensable mix of material that can be rolled into a ball or rope, suitable for use as an insulating base.

Sedative—to soothe or act in a sedative manner; to relieve pain.

Shearing force—force applied when two surfaces slide against each other or in a twisting or rotating motion.

Shelf life—the useful life of a material before it deteriorates or changes in quality.

Silane coupling agent—a chemical that helps to bind the filler particles to the organic matrix.

Silicone, addition—a silicone rubber impression material that sets by linking of molecules in long chains but produces no by-product. It is commonly known as polyvinyl siloxane and is the most popular material for crown and bridge procedures because of its accuracy, dimensional stability, and ease of use.

Silicone, condensation—a silicone rubber impression material that sets by linking of molecules in long chains but produces a liquid by-product through condensation.

Smear layer—a tenacious layer of debris on the enamel or dentin surface resulting from cutting the tooth during cavity preparation. It is comprised of fine particles of cut tooth structure, bacteria, and salivary components.

Soft liner, long-term—a soft material that lines a denture for use in patients who have problems with hard-acrylic denture bases. It is expected to last 1 to 3 years.

Soft liner, short-term—a soft provisional material that lines a denture for a short period of time to improve tissue health. It is also called a tissue conditioner and, it typically lasts from a few days to a few weeks.

Sol—a liquid state in which colloidal particles are suspended. Through cooling or by chemical reaction it can change into a gel.

Solder—an alloy used to join two metals together or to repair cast metal restorations.

Solubility—susceptible to being dissolved.

Stiffness—a material's resistance to deformation.

Strain—distortion or deformation occurring when an object cannot resist a stress.

Substantivity—property of a material to have a prolonged therapeutic effect after its initial use.

Surface energy—the electrical charge that attracts atoms to a surface.

Surfactant—a chemical that lowers the surface tension of a substance so it is more readily wetted. For example, oil beads on the surface of water, but soap acts as a surfactant to allow the oil to spread over the surface.

Syneresis—a characteristic of gels to contract and squeeze out some liquid which then accumulates on the surface.

Tarnish—discoloration resulting from oxidation of a thin layer of a metal at its surface. It is not as destructive as corrosion.

Temporary—materials expected to last from a few days to a few weeks.

Tensile force—force applied in opposite directions to stretch an object.

Therapeutic agents—materials used to treat disease.

Thermal conductivity—the rate at which heat flows through a material.

Thixotropic—property of a liquid to flow more readily under mechanical force.

Toughness—the ability of a material to resist fracture.

Toxicity—the degree to which a substance is poisonous.

Translucency—varying degrees of light passing through and being absorbed by an object.

Transparent—light passing directly through an object.

Trimming—the process of removing excess hardened gypsum from the cast for ease in working with the cast and appearance in presentation.

Triturator (amalgamator)—a mechanical device used to mix the silver-based alloy particles with mercury to produce amalgam.

Ultimate Strength—the maximum amount of stress a material can withstand without breaking.

Value—how light or dark a color is. A low value is darker and a high value is brighter.

Varnish—a thin layer placed on the floor and walls of the cavity preparation to seal the dentinal tubules and minimize microleakage.

Viscosity—the ability of a liquid material to flow.

Vitality—a life-like quality.

Water sorption—the ability to absorb moisture.

Wax pattern—a duplicate of the restoration carved in wax.

Wet dentin bonding – bonding to dentin that is kept moist after acid etching to facilitate penetration of bonding resins into etched dentin.

Wetting—the ability of a liquid to wet or intimately contact a solid surface. Water beading on a waxed car is an example of poor wetting.

Working casts—casts generally made from one of the dental stones and are strong enough to resist the stresses of fabricating an indirect restoration or prosthesis.

Working time—the time permitted to manipulate the material in the mouth.

Yield strength—the amount of stress at which a substance deforms.

Zinc oxide eugenol—a hard and brittle impression material used in complete denture procedures. A variation of this material is used as a provisional filling material.

Zinc oxide eugenol cement—a cement generally used as a provisional material or to temporarily cement provisional coverage.

Zinc phosphate cement—the oldest of the cements; used primarily for permanent luting.

Zinc polycarboxylate cement—the first cement developed with adhesive bonds; used primarily for permanent luting.

INDEX

Page numbers followed by *f* indicate figures; page numbers followed by *t* indicate tables

Fluoride (*Continued*)
 erosion protection, 92
 gels containing, 20, 93–94, 99t
 glass ionomer release of, 73–74, 177
 ingested, 93
 in-office application of, 93–94, 94f, 95t
 over-the-counter rinses containing, 94, 95t
 prophylaxis pastes, 94
 rinses containing, 92
 safety of, 94–95
 toothpaste containing, 94
 topical versus systemic effects of, 91–92
 varnishes, 93
Fluorosis, 90–91
Food and Drug Administration, 5
Force
 compressive, 7–8
 elastic modulus, 20
 principles of, 8–9
 shearing, 7–8
 sources of, 8
 tensile, 7–8
Free radical, 250–251

G
Gag reflex, 204–205
Galvanic shock, 10, 128
Galvanism, 7, 10, 129
Gamma-2 phase, 124, 127
Gauge, 125, 137
Gel
 definition of, 196
 fluoride, 20, 93–94, 99t
Glass ionomer cements
 biocompatibility of, 73
 chlorhexidine gluconate effects, 93
 clinical uses of, 73–74
 color of, 73
 definition of, 61, 73
 fluoride release from, 73–74, 177
 history of, 182
 hybrid, 61, 74–75, 177t, 183
 lamination technique, 74
 liners, 74
 luting cements, 73
 mixing of, 192–193
 properties of, 73, 75t, 177t, 182–183
 resin-modified, 183
 restorative materials, 73–74
 wear resistance of, 73
Gloves, 28
Gold alloy
 classification of, 133–134, 134t
 history of, 3
 insolubility of, 9
 malleability of, 20
 polishing of, 163–164
Gold solder, 136
Grit, 156, 158, 158f
Gypsum products
 abrasion resistance of, 232, 233t

Gypsum products (*Continued*)
 cast pouring of, 236–237, 243–245
 chemical properties of, 231–232
 classification of, 233–234
 cleanup of, 237
 dental stone
  definition of, 231–232
  high-strength, 234
  properties of, 234
 detail of, 233
 dimensional accuracy of, 233
 hardness of, 232–233
 impression plaster, 233
 infection control measures, 237–238
 manipulation of, 234–235, 236t
 mixing of, 235, 242
 model plaster, 233–234
 particles, 232
 physical properties of, 232–233, 233t
 production of, 232
 properties of, 231–233, 233t
 proportioning of, 234–235
 retarders of, 236
 selection of, 234
 setting expansion of, 233
 setting time, 235–236
 solubility of, 233
 spatulation of, 235–236
 storage of, 237
 strength of, 232–233, 236t
 viscosity of, 236t
 water/powder ratio of, 234–235
 working time for, 235, 236t

H
Hand protection, 28
Hard liners, 259
Hardness
 abrasives, 157
 definition of, 18, 20
 Moh scale, 157–158
 provisional restorations, 278
Hazard communication program
 chemical labeling
  description of, 32, 34
  guidelines for, 36
  National Fire Protection Association system, 35, 35f
  sample, 35f
 components of, 32–36
 coordinator of, 36
 employee training, 36
 material safety data sheets
  definition of, 26, 32
  explanation of, 32t
  labeling, 40
  sample, 33f-34f
 outline of, 35
Hazard communication standard, 31–36
Hazardous chemicals
 definition of, 26–27
 ingestion of, 27–28

Hazardous chemicals (*Continued*)
 inhalation of, 27
 skin exposure to, 27
Hazardous waste, 31
Heat-cured acrylic resins
 polymerization of, 255
 properties of, 252t, 252–253
Hemihydrate, 231–232, 232
High noble alloy, 124, 133
High-copper alloys, 128–129
High-strength base, 173–175, 174t
High-velocity evacuation, 37
Home bleaching, 103–104, 115–117
Hue, 7, 13, 79
Hybrid composite, 61, 65, 75t
Hybrid glass ionomer, 61, 74–75, 177t, 183
Hybrid layer
 definition of, 42
 formation of, 47
Hydrocolloid(s)
 definition of, 196, 198
 irreversible
  composition of, 201, 202t
  definition of, 196
  dimensional stability of, 202
  disinfecting of, 216, 217t
  dispensing of, 203
  impression making using, 202–205, 205t
  mixing of, 203–204
  permanent deformation of, 202
  setting of, 201
  tear strength of, 202
  uses of, 201
  working time for, 201
 reversible
  application of, 199–200
  composition of, 198–199, 199t
  definition of, 196
  delivery methods, 199–200
  disinfecting of, 216, 217t
  hydrophilicity of, 200
  properties of, 200–201, 213t
  viscosities, 199
Hydrocolloid conditioner, 199
Hydrodynamic theory of tooth sensitivity, 42, 50–51
Hydrofluoric acid, 49
Hysteresis, 196, 200

I
Ignitable, 26, 31
Imbibition, 196, 207
Implants
 antibacterial agents for, 142
 brushing of, 141, 141f
 denture supported by, 140f
 description of, 137–138
 endosseous, 125, 138–139
 failure of, 143
 home care of, 141–142